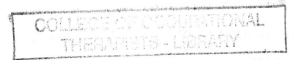

Choosing Assistive Devices

of related interest

Manual Handling in Health and Social Care
An A-Z of Law and Practice
Michael Mandelstam
ISBN 1 84310 041 X

Equipment for Older or Disabled People and the Law
Michael Mandelstam
ISBN 1 85302 352 3

Law, Rights and Disability
Jeremy Cooper
ISBN 1 85302 836 3

Disabled Children and the Law
Research and Good Practice
Janet Read and Luke Clements
ISBN 1 85302 793 6

Care Services for Later Life
Transformations and Critiques
Edited by Tony Warnes, Lorna Warren and Mike Nolan
ISBN 1 85302 852 5

The Care Homes Legal Handbook
Jeremy Cooper
ISBN 1 84310 064 9

Care Practice and the Law, 2nd Edition
Michael Mandelstam
ISBN 1 85302 647 6

Choosing Assistive Devices

A guide for users and professionals

Helen Pain

Lindsay McLellan

Sally Gore

Line drawings by Sarah Ifield

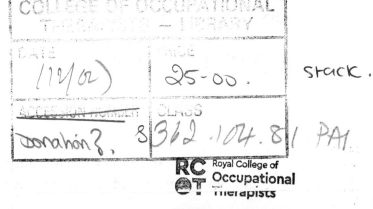

Jessica Kingsley Publishers
London and Philadelphia

First published in the United Kingdom in 2003
by Jessica Kingsley Publishers Ltd
116 Pentonville Road
London N1 9JB, England
and
325 Chestnut Street
Philadelphia, PA 19106, USA

www.jkp.com

Copyright © 2003 Helen Pain, Lindsay McLellan and Sally Gore
Illustrations © Sarah Ifield

Library of Congress Cataloging in Publication Data
Pain, Helen, 1950-
    Choosing assistive devices : a guide for users and professionals / Helen Pain,
Lindsay McLellan and Sally Gore
        p.cm.
    Includes bibliographical references and index.
    ISBN 1-85302-985-8 (alk. paper)
      1. Self-help devices for people with disabilities--Evaluation. I. McLellan, D. Lindsay.
    II. Gore, Sally, 1952- III. Title.

RM698 .P355 2002
617'.03--dc21   2002025465

British Library Cataloguing in Publication Data
A CIP catalogue record for this book is available from the British Library

ISBN 1 85302 985 8

Printed and Bound in Great Britain by
Athenaeum Press, Gateshead, Tyne and Wear

CONTENTS

ACKNOWLEDGEMENTS   8

PREFACE   9

PART I

CHAPTER I Introduction   13

    1.1 Background   13

    1.2 The purpose and range of this book   18

        Summary of section 1.2   19

    1.3 The process used in this book   20

        Summary of the process   25

    1.4 Getting information about assistive devices   25

        References   32

CHAPTER 2 Methods used in Evaluating Assistive Devices   35

        Introduction   35

    2.1 Classification of evidence   35

    2.2 Informal evaluations   36

    2.3 Focus groups   37

    2.4 Delphi technique   38

    2.5 Surveys   39

    2.6 Formal trials   42

        Summary   45

        References   46

PART 2

CHAPTER 3 Seating   **51**

    Introduction   51

  3.1 The importance of good seating   52

  3.2 Standard seating needs   55

  3.3 Special seating needs   65

  3.4 Pressure distributing products   88

    Key points   100

    References   101

CHAPTER 4 Toileting and Continence   **115**

    Introduction   115

  4.1 Difficulties once at the toilet   120

  4.2 Not getting to the toilet to pass urine   148

  4.3 Problems with bowel continence   159

    Key points   160

    References   161

CHAPTER 5 Bathing and Showering   **171**

    Introduction   171

  5.1 Keeping ourselves clean   172

  5.2 Bathing   180

  5.3 Showering   214

    Key points   234

    References   235

CHAPTER 6 Assisted Moving and Handling   **243**

    Introduction   243

  6.1 Devices to assist your independence   246

  6.2 Devices to assist when someone helps you   255

  6.3 Care assistant operated devices that do the task for you 263

  6.4 Self-operated devices that do the task for you   279

  6.5 Cleaning and maintenance   288

    Key points   290

    References   291

PART 3

CHAPTER 7 Conclusion   **301**

       Introduction   301

  7.1 The decision-making process   301

  7.2 Product design   304

  7.3 The impact of the environment   305

  7.4 Implications for information providers   306

  7.5 Implications for assistive device providers   307

  7.6 Implications for research   309

  7.7 Implications for education and training   310

  7.8 Hopes for the future   312

       References   313

Appendix I   Decision-making and problem-solving   **317**

       References   319

Appendix II   Organisations Involved in assistive Technology   **321**

Appendix III   Glossary   **323**

Appendix IV   Literature Search Strategies   **327**

SUBJECT INDEX   329

AUTHOR INDEX   333

Acknowledgements

We would like to thank those who have reviewed chapters of this book in draft form, for their interest, encouragement and invaluable comments and advice:

Kay Day, Dip COT SROT, Dialability, Oxford

Mandy Fader, PhD RN, Disability Equipment Assessment Centre at University College of London

Susan Farr, Dip COT SROT

Peggy Frost, MSc Dip COT SROT, Derby Disability Equipment Assessment Centre

Jani Grisbrooke, MSc BA(Hons) DipCOT SROT, Lecturer in Occupational Therapy, School of Health Professions and Rehabilitation Sciences, University of Southampton

Cheryl Honeycombe, Dip COT BSc(Hons) SROT

Susan Jackson, MSc MCSP SRP, Lecturer in Rehabilitation, School of Health Professions and Rehabilitation Sciences, University of Southampton

Julian Pearce, MSc MSCP SRP, Lecturer, School of Health Professions and Rehabilitation Sciences, University of Southampton

Susan Strong, Dip COT SROT, Southampton Wheelchair Service

Helen White, RGN, RHV, Director PromoCon

Lesley Wilson, BNSc(Hons) RGN, Southampton Continence Advisory Service

Helen Pain would like to give special thanks to her family who have been very supportive and provided lots of encouragement.

We would also like to thank Sue Wilkin, Medical Devices Agency, for her encouragement in the initial phase of planning this book, and staff in the Southampton Disability Equipment Assessment Centre for their support and patience, particularly as the book was nearing completion.

Preface

The authors have worked in the field of assistive device evaluation for more than ten years. Over that time they have become increasingly aware that there is little evidence to support practitioners and users in their choice of device to meet the specific requirements of a situation. There is much written about factors to throw into the equation, but no formula to solve the messy puzzle that is generated.

The need to begin the process of mapping possible solutions to such problems was the driving force behind writing this book, which attempts to bring together researched evidence and professional knowledge in a systematic way so as to create decision pathways or guidelines. Once a set of requirements has been identified, the guidelines can be applied to help select the device that is most likely to meet it.

The guidelines are not hard and fast recommendations. Even if they had undergone extensive field trials and were refined further, the individual nature of each situation would inevitably mean that the guidelines would still need to be applied flexibly and sensitively. They should therefore be regarded as collections of evidence ordered in a sequence that is logical for most (but doubtless not every) situation, and be used systematically to identify possible solutions. They seek to enhance, not circumvent, the professional advisers' role, and provide practitioners with evidence to support their practice. We believe that they will also help staff new to working in this field to develop their expertise more quickly and to apply the principles developed here to solving new problems.

Another force that brought this book into being was appreciation of how daunting the choice of assistive devices (ADs) can seem to those who require them. People who have newly acquired disabilities, and/or whose disabilities are complex, often look to professionals to guide their choice, simply because they feel unqualified to enter into the decision-making as an equal partner. We do not feel this is right, and hope that this book will facilitate the decision-making partnership, either by a potential AD user working through it first, or through its use as a workbook jointly with a professional.

Throughout the text, the potential user of assistive devices is addressed as 'you' because it is appropriate that practitioners should try to put themselves in users' shoes when negotiating solutions with them.

Part One

Part One

Chapter 1

Introduction

1.1 Background

If you have a disability and find a task difficult, you are faced with a choice. Broadly speaking, you either avoid the task, get someone to do it for you, or find a gadget to help you do it. If you decide a gadget would be your preference, finding the one that is best for you is not always easy.

First, you have to know where to look. In recent years, many products have become available in ordinary shops that a person with a disability can use with ease. This has been possible because of improved design and an increased awareness of people's differing needs. In addition to the gadgets in general retail outlets, there is a wide range of more specialist products, which are available through specialist suppliers, mail order and equipment provider services. Equipment provider services in the UK are either statutory, run by health and social services, or are charitable organisations such as the Red Cross. The specialist products are commonly called *assistive devices* or *assistive technology*. In the UK, such specialist products are also often called *equipment*, *adaptive equipment* or *disability equipment*. The term *assistive device* is widely used throughout the world and so will be used in this book.

Second, you have to choose a product that will match your requirements. For many this is either a trial and error exercise, or else one looks for advice from someone with experience. This book attempts to make the choice more systematic and transparent.

Third, you have to incorporate the gadget or assistive device into your everyday life. This may require familiarisation and adjustment over a period of time.

1.1.1 What is an assistive device?

Precise definitions of assistive devices vary slightly, but the European HEART project (Horizontal European Activities in Rehabilitation Technology) (1993–5) defined assistive technology as:

> any product, instrument, strategy, service and practice, used by people with disabilities and older people – specially produced or generally available – to prevent, compensate, relieve or neutralise the impairment, disability or handicap, and improve the individual's autonomy and quality of life. (Jensen 1999, p.80)

The focus of this book is helping you to select products that are on the specialist market, so *assistive device* will refer to these. Products that are generally available, though included in the HEART definition, will here be termed *non-specialist devices*.

Some authors further divide assistive devices into *tools* and *appliances*. A *tool* assists the user to do a task, so 'effective operation is usually dependent on the operator' (Vernardakis, Stephanidis and Akoumianakis 1994, p.205); an *appliance* replaces a function, for example a raised toilet seat reduces the need to bend the hips and knees further than is desirable. These categories are not always clear-cut so in this book, no such distinction is made.

1.1.2 Who uses assistive devices?

Census and survey information tell us that 14 per cent (over 6 million 20 years ago) of the UK adult population have some special needs related to disability (Martin, Meltzer and Elliott 1988), and 3 per cent of children (Bone and Meltzer 1989), although not all of these will use assistive devices (ADs) (Grundy *et al.* 1999; Martin, White and Meltzer 1989), see table 1.1.2.

The number of ADs used increases with age (Mann *et al.* 1999; Sonn 1996) which reflects the greater numbers of people with some physical impairment. Therefore numerically the largest group of AD users are aged 70–79 years, but looking at AD users within each age group, the proportion is highest for those over 80 years.

Table 1.1.2 Estimates of the number of disabled adults in the UK by severity. All numbers represent thousands

Severity category	Age								
	16–19	20–29	30–39	40–49	50–59	60–69	70–79	80 and over	TOTAL
10	5	13	9	7	11	22	47	97	210
9	6	13	11	15	31	64	86	138	365
8	5	18	22	26	40	64	104	117	396
7	6	20	26	35	49	81	124	145	486
6	9	31	31	43	61	87	158	125	545
5	12	31	42	51	95	148	182	147	708
4	7	37	47	59	96	155	187	117	704
3	5	28	45	52	110	175	218	117	750
2	4	28	31	58	112	227	268	111	840
1	15	45	78	107	187	311	313	141	1198
TOTAL	76	264	342	453	793	1334	1687	1254	6202

Reproduced with permission from Martin *et al.* 1988, *The prevalence of disability among adults*, National Statistics, © Crown copyright 2001.

The measures of disability used are the Office of Population Census and Surveys, now ONS (Office for National Statistics), Disability Scales (see Martin *et al.* 1988) in which severity category 1 denotes minor disabilities and category 10 denotes severe and complex disabilities.

1.1.3 Where are assistive devices used?

Assistive devices will be used in hospitals, residential care homes and in people's own homes. Some of the issues affecting choice of product will vary from setting to setting. For instance, a mobile commode used in a hospital ward will need to be robust, with seat height suitable for an average person, but one for use in a person's home will also have to be of a width that will pass through specific doorways and should have a seat height that is optimal for the user.

In the UK, the numbers of people who live in residential accommodation are about 109,000 adults under the age of 70 (3% of the disabled population for this age group) rising with age to 217,000 of age 80 years and older, representing 17 per cent of the disabled population for this age group (Martin *et al.* 1988).

Most people with disabilities thus live in the community, in housing with a range of facilities. In the UK, almost all homes have an inside toilet (of pedestal design), but in many there will only be one, and that one will be upstairs. Baths are usually upstairs too, and will normally stand on the floor rather than be sunken. Shower facilities are not common in older houses. An over-bath shower is more common than a separate shower, owing to limited available space.

Access to front doors frequently takes the form of steps leading up from street level to the door. It was only in 1999 that regulations (Department of Environment 1999) came into force that required new buildings to be accessible for wheelchair users.

Within the home, fitted carpets are commonplace in bedrooms and living rooms. Central heating is fairly standard, but many older houses have not had it fitted, especially if the occupant is elderly. It is within this type of environment that assistive devices are used within the UK community.

However, it is assumed in this book that in hospitals and residential homes, toilets are available on each level of the building, that both showers and baths are available, and that level access to such facilities is usual.

1.1.4 How are assistive devices obtained?

In the UK the majority of assistive devices (ADs) are loaned to users by authorities such as the social services for daily living devices, and the National Health Service for wheelchairs and nursing equipment. Provision of a device is dependent on an assessment by someone from the relevant authority. Additionally, the Red Cross is a major source of ADs for short-term loans. A potential user normally has to have a recommendation for a device, for example from their doctor, nurse or occupational therapist. A few charities that focus on specific conditions also loan ADs, or can be approached for a grant to enable a purchase.

Disabled people are increasingly purchasing ADs for themselves. Advice and guidance about what might meet your needs are available from books, websites, demonstration centres and specialist shops (see section 1.4 *Getting information about assistive devices*).

Second-hand devices can be purchased through some commercial suppliers, for example reconditioned stair lifts. Advertisements of second-hand products can be found on some websites and in some journals (see section 1.4 *Getting information about assistive devices*).

1.1.5 Choosing the right device

If you want a gadget or assistive device to help with an activity, choosing one can be complex because of the many different things that have to be taken into consideration:

- your requirements

- the requirements of others in the household

- the requirements of any people who give you personal assistance (termed *care assistants* in this book)

- the way the assistive device will fit into your lifestyle

- the way it will fit into the environment in which it will be used.

Good information about all these areas will enable you to choose a product that proves successful. Time and care spent in gathering this information is therefore time well spent. If you make a choice without considering all the relevant factors you are more likely to be dissatisfied with the product, and hence use it infrequently or not at all.

It is a well-researched fact that when choices are not clear-cut, finding the best solution is far from easy. Weighing up lots of information objectively is difficult. A brief review of the literature is given in Appendix I. Those of you who are experienced will already have a stock of ready-made solutions that have proved reasonably effective in the past. If you are new to the subject you may well feel overwhelmed, and look to an expert to decide for you. A middle way is for an experienced practitioner to work together with you through the decision-making process.

1.1.6 Review after provision of an assistive device

Once an AD has been chosen, and seems effective, you will have to incorporate its use into your everyday life. But however appropriate the choice, regular reviews of how well ADs continue to meet your needs should be done. The frequency of these will depend on your condition, so if your requirements are likely to change, reviews need to be more often than if your condition will not change for years. The expected life of an AD will also affect the need for review, so if for example you have uncontrolled movements, the chair you use regularly should be reviewed sooner than for a person who sits still all the time.

1.2 The purpose and range of this book

There are many publications that explain what needs to be included in the course of assessment for an AD. There are also several models linking the components of the assessment together (e.g. Bain 1998; Law *et al.* 1996; Mann and Lane 1995). Some of this literature helps with prioritising the mass of information that is available, but little addresses how to connect the information gathered to the product which will provide the best match between person and product, supporting guidance with evidence. It is this small but vital focus in the acquisition of an AD that this book addresses.

Information about the interaction between person and product, and what affects the usefulness of an assistive device (AD) is reviewed and collated in this book in the areas of seating (not including wheelchairs), toileting, bathing, showering, assisted moving and handling.

The book sets out to help you through the process of choosing a product that is going to work for you, in your situation. For each person, the features in the assistive device that are right for them will be different from those right for another. It is therefore a workbook, not a 'best buy' guide. It aims to bring together evidence that:

- highlights things that need thinking about

- provides guidance on what AD to look out for

- indicates what combination of features might best meet your particular needs.

It draws on research results and other published material, and guides your decision-making rather than presenting a ready-made solution. Although there is a reasonable body of information for some topics, much of what follows has been drawn from professional opinion and experience rather than systematically collected data. Research studies vary widely in how much confidence can be placed in their findings. They should therefore be used in the knowledge that they may not be fully applicable to your current situation. Unlike surgical procedures, which once done cannot be undone, ADs can usually be tested out, and sometimes themselves be adapted, to ensure a good match with your (the user's) requirements.

This book is for those who want to unpick the decision-making process and understand reasons for choosing a particular product, and who want to know what published work has to say.

1.2.1 What this book does not do

This book does not provide detailed descriptions of individual products currently on the market. It does not seek to compete with information and guidelines written specifically for the users, but rather to examine the evidence which may provide greater detail about what has been found to work well for people and why.

Summary of sections 1.1 and 1.2

- An assistive device is one option when a task is difficult.

- The number of people using devices increases with age.

- Although the majority of devices in the UK are loaned, an increasing number of products are being purchased privately.

- Choosing the right assistive device is a complex task because of the many factors that must be considered.

- Details of the following must be considered:

    o your (the user's) requirements

    o the requirements of others in the household

    o the requirements of the care assistant (if applicable).

- The following must also be taken into account:

    o how the assistive device will fit into your lifestyle

    o how the assistive device will fit into the environment in which it must be used

    o how effective the assistive device is.

- People are not good at judging between so many things at once.

- This book therefore seeks to help by:

    o providing a structure to guide you through the process

    o suggesting what should be thought about

    o using evidence to provide guidelines on what features you should find helpful.

1.3 The process used in this book

Working methodically through a process step by step will help when you are choosing an assistive device. The process that will be followed in this book is shown in Figure 1. 3.

Stage 1 Information gathering

Information is needed about your difficulties, and those of any *care assistant*[1] involved. If the disability has been a sudden event, for example a stroke or accident, finding out what problems will be encountered is part of the information-gathering process, but if the onset has been gradual, then a problem or set of problems will already be known.

Through defining the causes of the problems, your requirements can be formulated; for example, if you fall sideways in a chair, this means the requirement will be for support when sitting.

The following aspects about yourself should all be considered as the picture of your requirements is formed:

- your physical abilities

- your ability to understand how to use something safely

- your preferences

- your expectations of a device

- your attitude to trying something different.

Whatever the stated difficulty or problem is, there may be additional ones that come to light as the information is gathered. These will also need to be analysed.

If a care assistant is to be involved in helping you to use the assistive device, he or she will also have particular abilities and preferences, and these too must be identified.

Usually an occupational therapist or other health or social services professional (termed a *practitioner* in this book) will have been asked to assist with the choice of assistive devices (ADs), as they are able to provide insights on possible courses of action and likely future needs. The latter is important if your requirements are likely to change: the practitioner's experience may help with defining additional features that will enable the chosen product to meet your requirements satisfactorily for many years.

---

1   See Glossary for definition of words in italics.

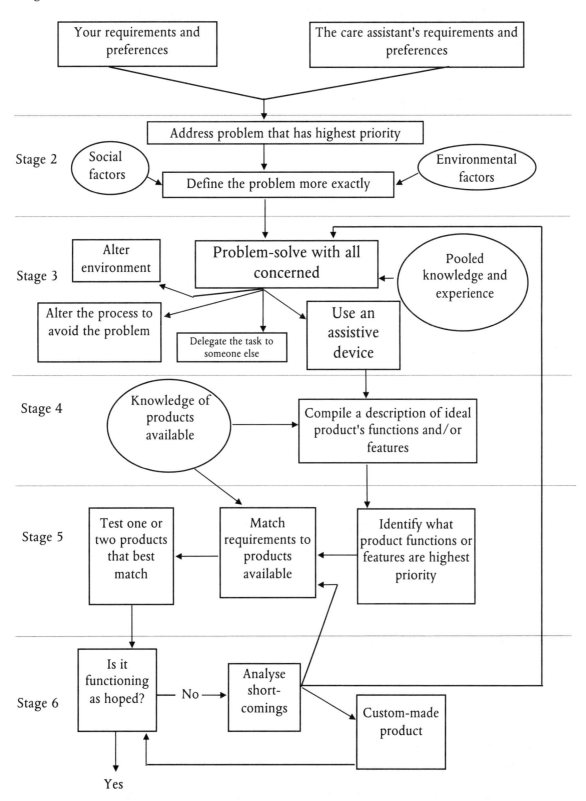

Figure 1.3 The process of choosing an assistive device to meet your (the user's) requirements.

People often already have a *solution* in mind. This forms part of the discussion but may have to be renegotiated if it proves impractical or better possibilities are identified. It is a positive advantage at this stage to keep an open mind about the options.

Stage 2 Refining the information

The next step is to identify the most pressing *problem* and to look at it in greater detail.

The problem may be caused by a combination of things. If the environment has become inaccessible, perhaps because of limited mobility, each area of difficulty in the environment should be recorded, for example stairs, steps, narrow doorways.

Each point of difficulty may need to be examined in detail, and this will include looking at the environment – the conditions, space and layout of the places where difficulty arises. Scale drawings using exact measurements are helpful when Stage 5 is reached and one is considering possible solutions, e.g. to ensure an AD fits in.

If an AD currently used is no longer suitable, its shortcomings should be identified.

The appearance of ADs may be important either to ease their acceptance, or if they are devices for constant use such as wheelchairs, to make the user feel confident socially.

Other social and cultural influences may also influence which ADs you consider acceptable or unacceptable, and these must be acknowledged in the decision-making process.

Stage 3 Deciding on the type of solution

Here the information gathered thus far is assessed against a range of possible solutions. Many will be rejected because they do not meet enough of the requirements, but it is worthwhile noting down the reasons for rejecting a suggestion, in case one wants to retrace the reasoning behind their rejection. Those that show potential should have both advantages and disadvantages noted against them.

You have intimate knowledge of the specific situation, and may have innovative ideas for solving your difficulty regardless of how much experience of assistive technology you have. Conversely, a practitioner has a fund of experience of similar situations, but is new to this particular one. Discussion is therefore fruitful to get the most ideas.

Possible solutions may involve altering the environment, for example moving house or adapting the current one. Another possibility would be to alter a process to avoid the problem, for instance selecting clothing which only has fastenings you can manage. Alternatively, you may wish to delegate a task such as shopping to another person instead of struggling with it.

Such solutions do not involve choosing assistive devices (ADs), whereas this book mainly focuses on situations in which an assistive device is the solution of preference. This does not mean that other ways of solving problems will not be needed *in addition to* an AD, especially in relation to physical alterations to the environment in which you live.

Stage 4 Identifying what type of assistive device you need

Having decided that an AD is wanted, a practitioner in the UK will be aware of what can be provided through the statutory services (the National Health Service or the local social services department). Each local area has slightly different rules about who is eligible for what type of AD. The amount of funds available for ADs also varies considerably, and there is often a long wait for funding to become available for certain products, whereas others may be in stock. This may affect the choice made.

Greater definition of the type of AD and the features it should have is now needed. Part 2 of this book provides information on a range of areas, organised to guide you through the process of deciding on what type of AD you need, and what features it should have in order to meet your own requirements and those of any care assistant who is involved with that activity.

Stage 5 Shortlist and test some assistive devices

An actual product may not be found that has all the features identified. The features should therefore be prioritised according to how essential they are to meeting your (the user's) requirements.

WHAT TO DO ONCE THE DESCRIPTION FOR AN ASSISTIVE DEVICE HAS BEEN COMPILED, WITH THE FEATURES PRIORITISED

Information about what products are available can be obtained from a variety of sources. There are places to go to see products or obtain advice; information is available in print through a number of sources, and is increasingly available on the Internet. Section 1.4 gives sources of information with a brief description of each. Products can then be considered to see which may be suitable. Start with the most important features and work through the possible products, eliminate the unsuitable ones, then continue with the other features until only two or three products which look suitable remain. These should be seen, handled and preferably given a trial in the environment in which they will be used.

Stage 6 Is it satisfactory?

A short test of most products enables you to tell whether they are going to be useful. Some products may take longer to assess fully, and it is worth asking if a manufacturer allows a trial period. This will give you time to get used to it: fine-tuning the adjustments may be necessary, for instance on a chair; you may need time to learn how to handle the controls; the room lay-out may need altering to position the AD most effectively for you; it may mean a new routine. All these things, as well as having to accept a new gadget in your life, will affect how you utilise a device (McCuaig and Frank 1991; Schweitzer *et al.* 1999).

If none of the products chosen at the end of Stage 5 solves the problem, other products can be tried, with the acknowledgement that some compromise of the ideal product description would then be necessary.

If no standard product solves the problems well enough, a custom-made product may be considered. Alternatively, a return to Stage 3 may be necessary, to generate more possible solutions that could then be explored.

To read in more depth about the theory behind this process

Appendix I reviews some literature about decision-making and problem-solving.

To find out who is involved with assistive technology and its evaluation.

Appendix II lists some organisations involved with assistive technology.

Summary of the process

Whatever assistive device you need, the process illustrated in Figure 1.3 should be used.

- Work through Stages 1 and 2: information gathering and refinement.

- Stage 3: Joint problem-solving to decide the best way(s) of tackling the problem. If ADs are considered a useful option, find the chapter concerning the area of activity you are looking at. The first part of it may give some background information when you are considering alternative approaches to solving the problem.

- Stage 4: If an assistive device is the preferred solution, continue working through the chapter to identity the features important to find in a product.

- Stage 5: Decide what features would be most important.

- Stage 5 continues with finding information about actual products. Possible sources of such information are listed below in section 1.4 *Getting information about assistive devices*. Match the information about specific products with the list of the features you require, so that two or three products that match them best can be trialled.

- Stage 6: Review how they work for you in practice. If they have shortcomings, these need to be identified so that some of the process can be worked through again to find a more suitable match with your requirements.

1.4 Getting information about assistive devices

1.4.1 Places to visit or contact

Disabled Living Centres (DLCs)

Now often called Independent Living Centres (ILCs). A network of demonstration centres where products may be viewed, and advice given. Disabled Living Centres Council (DLCC) will advise which DLC is nearest. Tel: 0161 834 1044

British Red Cross

National Headquarters
Tel: 020 7235 5454
Look in Yellow Pages for local centres, which provide assistive devices for short-term loan.

Retail outlets

Look in Yellow Pages under Disabled equipment for local outlets.

Exhibitions

NAIDEX
Tel: 01203 426520; www.naidex.co.uk

Independent Living Shows
Tel: 01275 831754

Continence

Continence Advisory Service
A network of centres throughout the UK. Your local service may be accessed via your family doctor (GP) or Health Centre, or ask the Continence Foundation (below) for your local contact.

Continence Foundation
307 Hatton Square
16 Baldwin Gardens
London EC1N 7RJ
Tel: (Monday – Friday 9.30–13.00): 020 7831 9831 or 0845 3450165
Helpline for advice and information

Enuresis Resource and Information Centre (ERIC)
Tel: 0117 9603060
Information and advice to children affected by bowel and bladder problems.

InContact
Tel: 020 7700 7035
An organisation for people affected by bowel and bladder problems.

PromoCon
Tel: 0161 8342001; www.promocon2001.co.uk
Helpline and centre where products are on display.

Hearing impairment

Royal National Institute for Deaf People (RNID)
Tel: 0870 6050123; Fax: 0870 6033007
Markets products for hearing-impaired people.

Sight impairment

Royal National Institute of the Blind (RNIB)
Tel: 020 7388 1266.
Markets products for sight-impaired people. Catalogue and some local centres.

Sexuality and disability

SPOD (The Association to Aid the Sexual and Personal Relationships of People
with a Disability)
286 Camden Road
London N7 0BJ
Tel: 020 7607 8851; www.spod-uk.org

1.4.2 Printed sources

GENERAL INFORMATION ON HOW TO FIND OUT ABOUT ASSISTIVE DEVICES

This is where to start if you know very little about assistive devices and what they
can offer the disabled person.

Department of Health (1996). *A Practical guide for disabled people*, HB6. Available
from PO Box 410, Wetherby, LS23 7LN.

The book covers organisations, benefits and entitlements to services, including
assistive devices. A list of all Disabled Living Centres is included; these you can
arrange to visit for advice and to have products demonstrated. In view of the publication date, contact addresses and telephone numbers may have changed.

Mandelstam, M., (1992). 2nd edition *How to get equipment for disability*. London:
Jessica Kingsley Publishers.

This covers entitlements to home adaptations, assistive devices and related
services. Different ways of obtaining products are explained, together with the
various pieces of legislation and official circulars that govern provision. The types
of assistive device obtainable from the NHS, social services departments, housing
education and employment services are described. There have been no substantial

changes since publication, but some details will have altered, and contact addresses and telephone numbers may have changed.

Mandelstam, M., (1996). *Equipment for older or disabled people and the law*. London: Jessica Kingsley Publishers.

This deals in detail with the mandate and constraints of statutory bodies with regard to providing assistive devices and home adaptations. It is useful to help you find out exactly what you are entitled to, what to do if things go wrong, and to see why such variation across the country is possible.

Browne, L. (1999) *If only I'd known that a year ago*. London: RADAR.

Information on a wide range of topics including obtaining assistive devices, written for newly disabled people.

INFORMATION ABOUT BROAD TYPES OF ASSISTIVE DEVICE AND RELATED ISSUES

Gradually more products are becoming available in shops that are of help in making daily tasks easier, but when the level of disability increases, an indication of the range of product types available through specialist firms is necessary.

RICAbility

24 Highbury Crescent
London N5 1RX
Tel: 020 7704 5200; www.ricability.org.uk
Several publications, with more being added regularly. Single copies available free.

Equipment for easier living (1995).
This provides very general information about the range of products on the market. It is not comprehensive but gives a good overview for domestic living.

Adapting your home (undated, *c*1998), in the series, 'Ability Guides'.
A good introduction to the possibilities, including types of assistive device.

Choosing products for bladder and bowel control (2001), in the series, 'Ability Guides'.
A leaflet explaining the causes, treatments and products for those with continence problems.

Children's continence products: a guide for parents and children (2001).

RADAR (the Royal Association for Disability and Rehabilitation)

12 City Forum
250 City Road
London EC1 8AF
Tel: 020 7250 3222; www.radar.org.uk

DETAILED INFORMATION ABOUT SPECIFIC PRODUCTS

If you know firms that supply products of interest to you, they will send details of them to you on request. Many offer demonstrations if the product is expensive. A number of firms offer a mail order service. Ensure that they will allow you to return the product if it is not suitable for your needs. If the product is designed specifically to address a difficulty that arises through impairment, you should be able to buy the product without paying VAT, and catalogues often have a declaration form in them to allow you to take advantage of VAT exemption.

RNID

Tel: 020 7296 8001
Mail order assistive devices for hearing-impaired people.

Medical Devices Agency

Tel: 020 7972 8360

Disability Equipment Assessment series (1992–98). Now called:
Disability Evaluation Reports (1998 to date). Divided into equipment for daily living, continence products, orthotics and prosthetics, mobility, pressure relief, moving and handling products. Reports are now becoming available on the web, see http://www.medical-devices.gov.uk

Various titles have been published, each reporting a detailed formal evaluation of a small category of disability equipment. There is a section near the beginning of each which gives guidelines for people when considering which product to choose. The information about specific products may not be applicable to current models even if the product is still available, as the manufacturers may have revised their products.

Disability Information Trust

Tel: 01865 227559.

Now subsumed under FAST, see section 1.4.3 below.

Various titles, each dealing with a larger group of assistive devices than the *Disability Evaluation Reports*, providing a brief comment about the majority of products within that group. Not every product available is described, and you must check the publication date as product ranges change quickly. Each section has an introduction that provides some guidelines.

DLF Hamilton Index

Tel: 020 7289 6111; www.dlf.org.uk

A comprehensive list of assistive devices, divided into sections according to product area. General guidance and advice is given at the beginning of each section, which is helpful. It is regularly updated so covers all products currently available in the UK. It is a subscription service which is available at most Disabled Living Centres (see above) and some health information centres.

RICAbility

24 Highbury Crescent, London N5 1RX
Tel: 020 7704 5200; www.ricability.org.uk

Various titles concerning specific groups of assistive devices. They include reports of evaluation projects commissioned by Ricability and summaries of evaluations conducted by others, and provide general guidelines to assist one's choice.

SECOND-HAND PRODUCTS
Disability Equipment Register

Tel: 01454 318818

A subscription service to buy and sell used products. Updated monthly. Available on Internet as well, see below.

DLF Factsheet on sources of second-hand products. Contact details in 1.4.3 below.

1.4.3 Internet or CD-ROM

GENERAL INFORMATION ON HOW TO FIND OUT ABOUT ASSISTIVE DEVICES
Internet

Try searching with 'disability equipment', 'assistive devices' or 'assistive technology'.

Disability information site www.disabilitynet.co.uk has a wide range of information including selling second-hand products. Much will be from the United States, and you may want to specify UK targets.

FAST (Foundation for ASsistive Technology) www.fastuk.org aims to bring together manufacturers, researchers, services providers and end users.

See also websites for organisations cited in the previous sections.

DETAILED INFORMATION ABOUT SPECIFIC PRODUCTS
Internet

Most manufacturers and many of the companies marketing assistive devices now have web sites. The number accessed through a general search (as above) may be daunting, so it may be better to find out a few firms through other means then look them up for more detailed information. www.enableme2.com is one of the sites that offer a range of information including products, but you have to bear in mind that the links to manufacturers are selective and limited.

www.abledata.com is an American database with information sheets, product information and a consumer forum.

DLF-DATA from the Disabled Living Foundation

286 Harrow Road
London W9 2HU; www.atlas.co.uk/dlf
Written enquiries or tel: 020 7289 6111

On-line by subscription or CD-ROM. There are some pages of guidelines and advice for choosing products, but the full catalogue of products is available only by subscription. This facility is available at some Disabled Living Centres and health information centres. They will help you to use it.

SECOND-HAND PRODUCTS

www.disabreg.dial.pipex.com
www.disabilitynet.co.uk
www.dlf.org.uk

References

For an explanation of the classification of evidence by category (* to ****), see Chapter 2, Introduction.

Bain, B. (1998) 'Assistive technology in Occupational Therapy.' In M. Neistadt and E. Crepeau (eds) 9th Edition *Willard & Spackman's occupational therapy*, pp.498–516. *Philadelphia: Lippincott.*
Describes a model that places the consumer at the intersection of environment, device and task.

Bone, M. and Meltzer, H. (1989) *The prevalence of disability among children.* OPCS surveys of disability in Great Britain, Report 3. London: HMSO.
Figures are based on a sample of 2025 people surveyed by post (n=1694) or personal interview (n=331). ****

Department of Environment (1999) Approved document 'Part M: access and facilities for disabled people.' *Building Regulations Amendment 1998.* London: HMSO.

Grundy, E., Alberg, D., Ali, M. *et al.* (1999) *Disability in Great Britain: results from the 1996/7 Disability follow-up to the Family Resources Survey.* Department of Social Security Research Report No. 94. Leeds: HMSO.
A survey of 5589 disabled people, of whom 23 per cent needed help with personal care at least weekly. This study did not specify the role of ADs nor whether having such devices affected people's need for personal assistance.

HEART (Horizontal European Activities in Rehabilitation Technology) (1993–5). *A programme funded 1993–1995 to survey the situation concerning assistive technology in Europe. Many initiatives have arisen from its recommendations. www.hi.se/english/heart.shtm. Accessed 7/10/00.*

Jensen, L. (1999) *Go for it!* Deliverable D05.4, Project DE3402. EUSTAT, European Commission. Accessible via www.siva.it/research/eustat/index.html

Law, M., Cooper, B., Strong, S. *et al.* (1996) 'The person-environment-occupation model: a transactive approach to occupational performance.' *Canadian Journal of Occupational Therapy* 63, 1, 9–23.
A model of how the person, occupation and environment interact.

McCuaig, M. and Frank, G. (1991) 'The able self: adaptive patterns and choices in independent living for a person with cerebral palsy.' *American Journal of Occupational Therapy* 45, 3, 224–234.

Mann, W. and Lane, J. (1995) 2nd edition *Assistive technology for persons with disabilities.* Bethesda, MD: AOTA.
The assessment process is described as having the Person, Environment, Tasks and Devices as components.

Mann, W., Tomita, M., Hurren, D. and Charvat, B. (1999) 'Changes in health, functional and psychosocial status and coping strategies of home-based older persons with arthritis over 3 years.' *The Occupational Therapy Journal of Research 19*, 2, 128–146.
Re-interviewed 61 people after 3 years; all were over 65 years old with self-declared arthritis. They reported an increase of 37 per cent in AD ownership, but did include a number of gadgets such as cordless phones and electric can openers that are not specialist devices. **

Martin, J., Meltzer, H. and Elliott, D. (1988) *The prevalence of disability among adults.* OPCS surveys of disability in Great Britain, Report 1. London: HMSO.
Based on a sample of 14,308 people surveyed by post (n=11,484) or personal interview (n=2824). ****

Martin, J., White, A. and Meltzer, H. (1989) *Disabled adults: services, transport and employment.* OPCS surveys of disability in Great Britain, Report 4. London: HMSO.

Survey data (see Martin et al. 1988 above) have also shown that the proportion of the disabled population using ADs increases with age, from 45 per cent for disabled adults under 50 years to 86 per cent for those above 74 years.

Schweitzer, J., Mann, W., Nochajski, S. *et al.* (1999) 'Patterns of engagement in leisure activity by older adults using assistive devices.' *Technology and Disability 11,* 103–117.

Sonn, U. (1996) 'Longitudinal studies of dependence in daily life activities among elderly persons.' *Scandinavian Journal of Rehabilitation Medicine* Suppl. 34, 1–35.

Surveyed 371 people who had consulted an occupational therapy service at 70 and at 76 years old; the number using ADs at 76 had increased from 78 to 175 (21% to 47%).

Vernardakis, N., Stephanidis, C. and Akoumianakis, D. (1994) 'Rehabilitation technology product taxonomy: a conceptual tool for analysing products and extracting demand determinants.' *International Journal of Rehabilitation Research 17,* 201–214.

Bibliography

ASSESSMENT

Neistadt, M. and Crepeau, E. (eds) (1998) 9th edition *Willard and Spackman's occupational therapy.* Philadelphia: Lippincott.

Maczka, K. (1990) *Assessing physically disabled persons at home.* Therapy in Practice Series, No.12. London: Chapman and Hall.

LEGAL ASPECTS OF USE OF ASSISTIVE TECHNOLOGY

Mandelstam, M. (2001) 'Safe use of disability equipment and manual handling: legal aspects – Part 1, Disability equipment.' *British Journal of Occupational Therapy 64,* 1, 9–16.

Mandelstam, M. (2001) 'Safe use of disability equipment and manual handling: legal aspects – Part 2, Manual handling.' *British Journal of Occupational Therapy 64,* 2, 73–80.

Chapter 2

Methods used in Evaluating Assistive Devices

Introduction

The guidelines set out in Part 2 of this book have been formulated by the authors, using published evidence and their professional experience. Each topic has been reviewed by at least two people with relevant experience (see Acknowledgements). Comments from reviewers were discussed between the authors and most were heeded fully. It is nonetheless still necessary to be aware of the strength of evidence that has contributed to the guidelines. Recording a detailed judgement for every piece of evidence used in compiling the guidelines set out in Part 2 would make them very confusing, so for clarity, a classification has been devised.

2.1 Classification of evidence[1]

The categories denote the degree of confidence you can place in a study's results. Evaluation of assistive devices encompasses a wide range of methods, each with its strengths and weaknesses, but in many cases, the method used in the research provides a guide to which rating will apply. We acknowledge this is an over-simplification, because confidence in the data will vary between one study and the next.

The authors have assigned evidence reviewed in this book to one of four categories using a star system (* to ****). These indicate the confidence with

---

1   Evidence classification using the star system appears in the right-hand column of tables in the book that summarise guidance

which the guidelines can be followed. These levels relate to the trustworthiness of the research and are based upon definitions published by Bandolier (1994):

Strong evidence **** The guideline is based either on *data* from the whole population, for example, a census of all people with a disability, or was drawn from a sample of a defined population such that one can be 95 per cent confident that the results accurately represent the actual population.

Some evidence *** The guideline is based on *quantitative* data from a group which was small in number or lacked sufficient description to guarantee confidence that it faithfully represents the type of person that you are interested in; or is a subgroup analysis with a statistically significant result; or is *qualitative* data from a sample that is well described and its analysis is trustworthy. Generalisation to those with similar characteristics has to be made with some judgement about how appropriate it will be in the particular situation in hand.

Evaluation of single products is *only* included in this category if there was clear comparison, e.g. with some other way of tackling the difficulty. This comparison would allow separation between the effect of testers being pleased to try anything at all, and real benefit from using the product.

Evidence requires care when applying ** The guideline is based on a single *case study* or qualitative data derived from a very small or poorly described sample. Because the data arises from particular individuals, applying it to those with similar characteristics has to be made with careful judgement. Sometimes qualitative data is reported from a subgroup of a quantitative study; this will usually be given a two-star rating.

Evaluation of single products usually falls into this category.

Guidance only* Anecdotal evidence with no indication of how it was gained; experts' opinion; authors' opinions formed from literature and professional experience. Consensus of professional opinion falls into this category but is a reliable source for a guideline provided the treatment or products have not developed since publication. The date of these references should therefore be noted carefully.

The following sections briefly describe methods used for assistive device evaluations and consider their merits.

2.2 Informal evaluations

If the evaluation findings concerning an assistive device (AD) are recorded as an opinion, it is not possible to determine whether it represents a balanced view, nor for whom the comments might be appropriate. The confidence you place in the information will depend on the experience of the evaluators, and their ability to resist bias.

Sometimes practitioners report having used the AD in the course of practice, but the users with whom it was tried are not described (e.g. Burdon and Craighead 2000). Sometimes a practitioner reviews a product, but there is no indication that a user's perspective was gained (e.g. Beresford 1999). Other articles are written by an expert in the field (e.g. Perr 1998).

Advantages	• Valuable information is presented, and authors of this type of article usually have considerable experience in their field.
	• You can expect the article to represent current best practice.
Disadvantages	• The possibility that it is biased, incomplete or not applicable to the situation in hand must be borne in mind.
	• The date of the article should be noted, because terminology, attitudes and devices may have progressed since publication.

Level of confidence with which the information can be applied to your situation: **guidance only(*)**.

2.3 Focus groups

For a focus group, between 8 and 12 people are invited to meet and discuss a topic. Topics that are particularly suitable for such discussions are those where opinions and attitudes are explored, or where pooled knowledge will enrich the debate. Each group usually lasts about an hour and a half, and a moderator ensures that the discussion includes all the areas that the *schedule* sets out. The researcher plans the schedule to help the group get started, tackle the core questions and summarise the discussion. Focus group members usually have not met beforehand.

To be confident that the results adequately represent the views of the specified population from which the group members have been recruited, several groups are convened, all with different members, until the researchers find that no new views are forthcoming. Lane *et al.* (1997) used focus groups in this way to define the characteristics of an 'ideal' battery charger for a powered wheelchair.

You have to discern from the way the research is reported whether the schedule and data analysis were unbiased or not.

Alternatively, this research method can be employed in the *pilot* phase to ensure that when the main study is conducted, all the important factors are included. For example, Pain and Pascoe (MDA 1998) conducted three focus groups with parents and their disabled child, and one with professionals, for them to try a selection of seating and then discuss the issues with regard to using them. The data were used to inform the topics in the questionnaire for the main user trials.

Advantages	• The opinions drawn from a group can be better than one from an individual because the discussion allows members to think things through more fully.
	• Information is gathered quickly (although recruiting and convening the group can be very time consuming).
Disadvantages	• It is not usually known what experience members have had of the devices under evaluation; therefore you cannot gauge what influence this has on their opinions.
	• The devices can only be tried out briefly and in the artificial setting of the group's meeting room. This will be more of a disadvantage for some devices than for others, depending on the environment in which they are customarily used. For example, an outdoor scooter would be disadvantaged, but a child's seat much less so.

Level of confidence with which the information can be applied to your situation: **some evidence (★★★)** if several groups have been conducted; **requires care applying (★★)** if only one or two groups were convened.

2.4 Delphi technique

Sometimes the pooling of people's experience with regard to a topic is required, but it is impractical to bring the participants together physically to conduct a focus group. The Delphi technique was developed by Delbecq, Van der Vean and

Gustafson (1975) before video-conferencing was possible, and requires the participants to respond to successive questionnaires (usually three) to explore the chosen subject and determine whether consensus can be reached. The participants (about 45 are recommended by Delbecq) are chosen because of their expertise in the subject.

The first round comprises an open question; the second is a ranking exercise using the response generated in the previous round; the third round usually asks a related question and requests comments on the results of the second round (MDA 2001a; Moore 1987).

Advantages	• The opinions of experts can be gained without having to bring them together.
	• Respondents are not influenced by peer pressure.
	• The feedback should enhance the respondents' replies.
Disadvantages	• Respondents will drop out at each round.
	• The level of knowledge about assistive devices (ADs) may not be known.

Level of confidence with which the information can be applied to your situation: **some evidence (★★★)** if at least 30–45 respondents began the survey; **requires care applying (★★)** if very few completed the final round, or if the selection criteria for the respondents is not described well.

2.5 Surveys

Surveys either ask a respondent at one point in time only, providing *cross-sectional* data, or return to the same respondent on more than one occasion, giving *longitudinal data*. Surveys may be conducted by post, telephone, via the Internet or face to face.

2.5.1 Postal surveys

A questionnaire sent by post has to be clear and concise, with unambiguous questions. The questions may have set responses from which respondents choose, or open questions to which respondents answer in their own words. A combination of these question types is frequently used: for example, Ryan, Rigby and

From (1996) sent a postal survey to 200 parents of disabled children to gain views about seating systems and ask for suggestions about design improvements. Posting a questionnaire on the Internet will be similar to a postal survey.

Advantages	• A wide geographical area can be covered.
	• Large numbers can be surveyed.
	• Data can often be analysed *quantitatively*, i.e. statistical tests can be applied.
Disadvantages	• Respondents may misunderstand the questions.
	• Interesting or ambiguous points cannot be followed up.
	• It is seldom possible to find out why people have failed to respond.

Level of confidence with which the information can be applied to your situation: **strong** (****) or **some evidence** (***) depending on the numbers surveyed, how the sample was chosen and the response rate; **requires care applying** (**) if the sample is further divided into subgroups, unless the result is statistically significant.

2.5.2 Telephone survey

An interview is conducted over the telephone. It would be usual to use a questionnaire, as Bentur, Barnea and Mizrahi (1996) did when following up purchasers of an assistive easy chair. The interviewers were not known to the respondents in this case, so the refusal rate (one out of 41) was remarkably low. Where the interviewer is known to the respondent, or where they knew a telephone follow-up was part of the study when they consented, refusal is uncommon. Finlayson and Havixbeck (1992) secured interview data from all respondents in a subgroup followed up by telephone in a post-discharge survey.

Advantages	• As for postal surveys, plus the facility to follow up ambiguous replies or explain questions that are not fully understood.

| | • It would be possible to record the number not wishing to respond as distinct from those unobtainable. |
| Disadvantages | • Fewer than for postal surveys, but questions or responses are more at risk of misinterpretation than with face-to-face interviews. |

Level of confidence with which the information can be applied to your situation: **strong** (****) or **some evidence** (***) depending on the numbers surveyed, how the sample was chosen and the consent rate; **requires care applying** (**) if the sample is further divided into subgroups, unless the result is statistically significant.

2.5.3 Face-to-face interviews

In face-to-face interviews, the interviewer has some control over how the questions are asked, what explanations are added, and whether the respondent is prompted to expand answers to open questions. A face-to-face interview can be very tightly structured, as in high street consumer surveys, or much less structured, for instance when attitudes or feelings are being explored. For example, Jensen (1993) wished to explore what influenced people in their decision to adapt their home, so used *in-depth interviews* which allowed respondents to speak freely about their experience.

Interviews are frequently used when conducting a study on the ownership and satisfaction with assistive devices, (e.g. Mann and Tomita 1998). A combination of surveys may be used, for example Gitlin, Levine and Geiger (1993) used face-to-face interviews with patients before discharge, but a series of three telephone interviews to follow these people up.

Video-conferencing between respondent and interviewer would be similar to a face-to-face interview.

Advantages	• Fuller information can be gained on open questions.
	• Interviewers can be trained to ensure all questions are answered fully.
Disadvantage	• The interviewer may unintentionally bias the respondent's answers.

Level of confidence with which the information can be applied to your situation: *Structured interviews*: **strong** (****) or **some evidence** (***) depending on the numbers surveyed, how the sample was chosen and the consent rate; **requires care applying** (**) if the sample is further divided into subgroups, unless the result is statistically significant. *In-depth interviews*: **some evidence** (***) or **requires care applying** (**) depending on the sample, quality of analysis and the trustworthiness of the conclusions or recommendations.

2.6 Formal trials

When a 'formal trial' is referred to in this book it means the testing of named products specifically for the research study. This contrasts with surveys that may ask current *users* about their experience with their assistive devices. The results of the tests are recorded in a planned and systematic way.

The setting in which the trials are conducted will affect the data. For example, testing a leg lifting device in a laboratory situation will not give any indication of how acceptable it would be in a user's bedroom (MDA 1999b). In contrast, the home setting provides data about compatibility in real bedrooms, but there are more environmental variations between users that may reduce the confidence with which one can compare one user's responses with another's.

The duration of each test also affects the data collected. Hawley, O'Neill and Webb (1999) described a case study of a ten-year-old girl with athetoid cerebral palsy who was given a single switch control device for driving her wheelchair. Her error rate ratio dropped from 0.45 over the first two weeks to 0.15 in the third month. If the trial had lasted only two weeks, the AD's effectiveness would have been reported in a much less favourable light. In contrast, a 30-minute test of an easy chair (MDA 1999a) was shown by piloting to give a reasonably accurate indication of how comfortable the user finds it.

Formal trials of ADs may be divided into three broad categories: technical and ergonomic testing and user trials.

2.6.1 Technical testing

Technical tests examine the performance of a product with regard to its strength, stability, durability, compressibility, etc. They may also include technical measurements such as dimensions and forces required to operate or move the product.

Manufacturers always undertake at least some technical tests before marketing a product, and should provide guidelines on maximum loads, correct use, care and maintenance of a product. These are seldom comprehensive, and often reported differently by each manufacturer, making comparison laborious or impossible.

Technical tests may be conducted by independent bodies in order to test the mechanical (MDD 1993) or performance characteristics of the products (MDA 2001b). Such tests may be conducted to determine any risks that may be incurred when people trial the products.

Advantages	• Provides information that enables judgement to be made about where and with whom the products may safely be tried.
	• Provides information on the mechanical and technical aspects of the products.
Disadvantage	• Does not relate to a potential user's needs.

Level of confidence with which the information can be applied to your situation: **strong** (****) or **some evidence** (***) depending on the tests used and how well they are described.

2.6.2 Ergonomic testing

Ergonomic tests examine how well the product is designed to fit the user, both physically and in its operation. The expertise of the assessors, the number of assessors per product and the environment used for testing will all affect the quality of the evidence gathered.

Hignett (1998) reported ergonomic testing of 12 mobile hoists, asking a range of professionals to use them on a *test circuit* in a hospital setting, with the same occupant, another professional, for every test. Each product underwent eight assessments. The results therefore are useful with regard to the advantages of various hoist features, but cannot help with performance over thresholds or carpeting, nor with how bona fide hoist occupants might feel.

| Advantages | • Provides information regarding how easy a product is to use. |
| | • Provides information that enables judgement to be made about where and with whom the products may safely be tried. |

Disadvantage	• The information usually concerns an 'average' person, so care must be taken when applying the results to those with particular needs.

Level of confidence with which the information can be applied to your situation: **some evidence (***)** provided the assessors are described and represent a range of expertise, otherwise **requires care applying (**)**.

2.6.3 User trials

A *user* is asked to test product(s), and information is collected through direct observation or from the user by means of a questionnaire. The length of the trial period and the setting in which it is tried will affect the data. If the user needs to gain skill or develop a technique to use a product effectively, a ten-minute test will not give an accurate indication of the product's effectiveness. Examples are given at the beginning of section 2.5.

If users try products out as part of a focus group, this book classifies this as a focus group trial (see section 2.3 above) and not a user trial.

Trials may be of a single product, or of several. With single product trials, it is important to know what product, if any, the user had immediately prior to the trial, as he or she will make comparisons and answer questions in the light of their experience. When a user tests several products, comparisons are made between them, and the data can be analysed on this basis. Thus, trials of several products by users give more robust data.

With products that are modular so that a different combination of components will be selected to suit each individual, direct comparisons between products can only be made intra-subject, i.e. on differences in performance that one individual notes. With devices such as these a *case study* approach may be used. It is possible to draw inferences from a series of intra-subject comparisons.

Qualitative comments may be gathered from the participants to add depth to data collected by closed questions.

Advantage	• Those testing the products can be selected to represent the range of requirements for which the assistive device has been designed.

Disadvantage
- Information that is of interest to services such as community equipment stores may not be gathered, for example concerning durability or ease of adjustment between successive users.

Level of confidence with which the information can be applied to your situation: *Quantitative data*: **some evidence** (★★★), usually quite strong if comparative testing has been undertaken by a range of users, or **requires care applying** (★★) if the sample is further divided into subgroups, unless the result is statistically significant, or the trial is of only one product. *Qualitative data*: **requires care in applying** (★★), but if the sample is comprehensive and the data can show that participants responded consistently, the evidence will be stronger.

Summary

The published evidence referred to in this book is classified into four categories. These indicate the trustworthiness of the study results and hence what degree of confidence the reader has when using the guidelines contained in Part 2 for a given situation.

Evaluations of assistive devices use a wide variety of methods. These include:

- informal evaluations, usually by an experienced professional

- focus groups, in which people discuss their views and experience of specific devices

- surveys, which can be by post, telephone or interview

- formal trials, where device(s) are tested in accordance with the study's protocol, and the outcomes noted in a systematic way. They may be technical, ergonomic or user-based trials.

References

Bandolier (1994) 'Assessment Criteria.' *Bandolier* 6, 5. On-line version accessed on 5/3/01 at www.jr2.ox.ac.uk/bandolier/band6/b6-5.html

We found no systematic reviews to meet the journal's criteria for the highest category (I). Therefore our **** is equivalent to category II; * equivalent to catagory V.

Bentur, N., Barnea, T. and Mizrahi, I. (1996) 'A follow-up study of elderly buyers of an assistive chair.' *Physical and Occupational Therapy in Geriatrics 14*, 3, 51–60.

Beresford, S. (1999) 'The Clos-o-mat shower toilet.' *British Journal of Therapy and Rehabilitation 6*, 7, 343–346.

Burdon, D. and Craighead, S. (2000) 'Seahorse sanichair for use by children and adolescents.' *British Journal of Therapy and Rehabilitation 7*, 7, 310–313.

Delbecq, A., Van der Veen, A. and Gustafson, D. (1975) *Group techniques for program planning: a guide to Nominal Group and Delphi processes.* Glenview, IL: Scott-Foresman.

Finlayson, M. and Havixbeck, K. (1992) 'A post discharge study on the use of assistive devices.' *Canadian Journal of Occupational Therapy 59*, 4, 201–207.

Gitlin, L., Levine, R. and Geiger, C. (1993) 'Adaptive device use by older adults with mixed disabilities.' *Archives of Physical Medicine and Rehabilitation 74*, 149–152.

Hawley, M., O'Neill, P. and Webb, L. (1999) 'A provision framework and software tools to aid the prescription of electronic assistive technology: results of a case study.' In C. Bühler and H. Knops (eds) *Assistive technology on the threshold of the millennium* pp.728–732. Amsterdam: IOS Press.

Hignett, S. (1998) 'Ergonomic evaluation of electric mobile hoists.' *British Journal of Occupational Therapy 61*, 11, 509–16.

Jensen, J. (1993) 'MS: a series of studies exploring the issues that influence the decision to structurally alter the home.' MSc Health Psychology. London: City University.

Lane, J., Usiak, D., Stone, V. and Scherer, M. (1997) 'The voice of the consumer: consumers define the ideal battery charger.' *Assistive Technology 9*, 2, 130–139.

Mann, W. and Tomita, M. (1998) 'Perspectives on assistive devices among elderly persons with disabilities.' *Technology and Disability 9*, 119–148.

MDA (1998) *Seating for young children with disabilities: an evaluation*, A23. London: Medical Devices Agency.

MDA (1999a) *Electric riser seats and chairs: an evaluation*, EL2. London: Medical Devices Agency.

MDA (1999b) *Leg lifters: an evaluation*, EL4. London: Medical Devices Agency.

MDA (2001a) *Bath cushions for people with severe disabilities: an evaluation*, EL6. London: Medical Devices Agency.

In addition to formal user trials, a Delphi survey was conducted with 30 people who had participated in the trials.

MDA (2001b) *Mattress elevators and pillow lifts: an evaluation*, EL7. London: Medical Devices Agency.

A formal trial of 16 mattress elevators and pillow lifts. Technical and ergonomic risk assessments were undertaken prior to user trials being conducted. One actuator overheated after a few minutes' use; this represented a potential hazard of burning the user, and the product was withdrawn. Ergonomic tests highlighted risks such as limb entrapment, and inclusion criteria were reviewed to ensure participants did not trial high-risk products without adequate assessment and warning.

MDD (1993) *Basic commodes: a comparative evaluation* DEA A5. Medical Devices Directorate. Norwich: HMSO.

The evaluation of 18 commodes included testing them against BS 4875 Part 1 and 2 Strength and stability of furniture, to Level 4 (severe domestic and general contract).

Moore, C.M. (1987) *Group techniques for idea building.* Applied Social Research Methods series Vol. 9. Newbury Park, CA: Sage Publications.

Perr, A. (1998) 'Elements of seating and wheeled mobility intervention.' *OT Practice 3,* 9, 17–24.

Ryan, S., Rigby, P. and From, W. (1996) 'Understanding the product needs of consumers of assistive devices.' *Canadian Journal of Rehabilitation 9,* 2, 129–135.

Bibliography

FOCUS GROUPS

Gitlin, L. and Burgh, D. (1995) 'Issuing assistive devices to older patients: an exploratory study.' *American Journal of Occupational Therapy 49,* 10, 994–1000.

Kitzinger, J. (1995) 'Introducing focus groups.' *British Medical Journal 311,* 299–302.

Stewart, D. and Shamdasani, P. (1990) *Focus groups, theory and practice.* London: Sage.

DELPHI TECHNIQUE

Sumison, T. (1998) 'The Delphi technique: an adaptive research tool.', *British Journal of Occupational Therapy 61,* 4, 153–156.

Part Two

Part Two

Chapter 3

Seating

Introduction

Before working through this section, it is important to do the following:

- Consider your (the user's) requirements, and the requirements of any care assistant or others in the household as applicable (see Chapter 1, Stage 1 in Figure 1.3).

- Have in mind the environment(s) in which the assistive device(s) will be used (Stage 2 in Figure 1.3); this may include decisions and arrangements for any necessary alterations to it.

This chapter guides you through the decisions about what categories of seating might be suitable, and helps to define what features you would want products to possess, within your preferred categories. This comprises Stage 4 in the process of choosing a product (see Figure 1.3). The examples give you an idea of how the Figures and Tables are used and may include additional things which could be tested or checked when trying out the selected two or three products (Stage 5 in the process described in Chapter 1).

The ideal before getting any product is to test it out, and with seating this is even more critical; a trial period of several days should be requested. Failing this, the minimum time advisable depends on the type of product, for example 20 minutes for easy chairs, a day or two for office or work seating, a couple of hours for pressure relief seating. If new skills have to be acquired in order to use the product effectively, much longer trials lasting several weeks could be needed.

Although this chapter does not include information about wheelchairs, the components of specialised seating are often fitted to wheelchairs and so are relevant to wheelchair users. Additionally, wheelchair users may wish to have alternative seating to their wheelchairs, to provide for different sitting positions and social or personal needs such as relaxation.

This chapter presents a review of different features and components of chairs and seats in relation to their functional performance and users' opinions. It is divided into standard or special seating needs. As a guide, if you can sit safely with no more support at your back than a dining chair provides, you probably do not need special support for seating. Pressure distributing products are covered in the final section in this chapter; these must be considered if you are not able regularly to change your position in a chair.

3.1 The importance of good seating

Most people sit for long periods each day, particularly if reliant on a wheelchair. Suitable chairs to encourage a good posture are therefore very important.

3.1.1 What is 'good' posture?

There is no ideal posture, but a good posture is one in which your weight is evenly distributed with no muscles over-working, and which enables you to do the task you want with the least fatigue. It should be easy to maintain eye contact when in conversation with others. The classic upright sitting posture with hips and knees at right angles, feet flat on the floor and the trunk more or less vertical (Figure 3.1.1) is not a suitable posture for many functional tasks (ten Haar 1999). Alternative postures, such as forward leaning, are being proposed for tasks such as writing, and a slightly reclined posture is desired by many when relaxing.

Lumbar support to keep pelvis upright and maintain the lumbar curve.

Hips and knees at 90°

Centre of mass

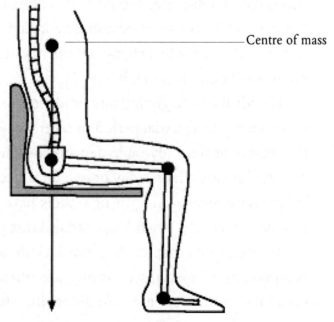

Figure 3.1.1 The classic upright posture

When you sit upright, your back muscles work to keep the pelvis upright and to balance your body over the ischial tuberosities (the bony points on your buttocks) and hip joint. A shaped backrest as in Figure 3.1.1 supports the spine's lumbar curve so that your muscles do not have to work as hard to keep the pelvis upright.

When choosing a chair, the first step in ensuring that it is comfortable and helps to maintain a good posture is to choose one that is a good fit.

3.1.2 A good fit?

Most chairs are designed to accommodate the 'normal' range of shapes, sizes and weights of adults, and will therefore suit 90 per cent of the population. However, even when your height and girth fall within the 90 per cent range, your body proportions may differ from the norm because of your disability. This could result in no chair seeming ideal. You may have to request particular dimensions or other features to ensure you can be seated in the best way possible. Some work has been done (Hobson and Molenbroek 1990) measuring people with cerebral palsy as an aid to good design, but the participants varied greatly in size and shape.

The usual recommendations to ensure a good fit are:

1. Height of seat from ground should be 25 mm (1in.) less than the measurement from the back of your knee to the ground, when seated with hips and knees at right angles in your usual footwear (Pheasant undated). However, if the seat is very soft, the seat height of the uncompressed cushion will need to be higher: measure from the *compressed* cushion.

   Too high a seat will result in the back of your legs pressing on the cushion edge, which will be uncomfortable and reduce circulation, as well as increase the likelihood of your ankles swelling. Alternatively, you slide forwards to get your feet to the floor, so slouching and increasing pressure on your sacrum (Collins and Shipperley 1999).

   Too low a seat will prevent the thighs from taking some of your weight, so increasing the pressure under your buttocks.

2. Depth of seat should be 25 mm (1in.) less than the measurement from the back of the buttocks to the back of the lower leg at the knee.

   Too deep a seat encourages slouching and makes your hips more liable to slip forwards.

Too shallow a seat puts more pressure on your *ischial tuberosities* because the thighs are not taking their usual share of your weight (buttocks and thighs take 75 per cent of your weight, Collins 2001).

3. Width of the seat should be 50 mm (2in.) more than your hip width in usual clothing (Pheasant undated), but a stool without armrests can comfortably be 50 mm *less* than hip width.

    Too wide a seat may mean you lean to one side, placing extra weight on that side and a strain on your spine (Collins and Shipperley 1999). Neither is advisable if you do not shift from side to side regularly.

The height of the seat above the floor is particularly important, and may need to vary from the recommendation either because it must match a table of fixed height, or because of difficulty rising (see subsection 3.2.1).

Other dimensions for which a choice is commonly available are backrest (height, contour, angle) and seat angle. These are discussed further in sections 3.2 and 3.3 because they need to be selected to fulfil particular functions, for example leisure, writing, or to meet special support requirements.

Children who find coping with adult seating difficult, but who do not need special seating (section 3.3) may benefit from a chair made to fit their measurements. Ensure adjustability for growth, by adjustable height legs, and a wider seat which initially can have side pads inside the armrests to fit the hips snugly.

3.1.3 Comfort

Comfort is subjective and therefore difficult to quantify. Most formal tests use a general comfort scale and/or a body part discomfort scale (e.g. Drury and Coury 1982). To compare the comfort of chairs, several are tried and the more comfortable one noted (le Carpentier 1969). Comfort may also be measured indirectly, for example by absence or reduction in pain, or decrease in fidgeting. The latter is probably a less reliable indicator than the others. Some propose that comfort has other qualities and is not just the converse of discomfort (Helander and Zhang 1997) and that both should specifically be measured.

Children as young as six can also be asked to discriminate between seating options (Rigby *et al.* 1996) provided they have real examples to try out.

Many factors contribute to comfort, but studies usually state that 20–30 minutes is required for an accurate judgement to be made (Atherton *et al.* 1979; Sweeney and Clarke 1992; MDA 1999). The dimensions, contours, backrest angle, upholstery and covering material will all affect the overall comfort. It is therefore helpful if users specify where discomfort is felt.

Comfort is also influenced by the task you are doing. You want different characteristics when relaxing in a chair than when writing or undertaking other tasks. When relaxing you want the chair to support you in such a way that gravity makes you sink into it. A slight rake in the backrest is usually desired, although women want less recline than men (le Carpentier 1969); further details can be found in Subsection 3.2.3 *Leisure seating*. Comfort will also be enhanced when the weight of the body is taken equally by buttocks and thighs. To achieve this the feet need to be supported at the height recommended in subsection 3.1.2. Softness of the chair seat *per se* may not provide comfort, because if muscle tone is low, your body will sink into an asymmetrical posture, potentially causing joint pain and in the long term soft tissue damage.

3.1.4 Deciding what type of seating is needed

In working through Figure 3.1.4, note down all the sections that you may need to look at. You may need more than one type of chair, for instance an easy chair and a chair for working.

3.2 Standard seating needs

'Standard' seating covers the basic requirements of support for the back, buttocks and thighs but excludes the special shaping and additional features that are reviewed in section 3.3.

Careful selection is important in order to achieve good posture, comfort and ease of sitting and rising.

3.2.1 Difficulties in getting up from a chair

The majority of times you get up from a chair, there is nothing in front of the chair, but sometimes there is a table, desk or work surface, so that you have to pivot first before rising, or push the chair backwards away from the work surface. To ease pivoting, a swivel chair is appropriate in some cases; an alternative is a fabric turning disc placed between yourself and the chair seat. If difficulty is experienced in pushing the chair back, a chair or stool on castors may help.

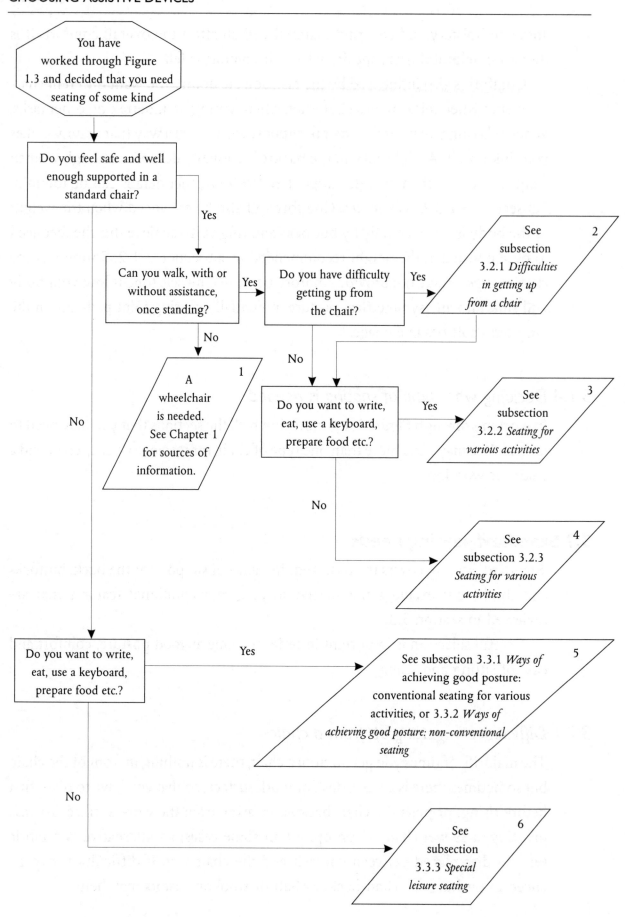

Figure 3.1.4 What type of seating?
(Section 3.4 'Pressure distributing products' should also be consulted if you sit for long periods.)

An example

Primrose has rheumatoid arthritis, and as well as being generally weaker than she used to be, she also has painful wrists, cannot lift her arms above her shoulders, and is wary of her knees buckling under her. She hates getting up from her easy chair because it makes her wrists and knees more painful. After sitting for long periods, she is then more stiff and when she does have to get up, it's even harder. She asked the social services what to do. An occupational therapist visited her at home, and they looked at Table 3.2.1 together.

- They experimented with higher seats by putting a raising unit under her chair. This didn't help much, because the seat sloped backwards a bit. The occupational therapist asked about other chairs in her house.

- Primrose showed her the one in her bedroom. This had a level seat, and they fitted some chair leg sleeves on it to make the seat higher. This proved a bit better, but getting up was still quite a painful process.

- A spring-assisted rising cushion was offered to Primrose. This made getting up easy, and she thought it would be the answer, but soon found that unless she placed a soft cushion at her back, she got low back pain. She had to return the loaned rising cushion.

- Her family clubbed together and offered to buy a new riser/recliner chair. They went to a shop that stocked several, and Primrose tried them all out. She found them all comfortable, and could press the buttons fairly easily. So she chose the one that had a pocket for the hand control that she could reach easily. The big pockets near the floor were too low.

- She was delighted with the chair, until one day as she lowered the chair after a visit to the toilet there was a loud crack. She hastily raised it again and looked under the chair. Her walking stick had fallen between the chair and its base frame, and been snapped as the chair went down.

- As she does not really need to use the mechanism to sit down, she now lowers the chair as soon as she has stood up and is steady on her feet.

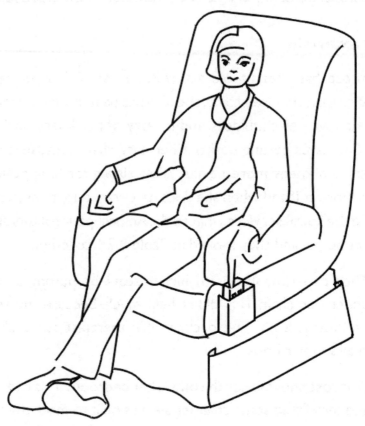

Primrose
Illustration 3.2.1a

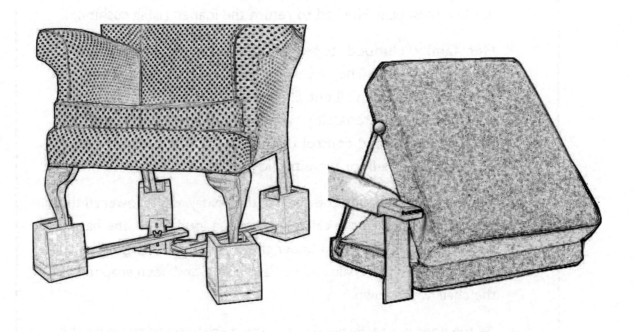

Chair raising unit
Illustration 3.2.1b

Spring-assisted rising cushion

Difficulty in rising from a chair is fairly common with increasing age or disability. Around 10 per cent of older persons may have difficulty in rising from a chair (Dunlop, Hughes and Manheim 1997), and in a sample from day centres for the elderly and a rheumatology outpatient clinic, the percentage reporting difficulty in getting up from their usual easy chair was 42 per cent (Munton *et al.* 1981).

Pain or weakness in the legs will make getting up from a chair more difficult. Too great a difficulty in rising may result in you reducing the number of times you move. This is not desirable, because staying in one position for long periods leads to more stiffness, weakness and pain, as well as increasing the risk of poorer circulation, swelling around the ankles and pressure sores (see also section 3.4).

Various strategies can be tried to reduce difficulty in rising. Leaning forward, tucking your feet back, rising with your head up, and using the armrests (Chan *et al.* 1999) all help to make rising easier (Laporte and Sveistrup 1999). It is therefore helpful to have chairs that are not boxed in right to the ground, so enabling your feet to be placed directly below your knees. The alternative is to shift your buttocks forward, which requires additional effort prior to rising. Maintaining momentum during the rise makes it seem easier, probably because less effort overall may be required, although this is not proven scientifically (Laporte *et al.* 1999). Finally, pausing between attaining a standing position and moving off is helpful to ensure balance is good, and any temporary faintness on getting up has had time to resolve (Munro and Steele 1998). All the studies conducted on rising difficulties have related to easy chairs, so see also subsection 3.2.3 *Leisure seating.*

Armrests enable you to share the effort of rising between your arms and legs (Munro and Steele 1998), and the design most helpful (see Figure 3.2.3) is:

- armrest height at about the level of your elbows when seated

- armrest length extends as far as the edge of the seat

- the end of the armrest is easy to grasp.

Quite frequently, people put an extra cushion on a chair to enable them to sit higher. This is potentially unsatisfactory because it may slip (Mann and Tomita 1998), and you tend to sink into the cushion more, so increasing the effort needed to get up. In addition the armrests will be relatively lower and so less helpful when rising, and any lumbar shaping of the backrest will be in the wrong place.

Table 3.2.1 Guidance on chair features that make rising from a chair easier

Possible solution	Factors in favour	Factors against
Higher seat height	Significantly improves the proportion of elderly able to rise independently (Weiner *et al.* 1993 *** Finlay et al. 1983 ***).	May need a footstool which is an extra hazard (Munro and Steele 1998*).
1. use chair raisers	Less expensive. Existing chair is retained.	Although there is a range of chair raisers, some chairs cannot be safely raised in this way with any standard raiser, so a carpenter would need to make a customised adaptation (Milne 1988**).
2. get new chair with seat height required	Can select contours, upholstery, etc. to meet your needs.	More expensive than chair raisers.*
Spring or pneumatic piston assisted	Reduces effort required (Wretenberg *et al.* 1993***). Footstool should not be needed (Munro *et al.* 1998*). No electricity supply needed.	Facility may not be used if insufficient instruction given (Bentur *et al.* 1996***). Spring-assist is not advised if you are prone to losing your balance or falling (Bashford *et al.* 1998*). May be a risk of finger entrapment between seat and chair frame on sitting down (MDA 1998c**).
1. cushion	Can be used on existing chair.	Benefit of lumbar contour will be lost because you sit higher.
2. chair	Lumbar contours will be in correct position.	More expensive than riser cushion.*
Electrically operated risers	Easy to operate.	Expensive. Risk of entrapment of items, animals, etc. between chair and seat base (MDA 2000**). Some are unstable when fully raised (MDA 1999**).
1. seat unit	You need to have good range of movement in your knees and little or no pain in your arms (MDA 1999**).	
2. chair	Suitable if you cannot bend your knees to 90° and/or have general weakness (MDA 1999**).	
Riser/recliner	Recline can be used to alter pressure distribution (ten Haar 1999*).	Does not appreciably reduce pressure under buttocks until reclined to 135° (Pellow 1999***).
	Suitable if you need to raise your feet level with your hips to prevent ankles swelling.	Not all leg supports rise sufficiently high to be effective in reducing swelling.*

Note: If you need to put your feet up but do not always want to recline at the same time, you will need a chair with two motors so the features can be operated independently. This increases the cost of the product.

Table 3.2.1 *Guidance on chair features that make rising from a chair easier* sets out the main ways to address difficulty in rising from a chair, in suggested order of consideration. Note, however, that other factors will affect your final choice, as indicated in the Table.

3.2.2 Seating for various activities

Seating needs will alter according to the task undertaken (Drury and Coury 1982). This section covers office and kitchen tasks, because these will encompass the majority of daily needs.

OFFICE TASKS

Provided a chair is basically a good fit, it should be comfortable enough (Helander and Zhang 1997). If you have a painful back you will place more exacting demands on design. The major goal is to keep the spine and neck in a position that does not strain the back mechanically but places the arms in the desired place. Whereas at rest you should have your centre of gravity over or slightly behind the ischial tuberosities (see Figure 3.1.1), for work tasks it should fall slightly in front (Myhr and von Wendt 1991). The problem with this is that often flexion occurs around the lumbar region rather than at the hips, and this puts more strain on the spine, so ways to reduce this have been investigated.

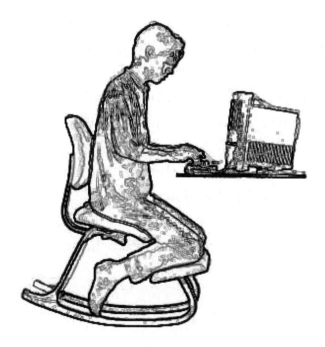

A Balans style chair
Illustration 3.2.2

The obvious thing to try first is to change the seat angle. A slight forward tilt (10–15°) does help to bring your upper body forward, so helping the spine stay naturally curved and reducing neck flexion (Brunswic 1984). The feet (or knees if the seat is a Balans type) must be supported so weight can be taken through them.

However, design criteria for office chairs for those without disabilities advise a forward seat angle of 0–5° (Grandjean 1980). If you have low back pain you would need to trial both Balans and conventional chairs to see which proved more comfortable; you may find the former comfortable (Greenfield 1986), but if a conventional chair design is chosen, an adjustable height backrest is advised (Sweeney and Clarke 1991).

Backrest designs are similarly contested, opinion being divided between a high backrest (Grandjean 1980) and a lower one to allow free arm movements. A lumbar pad is recommended. An evaluation of a prototype (Drury and Coury 1982) produced responses from users that indicated a backrest should be adjustable in rake and height and have a spring to accommodate a user suddenly leaning back.

KITCHEN TASKS

Many people prefer to sit when undertaking kitchen tasks, either because they are unable to stand for the length of time required, or because they feel unsafe tackling an additional task when standing.

The work surfaces in most kitchens are designed for people to use when standing. If you are a wheelchair user, chairs of standard height will not be satisfactory unless the kitchen has been adapted for you. High stools or adjustable-height office chairs are the common solutions. Whether you are a wheelchair user or not, the height between your elbows and the work surface is the important measurement. The height must be sufficient to allow comfortable use of the work surface with the elbow 88–122 mm (3.5–4.7 in.) above the surface (Pheasant undated). Ideally the elbow room should be adjustable because different tasks have different optimal heights (Pheasant undated): smallest elbow-to-surface height for use of sink, highest for tasks needing downward pressure such as rolling pastry. Adjustable-height stools make this possible.

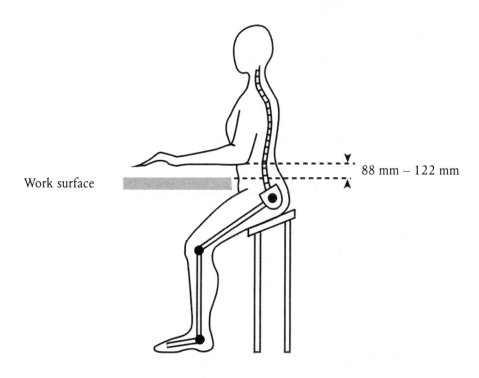

Work surface

88 mm – 122 mm

Figure 3.2.2 Elbow clearance at kitchen work surface

Table 3.2.2 Guidance on features of high seat chairs and stools for kitchen tasks

Your disability	*Chair feature*	*Guideline*	★
Low back pain	Seat	Sloping forwards often preferred.	★★
Rheumatoid arthritis, or osteoarthritis of lower limbs	Backrest	Preferred chairs with backrest.	★
	Armrests	Preferred to have armrests, or a wider seat so could push up from seat.	★★
Stroke	Backrest, armrests	Preferred to have these.	★★
Multiple sclerosis	Legs	Stable design.	★
Elderly	Seat	Lower than for younger people.	★
All users	Adjustments	Should be easy to reach and use.	★

Source: Greenfield 1986.

3.2.3 Leisure seating

If you have a disability or are elderly you may spend more time in a leisure chair than other people. The comfort of such chairs is therefore of particular importance. The chair must also be easy to get in and out of (see subsection 3.2.1 above) and if you move very little, it should incorporate pressure relieving seating (see section 3.4 below). The designs that provide comfort may impede getting up, and higher seats are not usually as comfortable (Alexander, Koester and Grunawalt 1996). Therefore a compromise will often be necessary.

Men tend to prefer a more reclined backrest and a less angled seat than women (le Carpentier 1969). More recline demands greater effort when preparing to rise to standing, so keeping the rake to 100–110° is recommended (Pheasant undated). A backrest with a convex lumbar curve and a concave curve for the upper body is ideal. Wings provide head support when resting. However, if you have people sitting to your side, as commonly occurs in rest homes, you will not be able to see them if the chair wings are too large (Ellis 1988).

People with ankylosing spondylitis were found to prefer good back and head support; those with low back pain wanted good lumbar support (Sweeney and Clarke 1992). It is important for the backrest to be of sufficient height on easy chairs, as participants in two studies reported insufficient head support on their chairs (Atherton *et al.* 1979; Mann and Tomita 1998).

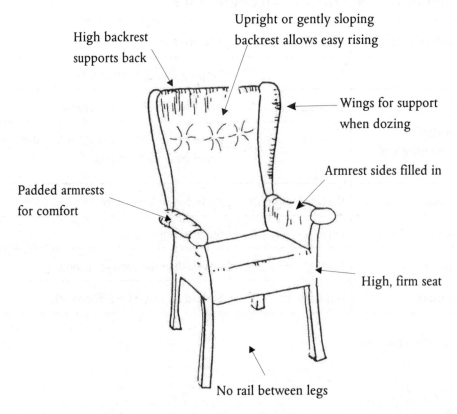

Figure 3.2.3 Features to look for in an easy chair. (Reproduced from Ellis 1998, 'Choosing easy chairs for the disabled.' British Medical Journal 296, 702. With permission from the BMJ Publishing Group.)

In residential settings, residents usually have 'their chair' in communal sitting rooms, so it can be chosen to meet that individual's needs. In hospital wards by contrast, chairs will be used by many different people. An audit has shown that only 50 per cent of staff on two rehabilitation and continuing care wards for the elderly were aware that seat height, depth and width were important (McCafferty *et al.* 2000). This audit also implied that the available chairs were not adjustable for height, so the only strategy for seating a patient at the appropriate height was to look for another chair.

It is therefore recommended that chairs used for a number of different people should be adjustable in height between 380 and 490mm (15–19.25in.) which should meet the needs of 90 per cent of the adult population (Pheasant undated). Although 380 mm is above the 5th percentile for women (355 mm, 14 in.) this may be acceptable for most because of their probable difficulty in rising from lower seats, unless their optimum seat height is not more than about 30 mm (1in.) less than the lowest seat height.

3.3 Special seating needs

You may be unable to maintain a good posture in standard seating. When standard seating is failing you, an assessment is needed to identify seating that is more suitable for you as an individual. Such an assessment includes identifying the tasks you wish to do, the posture best for you to undertake those tasks, the best posture for you to relax in, the environment in which the seat will be used, and any care assistant perspectives. Your individual preferences about the style and appearance of the chair will also be important when the final choice is made. Having considered all these things, you may decide you need more than one chair, for example one for leisure and one for work.

As your requirements become more complex, you will usually be assisted in the assessment process by a physiotherapist or an occupational therapist. Assessment is a skilled job, and the therapists 'ultimately rely on observational skills, evaluation results, the ability to try the client in a number of positions … and also rely on input from the client' (Trefler and Taylor 1991, p.220). The evaluation the authors speak of is the hands-on assessment of the client, rather than a descriptive evaluation of a chair's features.

A comprehensive seating assessment will include finding out exactly what happens to joints and muscles both seated and lying. The ways that practitioners do such assessments have been documented by many (e.g. Fife *et al.* 1991; Hastings 2000; Healy, Ramsay and Sexsmith 1997, Johnson Taylor 1987; ten

Haar 1999; Trefler and Taylor 1991). The starting point is the pelvis, and ideally this should be upright, level and straight. The support needed for the body and head cannot be determined until the pelvis is supported in the best way possible.

The goals for seating a person with special seating needs are more detailed than those for a standard 'good posture' (see subsection 3.1.1). The more detailed goals are to:

- provide a safe and functional position

- provide comfort

- improve head control

- decrease abnormal muscle tone

- delay or reduce contractures etc.

- increase independence

- assist care assistant's task (Hulme *et al.* 1987; Letts 1991; Trefler and Taylor 1991; Collins 2001).

Leaving a person who cannot sit upright without adequate support has a detrimental effect both functionally (e.g. Hulme *et al.* 1983; Deitz and Crepeau 1998) and physically, in that potentially avoidable deformities could develop over time. The consequences of poor seating are potentially great, risking the reverse of all the goals stated at the beginning of this section, and increasing the risk of pressure sores. 'Every person who spends a significant portion of their day in a sitting position deserves a seating system that accomplishes optimal support in socially acceptable positions' (Healy *et al.* 1997, p.706).

REASONS FOR NEEDING SPECIAL SEATING

Special support needs arise when various components of your body are not working quite as they do normally.

If your muscles do not work well enough to hold your body upright, they may be low in tone ('flaccid' or 'floppy'). This means that they cannot resist the pull of gravity, so only the skeleton can do this, and pressure is put on each joint in the direction that the body's weight (or mass) is acting. It is therefore vital to ensure that this pressure is directly through the joint, as this is the way the joint is designed to function. Prolonged pressure in other directions will eventually damage the joint.

If some or all of your muscles are high in tone ('tight' or 'spastic'), there is the same need to achieve pressure through the joints in the right direction, but this may be achieved by a different approach because the effect of positioning varies from one person to another. Each person's pattern of involuntary muscular activity will pose different challenges to attaining a good posture, although a common approach is possible for many people (see subsection 3.3.1 below).

When a person has not been able to sit in a well-supported posture, joints yield to the pressures on them, assume a different position and eventually stiffen up. Before stiffening up has occurred, it is possible to correct the problem and avert long-term damage. If the joints are stiff, seating has to accommodate this, although treatment to loosen them is sometimes suggested.

ASSESSMENT TOOLS

Any recommendation of the types of seating and support that may meet particular needs obviously must use some descriptions of those needs, and for this purpose standardised assessment tools are often used (e.g. Fife *et al.* 1991; Mulcahy 1986; Mulcahy *et al.* 1988; Myhr and von Wendt 1991). Such tools also enable evaluation of the seating devices by describing posture before and after their provision, although either they tend to be insufficiently specific or the *inter-rater reliability* is not good.

3.3.1 Ways of achieving good posture: conventional seating for various activities

Most of the literature assumes that seating systems will be part of a wheelchair, but many of the components could equally be for static seating, and on that basis are reviewed here. Static seating with the range of components that is described is mainly found for children, but there are products for adults, especially modular leisure chairs (see subsection 3.3.3).

The assessment process and the principles behind this are not evaluated here, but some of the strategies used to improve or support posture are summarised and the evidence for the effectiveness of seating and seating features that are used is reviewed.

Conventional seating implies a basic chair shape; non-conventional seating is considered below (subsection 3.3.2). Variations may be needed according to the activity, such as eating, use of computer, wheelchair operation, and all types of activity requiring the hands.

To achieve a good sitting posture, it is generally agreed that there should be one approach for those with low muscle tone (floppiness), described mainly for those who have spinal injuries, and another for those with high muscle tone (spasticity), described mainly for those with cerebral palsy or other neuro-motor problems. Each person should be assessed individually, and whilst the seat and lower back support would be provided for all, other features would be recommended only if considered necessary.

LOW MUSCLE TONE

When your back muscles are floppy, it is usually not possible to sit upright without the support of a backrest. Unsupported sitting is either impossible or else the pelvis tilts backwards or forwards until the ligaments around the spine's joints hinder further movement. Support is needed to work with gravity to provide stability in sitting (ten Haar 1999). Figure 3.3.1a illustrates how a good posture may be achieved, indicating where there are discrepancies between experts.

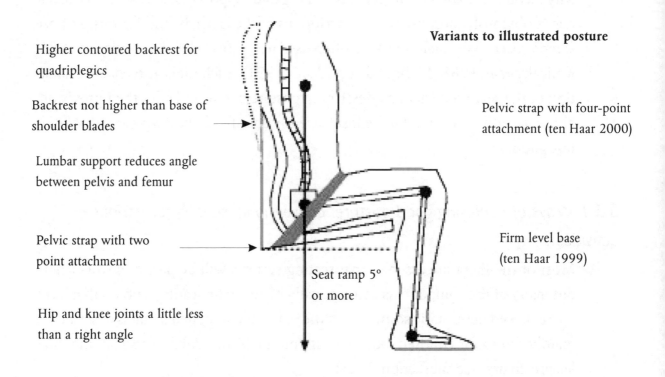

Higher contoured backrest for quadriplegics

Backrest not higher than base of shoulder blades

Lumbar support reduces angle between pelvis and femur

Pelvic strap with two point attachment

Hip and knee joints a little less than a right angle

Variants to illustrated posture

Pelvic strap with four-point attachment (ten Haar 2000)

Firm level base (ten Haar 1999)

Seat ramp 5° or more

Figure 3.3.1a Special support in conventional sitting for people with low muscle tone
Note: this Figure should be read in conjunction with Table 3.3.1a.

A sloped seat reduces forward slipping. It should be noted that biomechanically, sloping the seat up towards the front also tends to tip the pelvis into posterior tilt (Turner 2001). The function of the vertical backrest is to counteract this force, so there will be pressure at the top of the sacrum (at the top of the pelvis – PSIS[1] level). It is important that this pressure is spread across the back to avoid points of high pressure (see section 3.4 below). To keep the pelvis snugly against the

1   PSIS: posterior superior iliac spine, which is the edge of the bone at the back of the pelvis.

backrest, a pelvic strap may be needed, particularly if the pelvis tends to fall forwards rather than backwards.

An example

Peter had a spinal cord injury at T2,3 which has left him with good arm strength, but difficulty in keeping an upright posture. When sitting, he tends to be 'C' shaped, with his pelvis tilted backwards, and the rest of his spine in a single curve, except that he then has to bend his neck back to balance his head. He wants to be able to work at his computer without getting neck ache.

When he went to the seating clinic for an assessment, the therapist found that no joints had limited range of movement, so he was asked to try a seat that was gently sloped up towards the front, with a backrest that came up to just below his shoulder blades, shaped to support the lower back's curve. He felt he needed to jut his chin out to balance, so the therapist decided his centre of mass was a little far back, and adjusted the backrest angle to be a fraction more upright.

This felt better, but after a few minutes, Peter's hips had slipped forwards a bit, so a pelvic strap was suggested. He did not like that idea at all, and said he would prefer to lift himself up and reposition his hips when necessary.

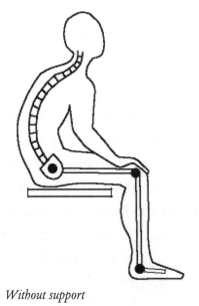

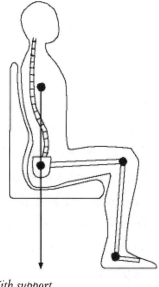

Without support

With support

Figure 3.3.1b Peter

HIGH MUSCLE TONE

When the muscles are tighter than is needed to achieve a good sitting posture, the aim of support is to encourage the muscles to relax, or to discourage them from tightening further. The muscles that are tight may be those that pull your joints straight or bend them, but for many it is the muscles that straighten the hips and knees that are tight, so the hips joints need to be bent to 90° or more to discourage the muscles from contracting. The ramped seat and pelvic strap reduce slipping, and the knees and ankles may need stabilising too (see Figure 3.3.1c).

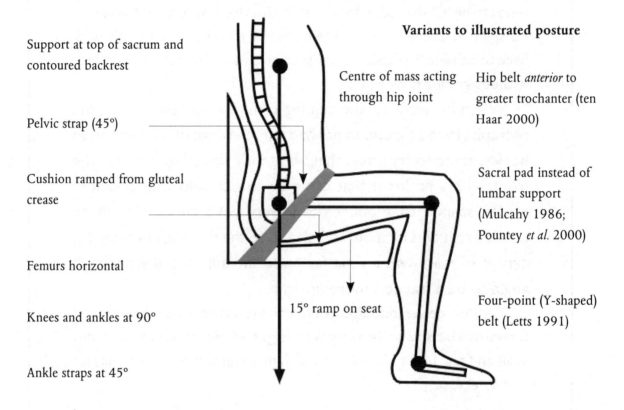

Variants to illustrated posture

Support at top of sacrum and contoured backrest

Centre of mass acting through hip joint

Hip belt *anterior* to greater trochanter (ten Haar 2000)

Pelvic strap (45°)

Cushion ramped from gluteal crease

Sacral pad instead of lumbar support (Mulcahy 1986; Pountey *et al.* 2000)

Femurs horizontal

15° ramp on seat

Four-point (Y-shaped) belt (Letts 1991)

Knees and ankles at 90°

Ankle straps at 45°

Figure 3.3.1c Special support in conventional sitting for people with high muscle tone. Note: This Figure should be read in conjunction with Table 3.3.1a

---

An example

James has cerebral palsy with spasticity and a tendency to extensor spasms. Without appropriate support, he arches over a chair and his feet tend to cross at the ankles. When the therapist assesses him, she finds that his joints are supple, so recommends a seat that is flat under his buttocks and sloped slightly up towards the front to ensure his femurs are horizontal. The backrest is vertical behind his sacrum, slightly curved inwards for his lumbar spine and outwards for his upper body. A pelvic strap keeps his pelvis upright.

For many people, more support is needed than that illustrated in Figure 3.3.1c, and ways of addressing these additional postural challenges are tabulated in Table 3.3.1a. These are usually part of a seating system for a wheelchair, but as mentioned above, some chairs, particularly for children, offer these components. Few of the components are mutually exclusive, so you may need a combination of things to solve the problem. Even with greater constraint, the aim should still be to enhance the ability to do tasks. This means the support must be sufficient to enable the user to move to do things, then be able to return to the 'at rest' posture (Fife *et al.* 1991; ten Haar 1999).

Table 3.3.1a How different components of special seating are used

Type of difficulty	Seating component	Guideline
Low muscle tone around the hips: pelvis tends to tilt backwards	Seat	Horizontal or slight slope upwards to front to reduce slipping. Contoured seat help to centre the pelvis.
	Pelvic strap	Attached so pull is just in front of the greater trochanter (bone at side of hip) (ten Haar 2000).
	Backrest	Lumbar support to hold pelvis upright; backrest no higher than base of shoulder blades.
pelvis tends to tilt forwards	Seat	Horizontal or slight slope upwards to front to reduce slipping.
		Contoured seat to help centre the pelvis.
	Pelvic strap	Attached at backrest and seat (four-point) so pelvis is pulled against the back support and prevented from slipping forwards (ten Haar 2000).
	Backrest	Lumbar support to support spine; backrest no higher than base of shoulder blades.
	Recline or tilt (periodic)	To help correct pelvic position.
	Working surface	Alternative to chest harness only for short periods to encourage acquisition of sitting balance (Mulcahy *et al.* 1988). The height should not be too high otherwise the shoulders are hunched (Letts 1991).

High muscle tone in lower limbs and around the hips	Seat	Ramped from gluteal crease (end of buttocks) to reduce slipping and keep femurs horizontal. Contours or pommel to keep legs apart.
	Pelvic strap	45° to pull across greater trochanter.
	Backrest	Lumbar support; alternatively a sacral pad to keep the pelvis upright (Pountney *et al.* 2000).
	Abduction *orthosis* or pommel	To stabilise hip joints and widen sitting base.
	Knee blocks	To stabilise the knees in a bent position and keep femurs in straight line with hip joints.
	Ankle straps	Essential if knee blocks used.
Trunk: scoliosis or asymmetry	Backrest	'Triangle of control' achieved by pads at hips and high on trunk on side away from apex and at apex (or just under rib that is joined to the vertebra at apex of spinal curvature: ten Haar 1999). A little backrest rake to relieve gravitational pull on the scoliosis (Trefler and Taylor 1991).
low muscle tone in upper trunk	Backrest	High contoured backrest with lumbar support. Slight backrest rake.
	Side support	If necessary to prevent falling to one side.
	Chest harness	Fixings to backrest should be level with top of shoulder.
	Recline or tilt	To provide rest for trunk muscles.
	Head support	Use only when necessary, e.g. in vehicles or when using a recline facility. Provide support only where it is necessary e.g. unilateral if that is sufficient. *Do not fix* head, e.g. with head band, unless there is no possibility of body slipping.
kyphosis (spine is bent so body comes forward)	Backrest	Recline or tilt slightly until line of vision is horizontal.
	Lumbar support	If the kyphosis is flexible, making the pelvis tilt forwards may encourage the upper spine to straighten (Pope 1996).
trunk rotation	Pelvic strap	Two- or three-point attachment: two points of attachment on forward hip.

Jerky movements	Seat and backrest	Minimise contours for those with athetosis to allow for movement (ten Haar 1999).
	Straps	Thigh straps may be suitable; ensure they do not dig into groin.
Asymmetrical movement	Seat and backrest	Provide maximum support, i.e. a moulded seat (Pope 1996).
Hard wear or misuse	All	Any user who tends to rock or pick will need a seating system designed to withstand expected misuse. A lengthened base, whether wheeled or static, will reduce the risk of tipping.
		Seating for those tending to self-harm must be carefully assessed and modified to minimise this risk.

The information above represents a consensus view among experts except where specific references are cited. Expert opinion includes authors such as the following (see Reference section): Cutter and Blake 1997, Deitz and Crepeau 1998, Hastings 2000, Healy *et al.* 1997, Letts 1991, Mulcahy 1986, Mulcahy and Pountney, 1986, Mulcahy *et al.* 1988, Pope 1996, Pountney *et al.* 1999, Swedberg et al. 1996, ten Haar 1999, 2000, Trefler and Taylor 1991, Zollars 2000.

The information above is applicable to children, with the exception of lumbar support if the child has not yet developed a lumbar lordosis (inward curve of the spine). The information is applicable to children, with the exception of lumbar support if the child has not yet developed a lumbar lordasis (inward curve of the spine).

For users and care assistants alike, such a range of components is daunting, and it is essential that everyone concerned knows why each component is included on an assistive seating device (ASD).

More examples

James (described above), finds that his legs still tend to straighten, shifting his hips away from the backrest. Some ankle straps to steady his feet are added and also knee blocks to prevent strain on his knee joints from the adductor spasms that pull his legs together. James feels very confined, but he gets used to it, and realises that he feels less tired and can do more when he is well supported.

Yvonne has spina bifida and has no feeling or movement from the waist down. She is 14 and beginning to be conscious of her looks. She feels short and dumpy, and thinks this might be partly due to the marked lumbar curve in her lower back. Her therapist is keen to improve her posture, and seizes the opportunity. Yvonne's pelvis is

---

tilted forward, but can be moved freely, whereas her upper spine has a roundedness (kyphosis) that cannot be straightened. Her therapist suggests a seat that is level under her buttocks with a slight upward slope towards the front, a backrest that is vertical to the top of her sacrum, then a slight lumbar curve, and a backward contour to accommodate her upper back. Once seated, Yvonne has a four-point pelvic strap that is attached to the seat and backrest and fits under her suprapubic catheter. She finds the weight of her upper body supported by the backrest curve, and is pleased at how discreet the lap belt looks. The seat has a gel pad under her buttocks, but is otherwise foam, with a small contour at the side edges to keep her legs from rolling outwards immodestly.

Yvonne is given the choice of colour for the seat and backrest cover and is highly delighted with her new system.

Amanda has cerebral palsy, and at 26 years, has developed a scoliosis and windswept hips to the left (both legs are skewed to one side). She had not been seen by a seating specialist since she left college at 19, and now the spine's curves cannot be straightened, and it is painful for her to try to straighten her legs. The therapist aims to support her comfortably but prevent further deterioration.

Amanda is given a seat that fits her hips very snugly, and the backrest has a pad at the apex of her curve on the one side, and another pad under her arm on the opposite side. A pelvic strap helps to keep her hips in place. Pads are fixed to support the left sides of her thighs to straighten the legs slightly.

Amanda tries these, but finds her hips really ache after a while, so she has to go back and explain that she cannot tolerate the seat for long periods. The pads are moved a little to the left, and this improves Amanda's tolerance to several hours a day, with which she is satisfied.

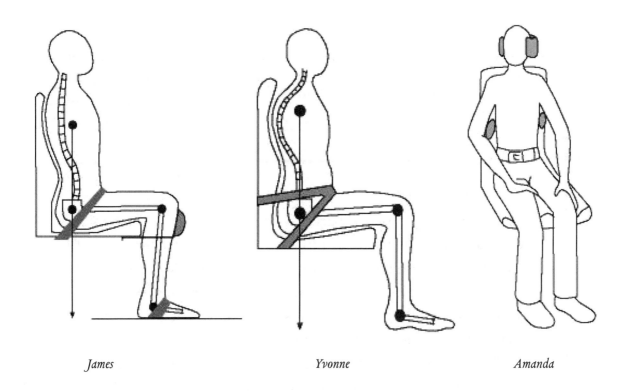

James   Yvonne   Amanda

Figure 3.3.1d James, Yvonne and Amanda

A reclining backrest or a *tilt-in-space* facility may be incorporated on a seating system to provide relief from an upright posture. See Table 3.3.3 *Advantages and disadvantages of special leisure chair features* for further information.

JERKY MOVEMENTS

When a person moves involuntarily, stabilisation rather than constraint is the aim (ten Haar 2000). The seating should allow some movement but be designed to encourage the body to return to position on relaxation. Comfort is also a key aim, but in practice is too often not achieved (Mann and Tomita 1998; Seeger, Caudrey and O'Mara 1984; Weiss-Lambrou *et al.* 1999).

An example

Trevor has athetoid cerebral palsy, and has never really felt comfortable in a chair, except for the sofa at home. He has broken more straps than he can count, and had a pressure sore at the bottom of his spine last year because of rubbing against the backrest. No one wants this to happen again now it is healed.

He and the seating specialist agree to try giving him as much room to move as is safe, so start with a flat seat that is a firm, pressure-distributing foam. The backrest is a soft foam, curved at the sides to nestle his trunk into the centre, built over a robust frame that will withstand the push backwards that Trevor frequently makes. He and the therapist discuss the extra stabilisation he will need: two options are thigh straps, or a tray across the wheelchair with foam underneath to limit the amount his legs can move.

Trevor tries the tray, and although it works quite well, he does not want to use the tray always. He wants to do without it when he goes out. So he uses the thigh straps mostly, and keeps the tray for when he uses his computer keyboard.

TYPES OF SEATING SYSTEM

A broad classification has been compiled (BSRM 1995):

- Fixed. The chair components cannot be altered.

- Adjustable.

- Modular. Various features are available that can be selected as needed and fitted to a basic design.

- Customised. Specially made to individual requirements. Includes moulded seats.

The last two types of seating system in particular are often called assistive seating devices (ASDs), and moulded seating is usually required for those who have fixed deformities. Modular and customised seating types will be considered in this sub-section.

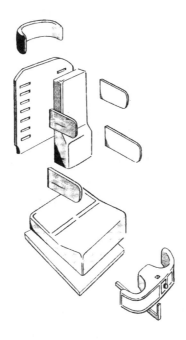

An example of components of a modular seating system
Illustration 3.3.1

The proportion of people needing this kind of seating is relatively small (1 per 1000 population: Lachmann, Greenfield and Wrench 1993) and in the UK these needs are almost exclusively met through the wheelchair services. The majority of children needing such seating have cerebral palsy, and the majority of adults have acute brain damage, multiple sclerosis or stroke (BSRM 1995). The other main group of users has spinal cord injuries.

If you need a special seating system you may feel you do not know enough to contribute to the selection of components, at least for your first seating system. If you want to become involved, ask to test out some of the possibilities for yourself, as this will give a real example for you to comment upon (Minkel 2000; Rigby *et al.* 1996). This is obviously not possible with moulded seats, but should be achievable for modular or adjustable seating.

Users with learning disabilities may take some time to get used to the new feel of a seating system, and their behaviour should be noted over the first few days to gauge their comfort and satisfaction with it.

CHOOSING AN ASSISTIVE SEATING DEVICE

An attempt has been made to guide the choice of ASD type (Trefler and Taylor 1991) based on the interaction between sensation, postural control and spinal deformity. People in the mildly affected group would have at least two of the following: normal sensation, 'good' postural control and mild deformity. Those in the most affected group would have at least two of the following: no sensation, severe deformity and 'poor' postural control. Trefler and Taylor's suggestions were modular seating for the mild group, customised or modular for the middle group and customised for the most affected group. Since this publication in 1991, the modular systems have become more sophisticated, and would probably be suitable for a high proportion in the two more affected groups.

More recently, Cutter and Blake (1997) have published a chart to assist in the choice of a supportive cushion, which can be summarised as: customised seating for people whose joints cannot be straightened to fit comfortably in standard shaped seating; modular seating for people who need 'high intervention' to sit them satisfactorily; seating for comfort if no special support is required, using a pressure distributing cushion if there are indications that one is needed (see section 3.4). Cutter and Blake state that modular seating systems will usually be satisfactory when the seating goals are 'few in number' (1997, p.124), and that whatever such systems are fitted to should be an integral part of the recommended solution. This is commonly a wheelchair, but some systems can be lifted off and fixed to a static base, so all aspects of the system's use have to be considered to ensure it will meet the practical requirements and lifestyle goals as well as the support needs.

It should be borne in mind that sometimes a compromise is necessary to achieve all the above. The seating system that is most ideal may be unsuitable in other respects, for instance you may not like it or find it uncomfortable, or a care assistant may lack confidence in how to adjust or fasten it, or it may make transfers in and out of your chair very difficult. In such cases, discussion and joint problem-solving will help to find a compromise that means the device will be of help and used regularly (Pope 1996).

Some studies have been conducted on the effectiveness of differing seating configurations. These have been with people who have different seating needs, and have examined different time periods resulting in different outcomes, so making the presentation of evidence difficult. On balance, the evidence to date relates mainly to children with cerebral palsy and a range of seating systems (e.g. Hulme *et al.* 1983; Hulme, Shaver *et al.* 1987; Hulme, Gallacher *et al.* 1987). Miedaner and Finuf (1993) considered that 'Clinical experience and recent studies imply that carefully selected and planned positioning can improve the functional abilities of individuals with neurologically related motor impairment' (p.177). Studies that have examined specific components of seating are presented in Table 3.3.1b, but owing to the many other factors that influence a child's development over time, no conclusions can yet be reached about the best ASD for a given person.

Table 3.3.1b Evidence concerning the effect of seating components

Seating component	User group	Outcome	★
Backrest angle	Cerebral palsy, spastic; 11 children.	Balance was better when backrest was at 90°: less muscle activity was recorded compared with the backrest at 75° or 120° (study by Nwaobi reviewed by Miedaner and Finuf 1993).	★★★
Seat angle various	Cerebral palsy, spastic; 6 adults and 6 controls.	Reaching ability not affected by seat angle (study by McPherson reviewed by Miedaner and Finuf 1993). Cf. Myhr 1994.	★★
	Cerebral palsy, spastic or athetoid; 13 children.	Quickest hand movements were recorded with 90° hip angle, with seat horizontal for those with spasticity, and 15° forward tilt for those with athetosis (studies by Nwaobi reviewed by Miedaner and Finuf 1993).	★★
backward slope	Cerebral palsy, spastic; 9 children and young adults.	A backward sloped seat (10° – 30°) improved performance with a joystick *only* if extensor spasm and flexor spasm about equal (Seeger *et al.* 1984).	★★
forward	Cerebral palsy, spastic; 1 child.	5° forward tilt reduced sway (McClenaghan 1989).	★★
	Cerebral palsy, mild-severe; 23 children.	Up to 15° forward tilt improved sitting ability and hand function (Myhr and von Wendt 1991).	★★★
Prone angle (stander)	Cerebral palsy, spastic diplegia; 10 children.	Simulated feeding was quicker, fine hand movements slower, than with horizontal sitting (Noronha *et al.* 1989).	★★
Contoured foam seat	Neurological impairments; 4 children.	Greater independence in sitting compared with standard seating (Deitz and Crepeau 1998).	★★★
Saddle seat, prone angle sitting; anterior and lateral trunk support	Cerebral palsy, spastic quadriplegia; 10 children.	Benefits 'physically and socially' were mainly qualitative and not demonstrated in the test data (Pope *et al.* 1996).	★★

3.3.2 Ways of achieving a good posture: non-conventional seating

The conventional basic chair shape does not enable the best posture for some people, particularly for activities such as feeding, playing games, using a computer, etc.

Departure from the conventional seat and backrest of everyday chairs has developed mainly in children's seating, predominantly to address the seating challenges that some people with cerebral palsy may face when attempting such activities. There are three types: straddle (or bolster) seats, prone angle seats and corner seats.

GENERAL CONSIDERATIONS WHEN SEATING A CHILD

- The more complicated it is to get a person into a seat, for example doing up straps, making fine adjustments, the less likely it is to be used. A lap belt is advisable for most users.

- Velcro fastenings are quick to fasten but catch on clothing when undone. Clips withstand greater pull. Clips that require the strap to be threaded through each time are not desirable in the long term because the strap frays (unless it is welded firmly at its end).

- A tray or table for young children should have a rim to stop toys and food falling over the edge.

- For use by several children, such as in a therapy or school setting, seating that is easy to alter and has a good range of adjustments is important.

(MDA 1998b)

STRADDLE SEATS

The idea of straddle seats arose many years ago (Cristarella 1975). Straddle seats aim to reproduce the benefits noted from people sitting on horseback: the pelvis is upright, the legs apart so that the hip joints are stable, and the hips are less flexed than in conventional seating. For those with tight hamstrings, it is easier to lean forwards because the hips are less bent and this enables the pelvis to move as you lean forward, rather than the spine bending (Brunswic 1984). For those who tend to have athetoid movements, the straddle position may be beneficial if the users are leaning forward slightly (Stewart and McQuilton 1987). There is mixed opinion about a straddle seat for those with a tendency to extensor spasms: it may make it worse (Myhr and von Wendt 1991; MDA 1995), but using kneeling pads to support the legs may alleviate extensor reactions (Stewart and McQuilton 1987).

Most seats are bolsters, but some are more like bicycle saddles with an exaggerated shape. The bicycle seat type can be found in products for adults. In a small study with children with spastic cerebral palsy, significant improvement in sitting up straight and in control of sitting posture were noted on a saddle seat (Reid 1996).

PRONE ANGLE SEATS

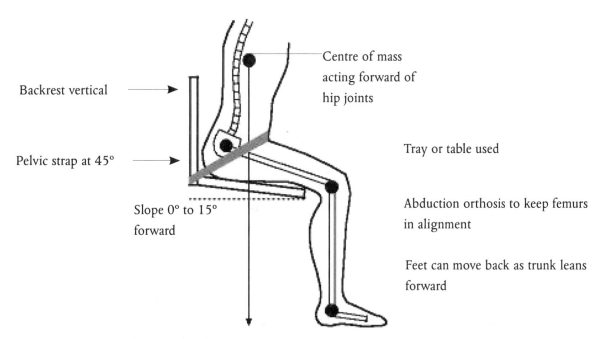

Figure 3.3.2a Forward leaning posture. For children with mixed muscle tone. (Myhr and von Wendt 1991; Myhr et al. 1995; McClenaghan 1989)

Sitting with a forward sloping seat encourages the centre of mass to come in front of the ischial tuberosities (see Figure 3.3.2a). As seen in subsection 3.2.2, office seating may have a forward sloping seat to encourage the spine to maintain its normal curves rather than become rounded like a C. This principle has been applied to children with cerebral palsy by researchers (Myhr and von Wendt 1991), and they suggested that this significantly improved postural control including the head, and had a positive effect on hand function. It is considered helpful for those with low muscle tone in the upper trunk and those with ataxia. Some with a mild tendency to extensor thrust may also benefit (MDA 1998b).

A seating system that incorporated both a straddle and prone angle seat was issued to children with cerebral palsy (Pope, Bowes and Booth 1994). Although no significant improvements could be reported, qualitative comments were made that the children benefited 'physically and socially'.

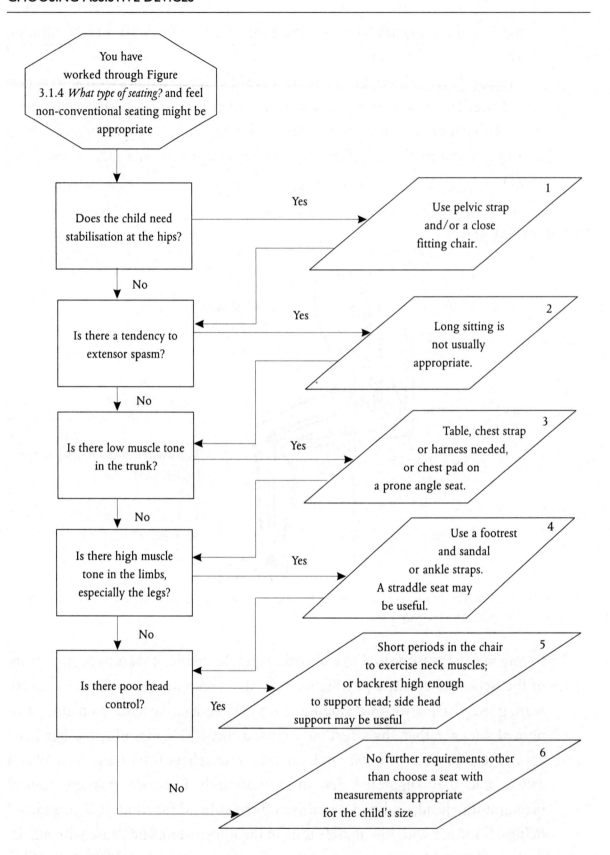

Figure 3.3.2b A guide to the choice of seating for a young child. If the user is older than five or six years, refer also to subsection 3.3.1 concerning other features that might be of help, for example knee blocks. (Adapted from MDA 1998b used with permission.) 'Seating for young children with disabilities: a comparative evaluation.'

An example

Andy was brain-damaged at birth, and by ten months he was unable to hold his head up or sit up. The therapists at the Child Development Centre explained to his mother that it was important for him to have a seat that would encourage him to sit up and start using his hands. They began working down Figure 3.3.2b together.

- Andy needed stability at his hips, so they knew he would need a pelvic strap, but he did not tend to extend (straighten) his hips involuntarily.

- His trunk was floppy (low muscle tone) so they noted the possibilities in slanted box 3.

- High tone was not evident in his legs.

- He had poor head control, so they decided to try short periods in a high-backed seat. A prone angle seat would have made it too hard for Andy to hold his head up, so an upright seat was needed.

A corner seat with a pelvic strap was tried, and a table adjusted to suit Andy's size. He sat in it well, and with the stability at his hips he was able to hold his head up for short periods. His mother put Andy in the chair two or three times a day, so that he gradually gained more head control, and started to show an interest in the toys that she put on the table.

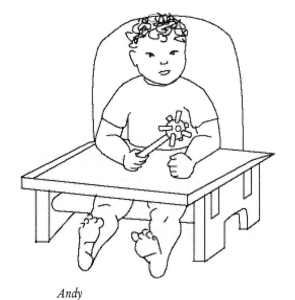

Andy

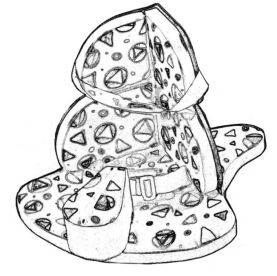

A corner seat

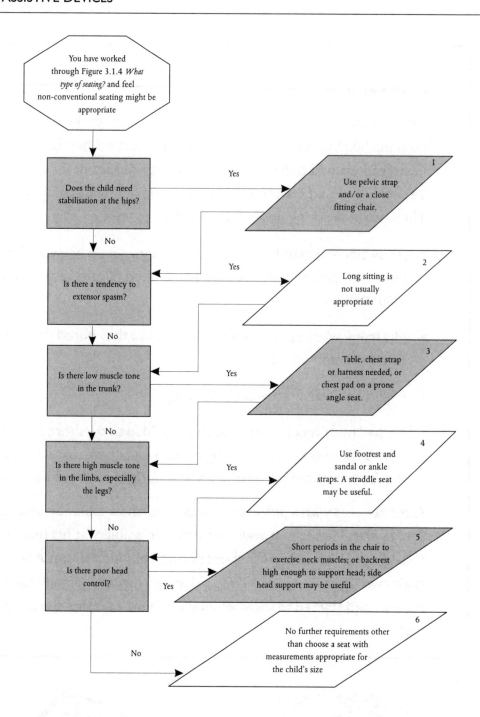

Andy's route through Figure 3.3.2b
Illustration 3.3.2

CORNER SEATS

Corner seats comprise two sides that meet centre back, and are usually floor level seats. Some versions have a flattened 'V' shape, so there is a backrest. They are designed to support a young child in a sitting posture so he or she can participate in age-appropriate activities. As the seat is on the floor the knees are usually straight, so this seating is not usually appropriate for those with a tendency to extensor spasm (MDA 1998b).

Table 3.3.3 Advantages and disadvantages of special leisure chair features

Factor	Advantages	Disadvantages
Usually offers a more relaxing and a less restricting sitting position than an ASD on a wheelchair	Relaxing. Comfortable.	If used for long periods, there may be a higher risk of complications such as hip dislocation, increased scoliosis.
Modular (optional features available)	It is usually possible to find all features necessary to suit your needs.	Some parts may be detachable so be prone to being lost; some may need regular readjustment; some may make the chair look less 'normal'.
Close fitting	Provides reasonable degree of support.	Makes getting in and out more difficult, especially if positioning of slings for hoisting is needed.
Upholstered	Comfortable. Blends in with other furniture.	Covers need to be removable for washing; this necessitates a reserve set, as upholstery material takes longer to dry. Covers can be fiddly to replace.
Castors	Chair can be moved fairly easily if unoccupied.	Deep pile carpets make moving difficult, as does the extra weight if the user is in the chair. The chairs are quite large and may not fit through doorways.
Straps	Many configurations available. May not be necessary if you are not going to attempt any activities. Lap belt most common.	Extra restriction detracts from the aim of a more relaxed position.
Tray	Enables meals or other activities to be undertaken in the chair.	Often attached across the armrests. When the latter are used for trunk support they may make the tray an unsuitable height.
Functional activities	50–81% of users had better reaching and grasping ability in these chairs compared with the minimum of support needed for their safety.	The ASD in a wheelchair may improve function further.

Recline	Allows rest periods without further manual handling.	Your buttocks will not be in the same position on returning to upright, so will need resettling.
Tilt-in-space	Hip angle opens.	Extensor spasm may occur as the backrest is lowered. Shoulders may hunch forward in an unconscious attempt to get upright.
	Especially useful if you are poorly but not ill enough to be confined to bed.	
	Bladder less constricted than in upright position; easier position for intermittent catheterisation (Cutter and Blake 1997; Lange 2000).	
	Useful for many users to provide resting position without the buttocks slipping out of place.	Must have integral footrest so this rises with the seat. If a tray is used it must be cleared or removed.
		You need to move away from work surface or remove items from tray attachment before tilting (Lange 2000).

Data drawn from MDA 1995 except where cited otherwise.

There is a consensus of opinion about the effect of recline (e.g. Trefler and Taylor 1991, Cutter and Blake 1997).

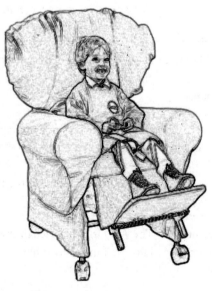 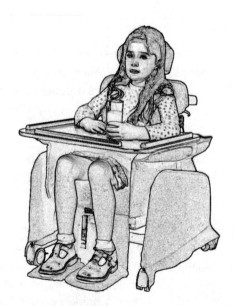

Modular leisure chairs
Illustration 3.3.3

3.3.3 Special leisure seating

No one wants to sit upright all the time, yet those who need special support to do so often have to remain in one position for long periods. Unless they have a recline or *tilt-in-space* facility, it is desirable that an alternative to the functional sitting posture is available. This may be a leisure chair. The leisure chair will need to provide more support than a standard easy chair in order to keep the user comfortable and safe.

The advantages of a leisure chair are twofold. First, it is a more relaxing and comfortable chair, and second it is a psychological and social symbol of leisure time. Leisure chairs are considered more 'normal-looking', so may enable the user to feel more part of the family than when using a wheelchair with an assistive seating device (MDA 1995).

As with standard easy chairs, it is important to sit in the chair for at least 20 minutes before deciding whether it is suitable or not. The advantage of the special leisure chairs is that they are all multi-adjustable, so minor alterations to maximise support and comfort can be made over a longer period of time once the chair is in full use.

When looking for a leisure chair, you want it to provide similar support to the special seating system, but using the features of an easy chair. Thus the armrests should be adjustable for height and width to stabilise the hips; the backrest needs to be malleable enough to provide the upper trunk support-needs; the wings or headrest should enable the head to stay in a comfortable position. A pressure relieving seat may be required.

Footrests are available on most of these chairs, and they help to keep your legs in the right position and can be adjusted in height so that the thighs take a share of the weight off your buttocks (see subsection 3.1.2). Footrests that are too high increase the pressure under the ischial tuberosities appreciably (MDA 1997a, see subsection 3.4.2).

Additional features such as tilt-in-space, straps and a tray may also be needed, and are usually available with these chairs. Table 3.3.3 below highlights factors to bear in mind when choosing a leisure chair, and is derived from a user evaluation of multi-adjustable leisure chairs (MDA 1995).

MULTIPLE USERS

These chairs are suitable for use by a succession of different individuals because they can be cleaned, and modular parts are available. However, they are not recommended for a group of concurrent users because adjustment to fit an individual takes time and skill. The chair should be left set up ready for use by a single person.

3.4 Pressure distributing products

3.4.1 The need for pressure relieving products

It is quite normal to shift your weight several times an hour when seated, and it is when this ability is lost that problems can arise. The effects of not moving are many, and may include reduced circulation and swelling of the lower legs, loss of calcium from the bones, weakness of muscles as a result of disuse, joint stiffness, and last but by no means least, pressure sores (decubitus ulcers).

The high incidence of pressure sores and the high cost of treating them (Burns and Betz 1999; Russell, Reynolds and Carr 2000) have stimulated the development of a range of pressure relieving and pressure distributing products. The process of choosing between them is no simple task, because each person responds to pressure differently, so there is no ideal cushion (Bishop *et al.* 1999; Pellow 1999). The way a cushion has been constructed can only be a guide to its actual performance. Small differences in performance may noticeably affect outcomes and it is unwise to choose your cushion purely according to how it has been made.

The main cause of a pressure sore, as its name implies, is pressure sufficiently high to stop blood from circulating to the skin and underlying tissue (Burns and Betz 1999). Research has suggested that blood stops getting through the smallest blood vessels at roughly 20–32 mmHg skin (or interface) pressure (Pellow 1999; Rithalia 1997a; Henderson *et al.* 1994).[2] An interface pressure of 60mmHg for an hour can cause changes that may lead to a pressure sore (Henderson *et al.* 1994). In practice, the measurement of pressure applied to the skin does not have a constant relationship to the pressure in the tissue immediately below. This relationship differs from person to person, and according to the part of the body. One recommendation for maximum interface pressures under the ischial tuberosities is 40 mmHg for people at high risk of sores to 80mmHg for those at low risk (Cutter and Blake 1997). This range demonstrates the reality that the same pressure at the skin may be tolerated by one person, but rapidly cause a pressure sore on another.

The skin interface pressure, which is measured by sensor cells placed between the person and the cushion is an indirect guide to what is going on underneath. 'There is insufficient evidence to determine an absolute threshold on the magnitude of pressure below which any particular person is at decreased risk of developing pressure ulcers' (Brienza *et al.* 2001, p.530).

---

2   mm Hg refers to the amount of pressure required to counteract the weight of a column of mercury of that height.

The pressures recommended as satisfactory in ensuring blood can flow to the skin range from lower than 32 mmHg (Collins 1999), to lower than 70 mmHg (Bishop *et al.* 1999). The wide range illustrates the variability between people, and that no magical figure guarantees effective pressure relief.

WHO IS MOST AT RISK OF PRESSURE SORES?

Because of the uncertain relationship between pressure and pressure sore development, the approach used is to assess people for their risk of getting pressure sores, and then to treat them with a range of interventions that will include some products that relieve or distribute pressure.

There are many other factors that affect susceptibility to a pressure sore, and these are incorporated into pressure sore risk assessments and guidelines. Factors known to increase the risk apart from unrelieved pressure include incontinence, heat and damp, malnutrition, poor sensation, thinness, increasing age, friction and shearing forces (Collins 1999; Wall 2000). The elderly and those with spinal cord injuries are therefore at higher risk of pressure sores, and interface pressures confirm this because they are much higher than in younger or non-paralysed people of similar body size (MDA 1997b; Minkel 2000).

Risk assessment scales have been devised to take these factors into account (e.g. Waterlow, Norton) and those with a high risk, i.e. who have several of the factors, should then be given special care. The validity of the scales has been shown by people with medium-high risk scores being significantly more likely to develop a pressure sore (Conine *et al.* 1994).

Guidelines for prevention and treatment of pressure sores have been available since 1985, but are mainly compiled by consensus amongst experts, and are based on 'little solid evidence' (Clark 1999, p.359; NICE 2001, para 6.1).

3.4.2 Strategies for pressure relief when seated

The most effective strategy is to get up, and allow circulation to flow back into the area that has been under too much pressure. A well-fitting chair (see subsection 3.1.2) will also help to distribute pressure as much as possible (Collins 2001; Collins and Shipperley 1999), by allowing the thighs to take some weight, and the feet too. The height of wheelchair footrests is critical, as a study showed that pressure under the ischial tuberosities is doubled when they are too high (MDA 1997a).

An example

Lee injured his spine in a road accident. His arms were not affected but he was not able to stand except with special support. He was given a Jay cushion (contoured foam with gel under his buttocks) for his wheelchair, and was taught to lift himself up regularly by bracing his arms, or leaning as far forwards as he could.

On a review visit to the spinal unit, the staff were disappointed to see that he had a small pressure sore on his sacrum. On questioning him, they discovered that Lee was spending many hours each day in an old arm chair. The occupational therapist called a few days later to look at it. Lee was slouched in the chair, a computer keyboard on his lap, monitor perched on a coffee table and the mouse on the chair arm.

When Lee got out of the chair, the occupational therapist discovered that the chair frame at the back of the seat could be easily felt, so realised it had been pressing on Lee's sacrum, causing the sore.

He could not be persuaded to sit in his wheelchair to use the computer, but agreed to search for a new easy chair. The occupational therapist recommended a pressure relieving facility in the chair seat as he would spend several hours each day in it. Together they selected possible products that had dimensions that fitted Lee, lumbar support and an option for a pressure relieving cushion.

Lee wanted a recliner and offered to contribute to the cost. This requirement left three possible products to try. Each of these was demonstrated, the occupational therapist and Lee insisting on a two-hour trial. (One firm only agreed to one hour.) None marked his buttocks or sacrum on inspection as he left the chair, so he chose the one that he felt was most comfortable and looked good.

Weeks of negotiation with local health and social services about the funding for the chair was eventually successful and the chair proved ideal for Lee.

When standing up is not possible, and the seat is as well fitting as possible, then additional strategies have proven to be of help:

- Lean forwards (Koo, Mak and Lee 1996). More effective than recline (Henderson *et al.* 1994).

- Lift the buttocks clear of the cushion by bracing the arms on the armrests. If your arms are not strong enough to do this, leaning forwards is better than leaning to one side which was shown to raise the pressure under the opposite buttock (MDA 1997a).

- Recline or *tilt-in-space* (the seat-to-backrest angle stays the same as chair reclines) by a minimum of 35° (Pellow 1999); 155° is more effective than 125° of tilt (Henderson *et al.* 1994). The tilt needed to reduce pressure sufficiently to be of benefit can rarely be calculated precisely, but 150° is likely to be of significant benefit (Pellow 1999).

- Use pressure distributing or pressure relieving products (see subsection 3.4.3).

A slouched posture increases the pressure on the sacrum (MDA 1997b) and under the buttocks (*ischial tuberosities*) (Koo *et al.* 1996). Lumbar support for those with spinal cord injury improved their sitting posture but did not significantly decrease the pressure under the ischial tuberosities (Shields and Cook 1992).

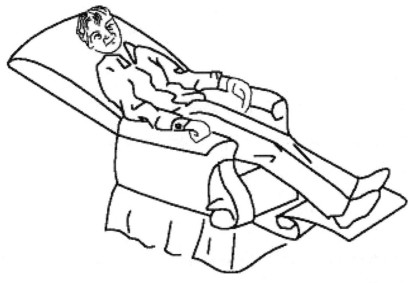

Lee
Illustration 3.4.2

3.4.3 Pressure relieving and pressure distributing products

A recent review by the National Institute for Clinical Excellence (NICE) has been conducted and guidelines updated on pressure sore prevention (NICE 2001).

NICE is currently undertaking a full review of evaluations of pressure relieving products. Evaluations related to seating are summarised in Table 3.4.3b *Some evaluations of pressure reducing cushions.*

In the community, awareness of the need for pressure relieving products is low (Wall 2000), and information about them for full-time wheelchair users is needed. For those that do have such products, usage rates are high (McGrath *et al.* 1985).

Pressure relieving products use foam, gel, air or liquid:

FOAM

- polyurethane foam, as is standard practice to use in easy-chair cushions

- layers of different grades of foam, usually a softer layer on top of a firmer

- foam that has vertical cuts across the top to assist areas with higher pressure on them to compress unhindered

- visco-elastic foam, which compresses a little more slowly, moulds to your shape more than standard foam, but is also slow to decompress when you move

- contoured foam. This is usually very firm, with raised edge and centre front to keep the thighs in good position

GEL

- gel cushion

- foam layer, with gel layer above

- contoured foam, with gel sac under buttocks

- gel sacs in a foam casing

AIR

- cushions made of stretch membrane with a valve to prevent over-inflation

- dry flotation: a matrix of interconnected bladders

- dynamic: a series of cells inflate and deflate in cycles. The configuration of cells varies, e.g. lengthways strips, crossways strips, both, H shape, square cells. One product has foam within the cells too

- dynamic: a series of cells as described above

- foam and liquid.

Most of these products have been designed to *distribute* pressure more evenly across the weight-bearing area, rather than allow it to concentrate under the bony ischial tuberosities. The dynamic ones seek to *relieve* pressure more actively by altering the areas that bear weight, so allowing blood to return to the tissues

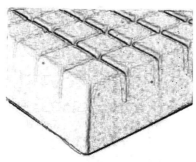
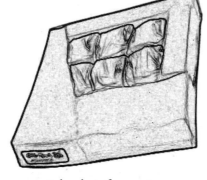
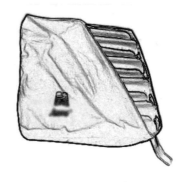

Foam with vertical cuts   *Gel sacks in foam casing*   *Dynamic cushion*

Illustration 3.4.3

regularly over the inflation–deflation cycle. Presentation of the pressure readings for these cushions is varied: a root mean square can be calculated to give an average reading (MDA 1997b, 1998a); the maximum and minimum can be quoted; the percentage time that pressure falls below a threshold, such as 20 mmHg, in a cycle (Rithalia 1997b). No research has yet been reported that compares the relative merits of dynamic pressure relief with reclining or tilt-in-space for the seated person on standard foam. Burns and Betz 1999 found a dynamic cushion's minimum pressure recording (upright posture) was significantly lower than that with a Jay cushion used at 135° tilt. This suggests that a dynamic cushion should provide better protection from pressure than tilt-in-space or recline, but more research is needed.

The type of material that a cushion is made from affects not only the pressure on the body, but also the temperature and moistness of the skin, postural stability and the ability to transfer. The factors in Table 3.4.3a below will be of different importance to each individual, so you should pick out those that would affect you most.

A number of product evaluations have been conducted, but how the factors above have affected cushion use and the users' opinion of them has not been included.

Table 3.4.3a Factors unrelated to pressure relief that affect cushion choice

Factor	Cushion type suggested	Guideline
Your sitting balance is not good	Foam, gel or mixture of the two	Air- and liquid-filled cushions are much harder to maintain your balance on (DLF 1999; Fletcher 1998).
You tend to get hot and sweaty	Gel or liquid	These fillings tend to draw heat away from the body (DLF 1999) They tend to encourage increased skin moisture (Cutter and Blake 1997), so a breathable (vapour permeable) cover is imperative.
You tend to feel the cold	Foam	Foam provides a little insulation, but does not increase skin moisture (Cutter and Blake 1997).
You need to transfer sideways	Foam or gel or mixture of the two	A firm, non-contoured surface eases the transfer (Collins 1998).
You have continence problems	Air or liquid	Easier to clean (DLF 1999).
You cannot cope with anything complicated	Foam, gel or mixture of the two	Dry flotation has to be checked for correct pressure regularly; dynamic cushions have to be plugged in (MDA 1998a).
You are sensitive to noise or vibration	Any non-dynamic construction	Quiet and no vibration (MDA 1998a).
You wish to minimise product problems and maintenance	Foam, gel or mixture of the two	Dry flotation has to be checked for correct pressure regularly; dynamic cushions have to be plugged in (MDA 1998a).

Evaluations have addressed the interface pressure or the incidence of pressure sores, and there must be caution in applying them for a number of reasons:

- Products change, and as the construction is only a broad indication of a cushion's performance, guidelines either have to be product-specific, or very general in nature.

- Trials have been conducted with user groups with different conditions and of differing age ranges.

- Different measures and methods have been used. With interface pressure measurements, readings using different instruments cannot be directly compared.

- Some evaluations have been conducted in a laboratory setting, some were field trials.

- The base on which the cushion is placed affects readings.

- Most evaluations have additional aspects that reduce one's confidence in the findings.

Table 3.4.3b Some evaluations of pressure reducing cushions

Trade name	Type of cushion(s) evaluated	Findings	Comment	★
Not specified	Contoured foam with air pockets under buttocks; 90% gel and 10% foam hybrid; two foam layers, contoured; gel layer over foam.	32 elderly ambulant people. No significant difference between the cushions' pressure readings (Bishop *et al.* 1999).	Averaged readings across four very different postures so masking true peak pressure for static sitting.	★★
Not specified	Various pressure reducing products (trial group) versus foam (control).	32 elderly wheelchair users in a residential setting. Pressure under ischial tuberosities significantly correlated to pressure sore development (p< 0.01). In trial group only 1 of the 6 ulcers coincided with peak forces; 7 of the 10 in control group coincided (Brienza *et al.* 2001).	25% of the trial group had 'protocol variances', which could have influenced the development of pressure ulcers. Various cushions in trial group allocated according to 'individual needs'.	★★★
Roho high profile; Jay2; ErgoDynamic	Dry flotation; contoured foam with gel under buttocks; H-shaped bladder dynamic cushion.	16 male quadriplegics; pressure measured under ischial tuberosities in wheelchair upright, tilted 135°. Comparing dynamic's minimum pressure when upright with the others' maximum pressure when reclined, the dynamic and Roho were similar, but the Jay significantly higher than the dynamic (Burns and Betz 1999).	Does not discuss the relative merits of dynamic versus tilt-in-space as methods of pressure relief.	★★★
Armchair with Karomed Transflo in seat	Gel sacs in foam casing (trial group); standard foam (control).	Chairs used by 506 in trial ward, 576 in control. Pressure sore incidence significantly less in trial ward (p< 0.0001) (Collins 1999).	Only a single product evaluation. Only one size of chair issued, so seat height not optimum for all.	★★★
Jay	Contoured foam with gel under buttocks (trial group); 4in. foam with stretch cover (control).	163 elderly wheelchair users in residential home. RCT. Significantly fewer developed pressure sores in Jay group (p< 0.05) (Conine *et al.* 1994).	Sacral sores were included although these may not have been related to the cushion. More dropped out of foam group because of discomfort than Jay.	★★★★
Various non-dynamic cushions including Nestor, Tempur-Pedic	30 surfaces including a sheepskin and a 'standard' armchair. Cushions of gel, gel and foam, hollow silicone fibres and air cells.	20 healthy young adults. Gels mostly performed more poorly than the armchair. Dry flotation type and Tempur-Pedic performed significantly better (p <0.05). Nestor poorer than armchair (Defloor and Grypdonck 2000).	Used 'maximum interface pressure' for calculations.	★★★

Various manufacturers including Roho and Jay	20 cushions and 3in. foam with PVC cover. Six were omitted from trial because they showed higher interface pressures with fit elderly people than the foam.[1]	33 users with flaccid or spastic paraplegia; or stroke. Roho and Jay performed best (MDA 1997a).	Concluded that structure alone does not predict performance. Quoting the mean pressure for dynamic cushions may mask their effect.	★★
CareFlex Hydro Tilt; Karomed Winchester with Transflo seat; Will Back with 'Unique' seat. Grant Alternating; Huntley Alpha; KCI Mediscus Astec; Parkhouse Alternating	3 armchairs with pressure relieving seats; reference armchair with foam. 4 dynamic cushions. Feather, fibre (cotton covers); foam (PVC cover).	12 fit elderly. Pressure under ischial tuberosities measured. 'Unique' (layered grades of foam) performed significantly less well than the other pressure relieving products, but better than the reference armchair (MDA 1998b).	Minimum dynamic pressure readings ranged from 20 to 36 mmHg, but mean pressure over cycle used (as in row above).	★★★
Roho high profile; Jay2; Special Health Systems Ultimate	Dry flotation; contoured foam with gel under buttocks; foam.	2 men with quadriplegia. Pressure measured under ischial tuberosities and sacrum, in upright, 35° and 45° tilt-in-space and 150° recline. Roho pressure reduction greater in lighter subject (Pellow 1999).	Pressures under right and left buttock can be markedly different. With pressure relieving cushions, recline or tilt-in-space will not appreciably reduce pressure further.	★★
HNE Alpha trancell, Talley BASE, British Astec Care chair, Pegasus Pro-Active	Dynamic	8 healthy adults on 4 dynamic cushions. Measurements under right buttock taken for a complete cycle of cushion pressure. Only Trancell and Care chair achieved 20 mmHg or less for part of the cycle (Rithalia 1997a).	Authors felt 30 mmHg might be a more suitable threshold.	★★★
Huntleigh Aura; Pegasus Proactive	Dynamic	RCT[2] 141 people with pressure ulcers treated on one of the systems. Healing rates calculated from size of ulcer on entry and healing time. Both systems effective in treatment of pressure ulcers (Russell *et al.* 2000).	No difference in nursing input, so authors conclude choice therefore rests on hire cost and maintenance issues.	★★★★
Roho High Profile, Roho Low Profile, Jay2, Flofit Flexseat, Invacare Pindot, Supracor Stimulite	Dry flotation; gel and foam; 'plastic'.	Interface pressures for 40 wheelchair users recorded, with sling seat (baseline) and the 6 cushions. Subjective measure of comfort revealed both Rohos significantly more comfortable than the others (p< 0.05). Pressures indicated these two were more effective for most users (Shechtman *et al.* 2001).	Results expressed as proportion of readings at each specified pressure range. This does not reflect the pressure gradient around the ischial tuberosities.	★★★

1. Nestor original, Obitus supercontour, spenco Omega 5000, sumed Luxor, Sumed system 93, Sumed Ultra 90

2. RCT randomised controlled trial

From these studies it is possible to discern that the majority, but not all of the specialised products are effective in reducing pressure damage, but to a widely varying extent. Dynamic cushions tend to be the most effective. Dry flotation (Roho high profile), the contoured foam with gel under the buttocks (Jay; Jay2) and some combination foams are the next most effective (MDA 1997b). As mentioned above, composition alone is not a sufficient guide to the pressure relieving properties of a cushion. Dry flotation is the most consistently effective type. The effectiveness of foams is less consistent. Ideally the individual products need to be evaluated comparatively (as in MDA 1997b) and a choice then made (Collins 1998).

PRESSURE RELIEVING PRODUCTS ARE ONLY PART OF THE SOLUTION

When using pressure relieving products, care must still be taken to reposition your body weight from time to time. The optimal interval between repositioning is still debated (Clark 1998). Ensure shearing is kept to a minimum, avoid creases in clothing and inspect the skin regularly (Collins 2001).

A TRIAL PERIOD IS IMPORTANT

If you are making a private purchase it is strongly recommended that you trial a cushion for a minimum of two hours, then make a visual inspection of the buttocks as well as making a subjective judgement of comfort. Again, comparison is needed, and 'test drives' of different cushions should be done as close together as possible while leaving enough time to recover from one test before starting the next one.

PRESSURE RELIEVING SEATING IN HOSPITAL AND RESIDENTIAL CARE

As mentioned in subsection 3.4.2, a chair of the right dimensions for the individual is an integral part of pressure sore prevention (Collins 2001). Too low a seat increases pressure on the ischial tuberosities, and too high a seat may cause swelling in the feet so increasing the risk of lower leg ulcers, and also encourages slouching which increases interface pressure under the sacrum (MDA 1997a). Being seated at the appropriate height is therefore the key. It may be counter-productive to place an additional pressure distributing cushion on a chair that was originally the correct seat height without adjusting the new seat-to-ground height accordingly. A chair ideally will have the chosen pressure distributing seat built in. Failing that, when you add a cushion the chair should be lowered by the cushion's thickness when compressed. If the cushion is for use in a wheelchair, the footplates can be adjusted upwards to maintain the optimal foot support height.

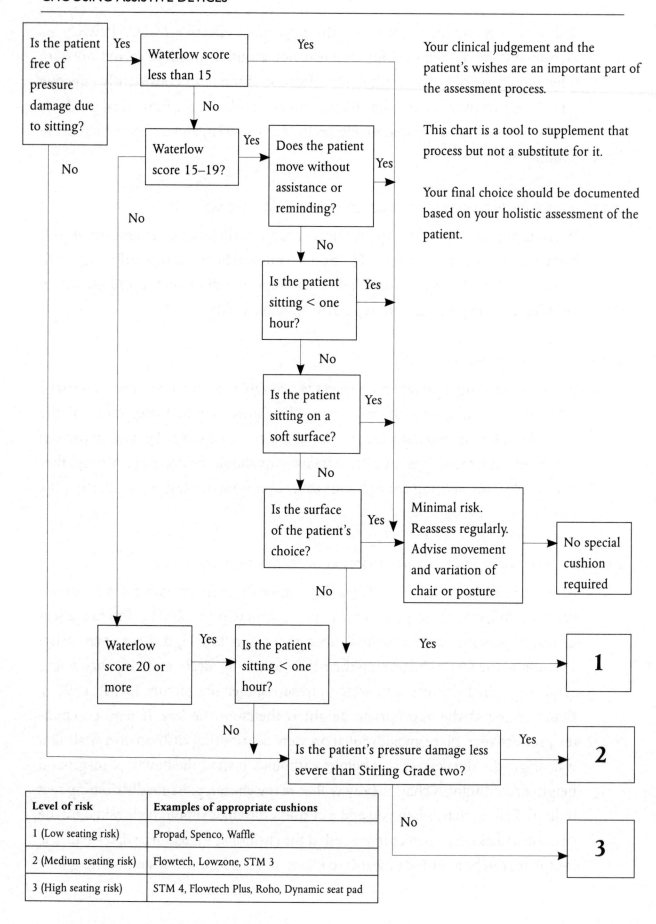

Figure 3.4.3 Pressure area care: flowchart for selection of cushions for seated patients. (Reproduced from Shipperley and Collins 1999, p.120.

People should be formally assessed for their risk of pressure sores using an assessment scale such as the Norton or Waterlow (Waterlow *et al.* 1996). In hospitals, a proportion of patients will not need special pressure distributing cushions, but an audit found that 59 per cent of those who should have had a special cushion did not (McCafferty *et al.* 2000). This illustrates one possible reason why incidence of pressure sores amongst those sitting for long periods is higher than for those confined to bed (cited in McCafferty *et al.* 2000).

The approach used by Shipperley and Collins (1999) is sensible: they chose a limited number of named products suitable for low, medium, and high risk (the last includes those with current ulcers). It is important to have different composition cushions within each risk bracket to accommodate differing needs listed in Table 3.4.3a that are not pressure related.

CUSHION USE AND CARE

Acquiring a pressure relieving or distributing cushion is only the first step: it will not be of use unless it is used, correctly positioned and maintained.

- *Comfort:* If it is not comfortable, you will probably not use it. McCafferty *et al.* (2000) found that patients often said they chose which chair to sit in on the grounds of comfort.

- *Positioning:* Some cushions can be positioned wrongly, such as contoured cushions. Errors will cause discomfort and increase the risk of pressure sores.

- *Covers:* The cover on a cushion can affect its performance: a two-way stretch, vapour permeable material is desirable because this does not inhibit the pressure distributing effect of the cushion, and reduces skin dampness. Any material including clothing between cover and skin must similarly be stretchy and vapour permeable otherwise the cushion will not be effective (Cutter and Blake 1997; Stockton 2000).

- *Adjustments:* Some cushions need adjusting, for example air pressure on dynamic cushions, or the amount of inflation for the dry flotation (Roho) cushion. Errors will increase the risk of pressure sores.

- *Maintenance:* If no one is willing to take responsibility for maintenance, a low-maintenance cushion such as a foam one should be considered. Even these need checking for deterioration, and will need replacing when the foam loses its resilience under the pressure points. 'Bottoming out' is an expression that refers to a cushion that is compressed to its full depth under the bony prominences, thus offering no pressure redistribution at all.

- *Review*: You should check regularly for any sign of pressure sore development[3] (Collins 2001). In addition, your needs and how the cushion is functioning for you should be reviewed from time to time.

Key points

This chapter has reviewed evidence concerning assistive devices (ADs) for seating. The first decision is whether you feel supported well enough in a standard chair. Postures are adopted for different tasks; a good posture is the aim, rather than an 'ideal' posture.

Standard seating needs

- Studies into difficulty in rising from a chair have shown that certain strategies are helpful, and choice of chair design and height can facilitate rising.

- For work tasks, a forward tilt on the seat can help to keep the spine in good position.

- For leisure, the backrest should be high enough to support the head.

Special seating needs

- There is broad consensus on the postures that seating should enable, but very little research reported on the effect of seating systems on users.

- Non-conventional seating has mostly been developed for children. Little research has examined for whom these products are useful.

Pressure relieving products

- Static sitting for long periods is the main cause of pressure sores.

- A well-fitting chair helps to distribute some of the pressure away from the buttocks.

---

3   The first stage is redness that does not clear when there is no pressure on it.

- People vary widely in the pressures measured under their buttocks, and in their relative risks of developing ulcers.

- Getting up regularly is the most effective way to prevent pressure sores.

- Special pressure distributing or relieving products are mostly better than standard upholsterer's foam, but still vary widely in their efficacy.

- The construction of a cushion alone is not sufficient guide to its efficacy.

References

Alexander, N., Koester, D. and Grunawalt, J. (1996) 'Chair design affects how older adults rise from a chair.' *Journal of the American Geriatrics Society 44*, 356–362.

Formal trials of an adjustable laboratory chair under ten conditions by two groups (29 fit elders, mean age 84, and 21 fit younger adults, mean age 23). They were videoed rising from five seat heights, armrest, seat cushion and seat and backrest angles. Subjective ratings of comfort and difficulty in rising were also recorded on five-point scales. Elders took significantly longer to rise (p 0.001 for most conditions) than younger adults. ******** *Neck flexion disproportionately greater in elders as seat is lowered (p 0.001). Addition of softer seat surface increased rising time, subjective difficulty in rising but increased perceived comfort amongst elders. However, with regard to comfort ratings, no details on how long they sat!*

Atherton, J., Chatfield, J., Clarke, A.K. and Harrison, R. (1979) *Easy chairs for the arthritic.* DHSS Aids Assessment Programme. Norwich: HMSO.

A pilot with 8 people who had arthritis or low back pain showed that the latter tended to know within half an hour whether a chair was uncomfortable, the former after 10 minutes. Therefore in formal user trials 20 people tested 10 chairs for 20 minutes each, and reported on comfort. Inadequate head support was reported in 104 of the 200 tests. Five testers had rheumatoid arthritis and they preferred padded arm support (17 complaints of lack of padding out of 30 tests of chairs with wooden armrests). Backrest rake also affected comfort, but it is difficult to know whether this was determined by disease, gender (see Le Carpentier 1969) or other factors. Vinyl covers were liked least; those with rheumatoid arthritis mostly preferred Dralon to woollen fabrics because it is less prickly. ******

Bashford, G., Steele, J., Munro, B. *et al.* (1998) 'Ejector chairs: do they work and are they safe?' *Australian Occupational Therapy Journal 45*, 99–106.

A survey of 16 current users of a chair with a spring-assisted rising seat hinged at the front, by personal interview. The sample had a range of diagnoses. Nine of these had a kinematic analysis of the user getting up, both with and without using the assisted rise. Of the 16, 12 felt it was easier to stand using the assisted rise. ****** *Impaired balance was considered to be a contra-indication. Those with rheumatoid arthritis or trunk weakness should find these seats helpful.* ***** *[Authors' note: because the assisted rise reduces the need for upper limbs to assist, so freeing them to act in a stabilising capacity (positioned on armrests with elbows well out), these contra-indications should not deter a person from testing a spring assisted cushion if it is considered potentially suitable.]*

Bentur, N., Barnea, T. and Mizrahi, I. (1996) 'A follow-up study of elderly buyers of an assistive chair.' *Physical and Occupational Therapy in Geriatrics 14*, 3, 51–60.

Forty-one of 54 purchasers of a chair with pneumatic piston assisted riser seat were traced. 40 agreed to an interview by telephone. The sample had a range of rheumatological and neurological conditions. Of those interviewed 38 were still using the chair, 33 'very satisfied' with it, 27 still using the assisted rise; 22 did not know the mechanism could be adjusted for strength of assist. This and general lack of instruction in use were the 'main' reasons for disuse. **

Bishop, S.A., Bulla, N., DiLellio, E. *et al.* (1999) 'The effects of low-cost wheelchair cushions and body type on dynamic sitting pressure in nursing home residents.' *Physical and Occupational Therapy in Geriatrics 17*, 1, 29–41.

Comparative formal user trial with 32 nursing home residents who each sat on four cushions on a standard wheelchair. Foam and gel mix; foam layers; contoured foam and air pockets; gel and foam layers. No statistical difference between the cushions, nor between pressure distribution under thin and obese subjects. Pressure readings for upright, side leaning and forward leaning were averaged.

Brienza, D., Karg, P., Geyer, M.J. *et al.* (2001) 'The relationship between pressure ulcer incidence and buttock-seat cushion interface pressure in at-risk elderly wheelchair users.' *Archives of Physical Medicine and Rehabilitation 82*, 529–533.

*Formal randomised trial with 32 elderly wheelchair users, mean age 85 years, who were assigned the same style wheelchair and randomly given pressure reducing cushion (PRC) or a foam cushion. Subjects left the study when they acquired an ulcer or when data collection completed (undisclosed period). Interface pressure recorded when subject adequately seated with respective cushion. Significant difference (p 0.001) between those who developed an ulcer and those who did not.*** *Risk assessment (Braden) scores* not *different between the ulcer/non-ulcer groups. Main criticisms: no definition of criteria for ulcer diagnosis; PRC varied according to clinician assessment; 25 per cent of PRC group had 'protocol variances' which confound the outcome.*

Brunswic, M. (1984) 'Ergonomics of seat design.' *Physiotherapy 70*, 2, 40–43.

*Formal trial with 22 people, aged 17–48 years, who sat on a rig which could be adjusted for seat inclination, without back support. A relationship was identified between lumbar flexion and hip flexion or knee extension. From these results the forward tilt seat with knee support is advocated.***

BSRM (1995) *Seating needs for complex disabilities.* London: British Society of Rehabilitation Medicine.

*This report includes a classification of special seating needs and systems, and notes that those with cerebral palsy are the largest group requiring special seating.**

Burns, S., Betz, K. (1999) 'Seating pressures with conventional and dynamic wheelchair cushions in tetraplegia.' *Archives of Physical Medicine and Rehabilitation 80*, 566–571.

Formal comparative user trial with 16 men with functional C4–C6 tetraplegia. Pressures under ischial tuberosities were measured when seated on Jay, Roho and dynamic cushions, in upright and 45° tilt-in-space positions, over one to six-minute periods. Dynamic cushion's minimum pressure when subjects were upright was significantly lower than the Jay when the chair was tilted, but not the Roho. ***

Chan, D., Laporte, D. and Sveistrup, H. (1999) 'Rising from sitting in elderly people: Part 2 Strategies to facilitate rising.' *British Journal of Occupational Therapy 62*, 2, 64–68.

*Literature review and expert opinion citing chair features and user strategies to make rising easier.**

Clark, M. (1998) 'Repositioning to prevent pressure sores – what is the evidence?' *Nursing Standard 13*, 3, 58, 60, 62, 64.

Searched the literature and found very little primary evidence. The origin of the two-hourly turning is unclear. Research suggests that even one hour might not remove the risk of pressure sore development. Tilting a person when recumbent to 30° by using pillows behind the back incurs less risk than when supine. **

Clark, M. (1999) 'Developing guidelines for pressure ulcer prevention and management.' *Journal of Wound Care 8, 7, 357–359.*

Literature review. Guidelines were first formulated in the Netherlands in 1985. In 1992 guidelines published in the USA contained 113 recommendations, but only 19 of these were supported by research data. The author comments that a factor in low adoption rates may be that many guidelines are based on experts' opinion rather than objective evidence.

Collins, F. (1998) 'Sitting pretty.' *Nursing Times 94, 38; 66, 68–70.*

Expert opinion reviewing biomechanics of sitting posture and describing types of pressure relieving cushions. *

Collins, F. (1999) 'An investigation into the contribution made by Winchester fireside armchairs in the prevention and management of pressure sores in the elderly acutely ill medical patient.' University of Brighton: MSc Clinical Life Sciences.

Controlled trial in two wards; trial ward had Winchester chairs with Transflo seats (n = 506 during trial period) and control had existing seating (n = 576). Significantly fewer pressure sores developed in trial ward (p = 0.0001). ***

Collins, F. (2001) 'Sitting: pressure ulcer development.' *Nursing Standard 15, 22, 54–56, 58.*

Cites the principles for good seating and advocates a well-fitting chair and cushion, plus regular inspection of the skin, to reduce incidence of pressure sores. *

Collins, F., and Shipperley, T. (1999) 'Assessing the seated patient for the risk of pressure damage.' *Journal of Wound Care 8, 3, 123–126.*

Basic guidelines (no supporting evidence) for a seat that provides a good fit and reasons why a poor fit can be detrimental. *

Conine, T., Hershler, C., Daechsel, D. *et al.* (1994) 'Pressure ulcer prophylaxis in elderly patients using polyurethane foam or Jay wheelchair cushions.' *International Journal of Rehabilitation Research 17, 123–137.*

Controlled formal trial with 163 elderly wheelchair users in long-term care who were randomly assigned to Jay or 4 in. foam with stretch cover. Significantly fewer pressure sores developed in trial group (p 0.05) than control. Interface pressure 60mmHg, Norton score 11, malnourishment, all significantly associated with development of pressure ulcers. ****

Cristarella, M. (1975) 'Straddling and sitting apparatus for the spastic cerebral-palsied child.' *American Journal of Occupational Therapy 29, 5, 273–276.*

Literature review and expert opinion on advantages of straddle seating. *

Cutter, N. and Blake, D.J. (1997) 'Wheelchairs and seating systems: clinical applications.' *Physical Medicine and Rehabilitation: state of the art reviews 11, 1, 107–132.*

Expert opinion underpinned with references. Includes reference to Ferguson-Pell's and Reswick and Rogers's recommendations for maximum interface pressures; comparison of recline versus tilt-in-space; cushion materials and their effects on skin; seat selection; solutions for positioning problems. *

Defloor, T. and Grypdonck, M. (2000) 'Do pressure relief products really relieve pressure?' *Western Journal of Nursing Research 22, 3, 335–350.*

Formal comparative trial with 20 healthy 19–45 year olds who sat on 30 cushion surfaces and pressures taken using a sensor mat. Sheepskin 'not appropriate' to use because of poor performance. **

Deitz, J. and Crepeau, E. (1998) 'Qualitative and quantitative research: joint contributors to the knowledge base in occupational therapy.' In N. Neistadt, and E. Crepeau (eds) *Willard & Spackman's Occupational Therapy* 9th Edition Philadelphia: Lippincott.

A description of K. Washington's PhD thesis. Formal trial of a standard high chair, first with foam pad, and second with contoured foam support (CFS) by four children with neuromotor impairment. A clinic observation period was followed by a four-week home trial of the last. Results showed better postural alignment in CFS. The home trial indicated that the parents valued the greater independence in sitting that the CFS provided. ★★★

DLF Fact Sheet (1999) *Choosing a wheelchair cushion.* London: Disabled Living Foundation.

Guidelines re choice of pressure relief cushion according to user needs. Also cites risk factors for pressure sore development.★

Drury, C., and Coury, B. (1982) 'A methodology for chair evaluation.' *Applied Ergonomics 13*, 3, 195–202.

A single office chair was evaluated using three methods: comparison with standards, subjective fitting, a trial of two and a half hours. For the last, a general comfort 11-point scale and a body part discomfort scale (three most and three least comfortable body parts) were administered every half hour. The chair broadly fell within recommended dimensions,★★★ *and performed fairly well. There were differences according to task, and an adjustable rake backrest was recommended because of the results.*★★

Dunlop, D., Hughes, S. and Manheim, L. (1997) 'Disability in activities of daily living: patterns of change and a hierarchy of disability.' *American Journal of Public Health 87*, 3, 378–383.

Longitudinal study over 6 years of 5151 people aged 70 years and over: difficulties with daily living activities were assessed, then analysed for pattern of onset. Initially, 10.6 per cent of the sample had difficulty with transfers which included rising from a chair; 6 years later this had risen to 13.5 per cent (men) and 17.9 per cent (women).★★★

Ellis, M. (1988) 'Everyday aids and appliances: choosing easy chairs for the disabled.' *British Medical Journal 296*, 701–702.

Expert opinion unsupported by references, but clear diagrams citing key features to seek. ★

Fife, S., Roxborough, L., Armstrong, R. *et al.* (1991) 'Development of a clinical measure of postural control for assessment of adaptive seating in children with neuromotor disabilities.' *Physical Therapy 71*, 12, 981–993.

The Seated Postural Control Measure (SPCM) was shown to have good reliability for all sections except the visual judgement of angles.

Finlay, O., Bayles, T., Rosen, C. and Milling, J. (1983) 'Effects of chair design, age and cognitive status on mobility.' *Age and Ageing 12*, 329–335.

All except 4 residents of 3 homes (n=92) who were included in one of two studies. 1. Survey of 61 residents who were assessed as able or unable to rise from 3 chairs . More could rise from the highest chair (seat height 445 mm) p .002.★★★ *2. Formal comparison of 31 residents rising from 2 chairs. Whole sample showed those who could rise without difficulty were younger (p .05) and those who did not benefit from higher seat tended to have greater cognitive deficit (p 0.02).*★★★ *Seat height and armrest height were not altered systematically, so conclusion about armrest height cannot be deduced from results.*

Fletcher, J. (1998) 'Pressure-relieving equipment: criteria and selection.' *British Journal of Therapy and Rehabilitation 5*, 3, 125–126, 128, 130.

Expert opinion. Comments mainly relate to pressure relieving products for beds, but rightly highlight that balance may be challenged by alternating-cell products. ★

Grandjean, E. (1980) *Fitting the task to the man.* New York: International Publications Service.

Ergonomically based design criteria. Includes recommendations for design of office seating. **

Greenfield, E. (1986) *Assessment of high stools and chairs for use in the kitchen or at a high workbench.* DHSS Disability Equipment Assessment Programme. Heywood: HMSO.

Formal user evaluation by 40 people with neurological, rheumatological conditions, or frail elderly. They tested all ten evaluation products, unless they were considered unsafe with that individual. Those with osteoarthritis preferred a backrest ** *or a wider seat so they could push up from it with their hands. Rheumatiod arthritis: probably preferred the same, plus a lightweight product.* * *Those with hemiplegia preferred a backrest, arms and a stable product.* ** *Those with MS probably wanted stability,* * *those with back pain an office chair, sloped seat or Balans style.* * *A sloped seat not recommended for those with visuospatial problems.* *

Hastings, J. (2000) 'Seating assessment and planning.' *Topics in Spinal Cord Injury 11*, 1, 183–207.

Expert opinion on seating for those with spinal cord injury. Description of aspects of wheelchair components and their usage. *

Healy, A., Ramsay, C. and Sexsmith, E. (1997) 'Postural support systems: their use, fabrication and functional use.' *Developmental Medicine and Child Neurology 39*, 706–710.

Expert opinion describing parameters for assessment, postural support and support system materials. * *Uses Trefler and Taylor's (1991) three categories of seating need.*

Helander, M., and Zhang, L. (1997) 'Field studies of comfort and discomfort in sitting.' *Ergonomics 40*, 9, 895–915.

Comparative evaluation of 20 office chairs by 10 fit women and 10 fit men used to refine a tool to measure comfort and discomfort. Discomfort affected by biomechanics but if a chair conforms to basic design criteria it will be adequately comfortable – unless the user has back problem. **

Henderson, J., Price, S., Brandstater, M. *et al.* (1994) 'Efficacy of three measures to relieve pressure in seated persons with spinal cord injury.' *Archives of Physical Medicine and Rehabilitation 75*, 535–539.

Formal comparative trial with 7 people with paraplegia and 3 with quadriplegia. Interface pressure readings taken under ischial tuberosities, in four conditions: upright, forward leaning, 35° tilt and 65° tilt. Significant reduction in pressure with 65° tilt compared with upright posture, but forward leaning was more effective. ***

Hobson, D. and Molenbroek, J. (1990) 'Anthropometry and design for the disabled: experiences with seating design for the cerebral palsy population.' *Applied Ergonomics 21*, 1, 43–54.

People with cerebral palsy (n=133) aged 2–55 years who were unable to walk were measured. **

Hulme, J.B., Poor, R., Schulein, M. and Pezzino, J. (1983) 'Perceived behavioral changes observed with adaptive seating devices and training programs for multihandicapped, developmentally disabled children.' *Physical Therapy 63*, 2, 204–208.

Postal survey of 130 people (aged 1–67 years) involved in an equipment project; 105 responded. Those who had received only a special seating device (n=33) were analysed; 85 per cent had cerebral palsy. Significantly more time interacting (p=0.004), sitting up (p=0.001) and improvement in self-feeding (p=0.005) since provision of seating device, *** *but the ratings were subjective retrospective perceptions.*

Hulme, J.B., Gallacher, K., Walsh, J. *et al.* (1987) 'Behavioral and postural changes observed with use of adaptive seating by clients with multiple handicaps.' *Physical Therapy 67*, 7, 1060–1067.

Follow-on study of those with a special seating device, from the above reference. Parent questionnaire (initial and last visits) and therapist observation about posture and function every six weeks, from three months before provision of an AD to six months after. Nineteen of 27 completed, mean age of child 2.4 years. All key aspects of *sitting posture improved with the AD (p=0.01), head control improved (p=0.01), grasp improved (p=0.02), time sitting increased (p=0.01).* ***

Hulme, J.B., Shaver, J., Acher, S. *et al.* (1987) 'Effects of adaptive seating devices on the eating and drinking of children with multiple handicaps.' *American Journal of Occupational Therapy 41*, 2, 81–89.

Same study as above reference: 11 children were also assessed for eating/drinking. Food and liquid retained more in mouth (p .01) enabling progression from puréed to chopped food, and bottle to cup, *** *but very small numbers.*

Johnson Taylor, S. (1987) 'Evaluating the client with physical disabilities for wheelchair seating.' *American Journal of Occupational Therapy 41*, 11, 711–716.

Expert opinion: assessment and prescription for seating. Uses Trefler and Taylor's three categories of seating need. *

Koo, T., Mak, A. and Lee, Y. (1996) 'Posture effect on seating interface biomechanics: comparison between two seating cushions.' *Archives Physical and Medical Rehabilitation 77*, 40–47.

Controlled study of ischial pressures of 6 males with paraplegia, 8 male controls were measured using the Oxford Pressure Monitor. Spinal cord injury subjects tend to flex lower spine more than controls; Roho cushion significantly more efficient at distributing pressure than foam (unspecified thickness) on ply base. The better pressure relieving properties meant that side leaning did not relieve pressure further, but forward leaning did. ***

Lachmann, S., Greenfield, E., and Wrench, A. (1993) 'Assessment of need for special seating and/or electronic control systems for wheelchairs among people with severe disabilities.' *Clinical Rehabilitation 7*, 151–156.

Users of a wheelchair service that had no sitting ability (n=215) were surveyed. Method vague, but 13 needed special seating who did not have it. **

Lange, M. (2000) 'Focus on: tilt and recline systems', *OT Practice 5*,10, 21–22.

Expert opinion comparing tilt-in-space and recline facilities. *

Laporte, D., Chan, D. Sveistrup, H. (1999) 'Rising from sitting in elderly people: Part 1 Implications of biomechanics and physiology.' *British Journal of Occupational Therapy 62*, 1, 36–42.

Literature review and expert opinion on mechanics of rising and effect of weakness and stiffness. **

Le Carpentier, E. (1969) 'Easy chair dimensions for comfort – a subjective approach.' *Ergonomics 12*, 2, 328–337.

Formal trial with 20 people who were distributed equally between sex and age (< 40 years; 40+). They were allowed to adjust an easy chair rig for seat height, width, depth, tilt and seat-to-backrest angle. Men preferred a larger seat-to-backrest angle than women (113° cf. 105°) *** *and the mean seat height plus seat depth measurement was 880mm (SD 35mm) for all.* *** *[Note the subjects were healthy younger adults.]*

Letts, R.M. (Ed) (1991) *Principles of seating the disabled* Boca Raton, Florida: CRC Press.

Goals of good seating, assessment and practical solutions. Features described will remain appropriate rather than the actual products owing to the market having developed since publication. * *Some literature to support recommendations but these are not reviewed.*

Mann, W. and Tomita, M. (1998) 'Perspectives on assistive devices among elderly persons with disabilities.' *Technology and Disability 9*, 119–148.

508 current AD users from a longitudinal study were interviewed. Respondents complained of chair discomfort (n=3) and an additional cushion slipping off the seat (n=1). **

McCafferty, E., Watret, L., Brown, C. *et al.* (2000) 'A multidisciplinary audit of patients' seating needs.' *Professional Nurse 15,* 11, 715–718.

Survey conducted on 8 rehabilitation or continuing care wards for the elderly. Staff were asked their views on seating via a questionnaire; 50% stated a chair should be of height and depth appropriate for individual, 14% felt pressure relieving cushions important. Of 161 patients interviewed, 57 per cent felt they were included in the choice of seating. Of 157 patients assessed for risk of pressure sores; 59 per cent with Waterlow score 10 did not have a special pressure relieving cushion; 8 per cent with minimum risk had a special cushion. **

McClenaghan, B. (1989) 'Sitting stability of selected subjects with cerebral palsy.' *Clinical Biomechanics 4,* 4, 213–216.

Formal trial with 6 people with spastic diplegia cerebral palsy (CP), aged 4.5–34 years, and 6 age-matched controls. They sat on an adjustable chair jig with seat horizontal and hips and knees at 90°, arms on table and feet supported with ankle neutral. Kistler force plate used to measure centre of pressure on seat. Those with CP sat with their centre of pressure significantly forward to the matched control p .05. *** *More sway as centre of pressure moved forward, in CP and controls. More weight placed through arms and feet when weight forward. A single case study report added to this study showed that a 5° forward tilt to seat reduced the sway and moved the centre of pressure towards the ischial tuberosities.* **

McGrath, P., Goodman, J., Cunningham, J. *et al.* (1985) 'Assistive devices: utilisation by children.' *Archives of Physical Medical Rehabilitation, 66,* 430–432.

Postal survey to 747; 502 responses. 100% usage of pressure relieving products. **

Mann, W. and Tomita, M. (1998) 'Perspectives on assitive devices among elderly persons with disabilities.' *Technology and Disability 9,* 119–148.

MDA (1995) *Upholstered chairs for children with disabilities: a comparative evaluation,* A16. London: Medical Devices Agency.

Formal comparative user trial with 29 children aged 5–18 years who each tested 5 multi-adjustable chairs. Improvements in upper limb function were noted in 50–81 per cent compared to when tested with minimum support for safety. A postal survey of current users was also conducted: 314 sent, 114 returned, 100 eligible. Tilt-in-space was deemed useful by the majority who had this facility. **

MDA (1997a) *The effects of posture, body mass index and wheelchair adjustment on interface pressure,* MDA/97/20. London: Medical Devices Agency.

Literature review cited that 70 per cent people of average to large build do not *have maximum pressures under their ischial tuberosities: there is a link between pressure gradients and body build rather than maximum pressure readings, with thinner people showing greatest gradients.*

Formal trial used Talley pressure monitor with 27 elderly ambulant people, 3in. foam cushion with vinyl cover in standard sling seat wheelchair, sitting in various positions. Mean pressure (88 mmHg) was significantly higher than that of younger adults. Interface pressure showed 100 per cent increase between footrests at lowest to highest adjustment. Slouched posture significantly increases sacral pressure but relieves very little from the ischium. *** *Plywood base under cushion produced the highest pressures under ischium. Side leaning with sling seat raised pressure under the* opposite *ischial tuberosity. No correlation between Body Mass Index and ischial pressures.* ***

MDA (1997b) *Wheelchair cushions static and dynamic: a comparative evaluation,* PS4. London: Medical Devices Agency.

Formal comparative user trial. The interface pressure under the ischial tuberosities of 12 elderly ambulant people, using a sequence of 20 wheelchair cushions plus a 3in. foam cushion with PVC cover, was measured. Six cushions had significantly higher mean pressures than the foam cushion used as reference. These were therefore excluded from tests by people with spinal cord injury or stroke. Flaccid paralysis results in higher interface *pressures (***); Roho high profile and Jay cushions were most effective in reducing interface pressures. Dynamic cushions' results were presented as a mean over the inflation cycle; these means did not differ significantly from the static cushion results. This, however, may not accurately reflect the clinical effect of these cushions.*

MDA (1998a) *Armchairs with special features to reduce interface pressure, alternating pressure cushions (mains powered), and supplementary cushions: a comparative evaluation*, PS5. London: Medical Devices Agency.

Formal comparative user trial. The interface pressure under the ischial tuberosities of 12 elderly ambulant people using the products which included feather and fibre pillows and cushions. Feather seat and pillow, fibre pillow all had similar interface pressure readings to the reference armchair. Dynamic cushions, gelsacs in foam casing and water-filled sacs gave significantly lower pressure readings.***

MDA (1998b) *Seating for young children with disabilities: a comparative evaluation*, DEA A23. Norwich: Medical Devices Agency, HMSO.

Formal comparative user trial by 40 children under 5 years who each tested up to 4 seats, either floor sitters, conventional chairs or straddle seats. Four of seven of those with high tone in their legs testing corner seats achieved a satisfactory posture. Up to four of the five with poor head control could sit satisfactorily for short periods in corner seats that gave good stability at the hips.**

MDA (1998c) *Self-lift chair: the Caithness, Cairngorm and Clansman*, Safety Notice SN9832. London: Medical Devices Agency.

A person was ejected from one of these spring-operated chairs. Warning given to ensure the spring loading is appropriate to user's weight. Also noted is risk of finger entrapment between frame and seat pad.

MDA (1999) *Electric riser seats and chairs: a comparative evaluation*, EL2. London: Medical Devices Agency.

Formal comparative user trial of 10 electric riser chairs and 5 riser seats. They were divided into 3 groups and tested by 45 people, each testing all chairs in one group. Range of disabilities, mean age 61 years. Used mechanism to sit; sat for 30 minutes; used mechanism to rise. From results, recommendation that those without limited knee flexion or/and upper limb weakness may benefit from seat unit; those with general weakness or/and limited knee flexion more appropriately should have chair.** Owing to potential for some chairs to be unstable when fully raised, user should only raise it sufficiently to facilitate standing.**

MDA (2000) *Electrically operated lift and recliner chairs: risk of entrapment*, Safety Notice SN2000(19). London: Medical Devices Agency. Accessed via www.medical-devices.gov.uk on 8/11/01.

Warning of risk of toddler or pet entrapment when chair is lowered.

Miedaner, J. and Finuf, L. (1993) 'Effects of adaptive positioning on psychological test scores for preschool children with cerebral palsy.' *Pediatric Physical Therapy* 5, 4, 177–182.

Formal trial with 12 children with spastic cerebral palsy who were tested using the Bayley scales in an optimally supported and minimally supported sitting position, six in one order, six in the reverse order. Significantly increased scores intrasubject for the optimally supported position (p 0.05).*** Literature review tabulated outcomes of previous studies.

Milne, J. (1988) *Assessment of chair and bed raising systems. Disability Equipment Assessment Programme.* London: Department of Health.

Formal comparative user trial of 13 raising systems. They were tested by 50 users (mainly over 70 years), who tried 1–3 products each. In a large number of cases the products could not be trialled because of technical difficulties or safety risks. A selection of raisers should be available to ensure the most secure fit is obtained.**

Minkel, J. (2000) 'Seating and mobility considerations for people with spinal cord injury.' *Physical Therapy* 80, 7, 701–709.

Literature review and expert opinion.* Divides seating needs of spinal cord injury (SCI) people into three (above C5; C5–T8; T9–T12). Several studies show that those with SCI sit with pelvis posteriorly tilted and have greater interface pressures under buttocks than non-SCI people. One study showed that increased lumbar support does not reduce interface pressure for SCI but does for non-SCI. Minkel suggests matching seat-to-backrest angle to that obtainable at hip joint; this differs from a reference (Zacharkow 1984) who suggested 95°.

Mulcahy, C. (1986) 'An approach to the assessment of sitting ability for the prescription of seating.' *British Journal of Occupational Therapy* 49, 367–368.

An early description of the Chailey Levels of Sitting Ability, see Mulcahy et al. 1988.

Mulcahy, C. and Pountney, T. (1986) 'The sacral pad – description of its clinical use in seating.' *Physiotherapy* 72, 9, 473–474.

Expert opinion. A small pad for use in conjunction with a ramped cushion (see next reference) and pelvic strap to prevent posterior rotation of pelvis in children who can anchor their bottom but have not yet developed a lumbar curve.*

Mulcahy, C. and Pountney, T. (1987) 'Ramped cushion' (letter), *British Journal of Occupational Therapy 50*, 3, 97.

Description of how to construct a cushion ramped upwards at 15° from the gluteal crease.

Mulcahy, C., Pountney, T., Nelham, R. *et al.* (1988) 'Adaptive seating for motor handicap: problems, a solution, assessment and prescription.' *British Journal of Occupational Therapy 51*, 10, 347–352.

Clinically developed seven-point assessment scale for children with cerebral palsy.**

Munro, B. and Steele, J. (1998) 'Facilitating the sit-to-stand transfer: a review.' *Physical Therapy Reviews* 3, 213–224.

Technical assessment. Use of armrests reduce mean maximum movements at hip and knee.**** Armrests also used to aid balance, and more pressure applied by older people. Raising seat height reduces effort required to stand,**** as does using assisted riser chairs.**** Munro and Steele counter the argument that assisted riser chairs cause leg weakness by quoting unpublished data that show vastus medialis and rectus femoris activity remained high when elders with rheumatoid arthritis used assisted riser seats; also that rising is a means to undertake other activities that themselves exercise the legs.

Munro, B., Steele, J., Bashford, G. *et al.* (1998) 'A kinematic and kinetic analysis of the sit-to-stand transfer using an ejector chair: implications for elderly rheumatoid arthritics.' *Journal of Biomechanics 31*, 263–271.

Formal trial with 12 elderly females who had rheumatoid arthritis and Barthel scores   80 . They were filmed standing up from two seat heights, with and without an ejector mechanism. Reaction forces under feet and hands were measured. The higher seat (540 mm) reduced forces significantly, as did the ejector seat used at either height.***

Munton, J., Ellis, M., Chamberlain, M. and Wright, V. (1981) 'An investigation into the problems of easy chairs used by the arthritic and the elderly.' *Rheumatology and Rehabilitation 20*, 164–173.

Survey; 561 questionnaires were administered in day centres or outpatient clinics. For these, 379 addendums were returned with usable chair measurements. Age range 20–91, with neurological (20%) as well as arthritic conditions; 97 per cent ambulant; 70 per cent had standard easy chair; 42 per cent had difficulty rising from their usual easy chair; 63 per cent used extra cushions.**

Myhr, U. (1994) 'Influence of different seat and backrest inclinations on the spontaneous positioning of the extremities in non-disabled children.' *Physiotherapy Theory and Practice 10*, 191–200.

Formal trial with 10 children, 4.2–9.5 years old who sat in 5 positions, and completed a standardised task in each. Videotaped and analysed. Spontaneous positioning of feet when reaching is usually posterior to knee joint until chair seat and backrest are reclined. Legs are then often extended when reaching. Backward sloping seat encourages posterior pelvic tilt and flexion of spine. ** *Small numbers, but biomechanically logical.*

Myhr, U. and von Wendt, L. (1991) 'Improvement of functional sitting position for children with cerebral palsy.' *Developmental Medicine and Child Neurology 33*, 246–256.

Formal trial with 23 children who had cerebral palsy (aged 2–16 years). They were observed in 6 sitting conditions, including the 'functional sitting position' (FSP). They were filmed and subsequently assessed using the Sitting Assessment Scale, and the centre of mass plotted relative to the fulcrum (ischial tuberosities). Head, trunk, foot and upper limb control were all better in the FSP (p .001). *** *On visual inspection, data seem to indicate that the critical element of the FSP is that the centre of mass is anterior to the fulcrum. The abduction orthosis and table had some additional impact but a comparatively small one.**

NICE (National Institute of Clinical Excellence) (2001) *Clinical guidelines for pressure sore prevention.* At www.nice.org.uk/pdf/clinicalguidelinepressuresoreguidancenice.pdf accessed on 24/7/01.

Noronha, J., Bundy, A. and Groll, J. (1989) 'The effect of positioning on the hand function of boys with cerebral palsy.' *American Journal of Occupational Therapy 43*, 8, 507,512.

Formal trial with 10 boys (mean age 12.5 years) with spastic diplegia. They performed the Jebson-Taylor hand function test in a standard seat and in a prone stander. No significant difference in scores, but speed was greater in prone stander (p=0.0004 **) *with simulated feeding, and slower for small objects (p* .03 **). *Function on slippery surface poorer. But tasks are unilateral, and the relative work height was different in the two conditions.*

Pellow, T. (1999) 'A comparison of interface pressure readings to wheelchair cushions and positioning: a pilot study.' *Canadian Journal of Occupational Therapy 66*, 3, 140–149.

Formal trial of three cushions and five seating positions with two males with C5 quadriplegia, (one incomplete lesion). Interface pressures measured under ischial tuberosities and sacral tip; 150° recline reduced pressure *** *the most in all but one of the readings. Even a slight tilt lowered pressure when using gel or foam cushion.** *The higher pressure reading under buttocks in the lighter subject was reduced by the Roho.***

Pheasant, S. (undated; c.1997) 2nd edition. *Bodyspace.* London: Taylor & Francis.

*Recommendations for seat height, depth and width based on data from a large sample representative of the general population.*****

Pope, P., Bowes, C. and Booth, E. (1994) 'Postural control in sitting. The SAM system: evaluation of use over 3 years.' *Developmental Medicine and Child Neurology 36*, 241–252.

*Longitudinal single product evaluation. Ten children with spastic quadriplegia, aged two to nine years, were issued with SAM (moulded saddle seat, prone angle seat, anterior and lateral trunk support) with optional powered wheelbase. Test battery on issue and three annual reviews. No significant improvements detected, but qualitative benefits reported both physically and socially.***

Pope, P. (1996) 'Postural management and special seating.' In S. Edwards (ed) *Neurological physiotherapy: a problem-solving approach.* London: Churchill Livingstone.

*Expert opinion on principles and ways of achieving postural control in sitting.**

Pountney, T., Mulcahy, C., Clarke, S. and Green, E. (2000) *The Chailey approach to postural management.* Birmingham: Active Design.

Expert opinion on principles and ways of achieving postural control in sitting. *It is implied that sacral pads used in conjunction with knee blocks and lateral pelvic support can be used with older children and adults, cf. Mulcahy and Pountney 1986.*

Reid, D. (1996) 'The effects of the saddle seat on seated postural control and upper extremity movement in children with cerebral palsy.' *Developmental Medicine and Child Neurology 38*, 805–815.

Formal trial of single product plus control condition. Six children with mild–moderate spastic cerebral palsy, aged four to eight years, able to sit on a flat bench without holding on, were tested on a flat bench and a saddle seat prototype: 40 minutes on each seat, repeated at another session in the reverse order. Sitting ability improved with the saddle seat (p   0.007). They sat up straighter on saddle seat (p   0.0005). *** Variability in response to saddle seat was wide. Effect on reaching not significantly different.

Rigby, P., Ryan, S., From, W. *et al.* (1996) 'A client-centred approach to developing assistive technology with children.' *Occupational Therapy International 3*, 1, 67–79.

User evaluation of 5 cushions by 84 children, aged 6–13, 50 of whom were current users of special seating systems; 58 had cerebral palsy. They tested, then rated their views using a three-face scale. At end, they chose their most preferred. A discussion group was held the following day. Some children consistently chose the smiling face, so their discrimination is questionable, but most children showed preference for the softer cushions, and the younger children chose brighter colours more frequently than the older. ** The authors conclude that children can reliably be canvassed for their opinions on AT provided they have concrete examples to evaluate.

Rithalia, S. (1997a) 'Assessment of pressure relief characteristics in alternating pressure air cushions.' *International Journal of Rehabilitation Research 20*, 205–208.

Comparative trial. Eight healthy adults had interface pressures under right buttock continuously measured for one cycle for each of four cushions. ** Few readings of   20 mmHg were recorded. Author felt that 30 mmHg may be a more appropriate threshold.

Rithalia, S. (1997b) 'Know how: alternating pressure relief.' *Nursing Times 93*, 46, 76–77.

Describes a method of reporting performance of dynamic pressure relieving cushions: as a percentage of time that the interface pressure is below a specified threshold, e.g. 20 mmHg.

Russell, L., Reynolds, T. and Carr, J. (2000) 'A comparison of healing rates on two pressure relieving systems.' *British Journal of Nursing 9*, 22, 2270–2280.

A randomised controlled trial (RCT) of 2 systems comprising a dynamic mattress and cushion each:141 met entry criterion of having a pressure ulcer and were entered over a period of 18 months. Both systems were effective treatment for pressure ulcers but no significant difference between them.****

Seeger, B., Caudrey, D. and O'Mara, N. (1984) 'Hand function in cerebral palsy: the effect of hip flexion angle.' *Developmental Medicine and Child Neurology 26*, 601–606.

Formal trial of the effect of seat angles by 9 children, aged 7–20 years, 6 with more extensor spasm than flexor spasm and 3 with extensor and flexor spasm rated equal. They sat in a wheelchair rig with seat angle at 0°, 10°, 20°, 30° (backward tilt). Used joystick for a computer response task. Measurements were taken of response times in all 4 seat conditions, on 4 occasions, in order predetermined by a Latin square. Seat angle did not significantly affect response speed for the extensor spasm group,*** but there was a significant difference in speeds between 0° and 30° for the 3 with flexor and extensor spasm. ** Seat angles of 10° and 20° were reported 'less uncomfortable' than the other conditions.

Shechtman, O., Hanson, C., Garrett, D. *et al.* (2001) 'Comparing wheelchair cushions for effectiveness of pressure relief: a pilot study.' *The Occupational Therapy Journal of Research 21*, 1, 29–48.

Formal comparative user trial. Pressure mat 46 cm square was used to measure interface pressures under 40 wheelchair users sitting on sling seat (baseline) and six pressure distributing cushions. Five-point scale of subjective comfort completed by 30. Roho significantly more comfortable (p   0.05) *** and more effective for most. **

*Those with higher Body Mass Index recorded greater percentage of higher pressures.*** [Authors' note: this is not the same as measuring under the ischial tuberosities.]*

Shields, R., and Cook, T. (1992) 'Lumbar support thickness: effect on seated buttock pressure in individuals with and without spinal cord injury.' *Physical Therapy* 72, 218–226.

*Formal trial of effect of lumbar support on 18 with spinal cord injury (SCI), 12 paraplegics, 6 quadriplegics, and 18 controls, mean age 27 and 35 respectively. Sat on jig with optical system to measure interface pressure under the ischial tuberosities. Knees 80° flexion, ankles 10° plantarflexion. Seat 10° backward tilt and 95° seat-to-backrest angle for 4 conditions of lumbar support (unpadded wood) 0, 25 mm, 50 mm, 75 mm thick. Pelvifemoral angle measured for each condition. The range of pelvifemoral angle was below that of controls, but lumbar support did increase these. No significant reduction in interface pressure *** for SCI but there was for controls, relieving up to 90 per cent of pressure under ischial tuberosities. Pressure gradient much higher for those with flaccid paralysis compared with controls.*

Shipperley, T. and Collins, F. (1999) 'A seating assessment tool for community use.' *Journal of Wound Care 18*, 3, 119–120.

*Clinically derived flowchart for differential prescription of pressure relieving cushions.**

Stewart, P. and McQuilton, G. (1987) 'Straddle seating for the cerebral palsied child.' *British Journal of Occupational Therapy 50*, 4, 136–138.

*Description and rationale for straddle seating. Observational improvement in upper limb function.**

Stockton, L. (2000) 'Guide to choosing the right pressure reducing cushion.' *Community Nurse 6*, 2, 33–34.

*Expert opinion. Need to consider cushions and cover. Stability and keeping moisture from the skin are also important.**

Swedberg, L. (1998) 'Low-tech adaptations for seating and positioning.' *OT Practice 3*, 9, 26–31.

*Expert opinion. Practical solutions to seating challenges.**

Sweeney, G., and Clarke, A.K. (1991) *An evaluation of office seating for people with arthritis and low back pain.* MDD/200/91 Disability Equipment Assessment. Norwich: HMSO.

*Formal comparative user trial of 15 office chairs, divided according to task specified by manufacturer: typing, computer, clerical. From pilot work, two-day trial considered sufficient. Thirty people tested the five chairs in one group (ten tests per chair). Varied reaction to most features, but adjustable height backrests were favoured.***

Sweeney, G., and Clarke, A.K. (1992) An evaluation of easy chairs for people with arthritis and low back pain. MDD/206/92 Disability Equipment Assessment. Norwich: HMSO.

*Formal comparative user trial of 15 chairs divided into 5 groups. Twenty tested all chairs in one group. Total subjects 100, aged 17–88. After piloting, 30 minutes considered sufficient for accurate judgement of comfort. Those with ankylosing spondylitis wanted good support for back and head; those with low back pain wanted good lumbar support.** Sit-to-stand was not assessed.*

ten Haar, B. (1999) 'Helping gravity help you: part 1.' *Posture and Mobility 9*, 21–24. (Newsletter of Posture and Mobility Group, England and Wales.)

*Based on lecture tour by T. Hetzel: expert opinion. Postural control should provide symmetry for rest, and allow movement into asymmetry for function (p.22). Emphasises that the seating design will vary according to the user's pattern of muscle tone as well as sitting ability.**

ten Haar, B. (2000) 'Helping gravity help you: part 2', *Posture and Mobility 11*, 5–9. (Newsletter of Posture and Mobility Group, England and Wales.)

Belts, footrests and harnesses. Advise tilt-in-space is used from an early stage in muscular dystrophy to discourage problems arising from anterior pelvic tilt.*

Trefler, E. and Taylor, S. (1991) 'Prescription and positioning: evaluating the physically disabled individual for wheelchair seating.' *Prosthetics and Orthotics International 15*, 217–224.

Expert opinion. Formulated a three-dimensional model to assist prescription: sensation, postural control and deformity as its axes.* *[Authors' note: the range of modular seating systems has improved since this publication, so the recommendations with regard to types of seating do not reflect the options available now.]*

Turner, C. (2001) 'Posture and seating for wheelchair users: an introduction.' *British Journal of Therapy and Rehabilitation 8*, 1, 24, 26–28.

Review of biomechanics of seating.*

Wall, J. (2000) 'Preventing pressure sores among wheelchair users.' *Professional Nurse 15*, 5, 321–324.

Survey of 10 wheelchair users with history of pressure sores, living in the community, aged between 18 and 65 years, with multiple sclerosis. Semi-structured interviews with users and carers about their views of why they developed a sore, and what one could do to prevent them. They felt static sitting and friction during transfers were main contributing factors.** *Lack of knowledge about incontinence; no comment from any participant about pressure relieving cushions.*

Waterlow, J., Vernon, M. and Gilchrist, B. (1996) 'The Norton score and pressure sore prevention.' *Journal of Wound Care 5*, 2, 93–99.

Three reviews of the original article (1962) in which the Norton risk assessment scale was reported. Includes some comments about the Waterlow risk assessment scale.*

Weiner, D., Long, R., Hughes, M. *et al.* (1993) 'When older adults face the chair-rise challenge.' *Journal of the American Geriatrics Society 41*, 6–10.

Formal trial of effect of different chair heights by 22 elders, mean age 72. They rose from a chair without arms, at a height 17-22in. at 1in. intervals, presented in random order. Recorded on motion analysis software. Eleven had difficulty rising from 17in.; only two had difficulty in rising from 22in. seat. Increased seat height significantly increases the proportion of elders who can rise from it.*** *Increased height decreased the degree of shoulder and hip flexion used in rising. However, subjects had to cross their arms, so impact of armrests not assessed. Also, the footrest prevented posterior movement of feet to assist rising.*

Weiss-Lambrou, R., Tremblay, C., LeBlanc, R. and Dansereau, J. (1999) 'Wheelchair seating aids: how satisfied are consumers?' *Assistive Technology 11*, 43–53.

Survey of 24 adults who had modular seating systems in a powered wheelchair, interviewed using the QUEST standardised instrument. Comfort was rated as most important but respondents were least satisfied (6 unsatisfied, 7 'more or less' satisfied) with comfort. Statistical tests showed that there were differences between men and women, and between those in residential accommodation versus community, but numbers for comparisons were low and findings should be viewed as tentative.**

Wretenberg, P., Arborelius, U., Weidenhielm, L. and Lindberg, F. (1993) 'Rising from a chair by spring-loaded flap seat: a biomechanical analysis.' *Scandinavian Journal of Rehabilitation Medicine 25*, 153–159.

Formal trial of product and control condition by nine healthy males and eight people with osteoarthritis awaiting knee surgery. They rose from seat with and without a spring-assist. The spring-assist reduced the knee moment during rising by approximately 40 per cent.***

Zollars, J. (1996) *Special seating: an illustrated guide.* Minneapolis: Otto Bock Orthopedic Industry.

*Comprehensive text on special seating needs: assessment and provision.**

Bibliography

Butler, P., Nene, A. and Major, R. (1991) 'Biomechanics of transfer from sitting to the standing position in some neuromuscular diseases.' *Physiotherapy 77,* 8, 521–525.

*Observational study of ten people; video-recordings were analysed and five compensatory strategies described. *** Concluded that such strategies must be taken into account when interventions are planned.**

Ebe, K. and Griffin, M. (2000) 'Quantitative prediction of overall seat discomfort.' *Ergonomics 43,* 6, 791–806.

*Subjective comfort ratings by 20 fit young men when seated on 3 grades of foam or wooden seat, under static and vibratory conditions. For static and low vibration conditions, the comfort is correlated more to seat stiffness (higher density foam more comfortable). *** But very short test times used.*

Fleckenstein, S., Kirby, R. and MacLeod, D. (1988) 'Effect of limited knee flexion range on peak hip moments of force while transferring from sitting to standing.' *Journal of Biomechanics 21,* 11, 915,918.

*Technical evaluation of ten normal subjects when rising from sitting, both with knee at 105° and 75° flexion. The movements were cine-recorded. Reducing the angle of knee flexion increased the hip extension moment *** but authors warned that reduced knee flexion may accelerate hip joint damage so advocate maintaining range of movement at this joint. **

James, L. (2001) 'Special chairs project.' Southampton Physical Disabilities Services & City Council. Report for Joint Equipment Stores: unpublished.

Postal survey: 41 questionnaires were returned from 55 sent to Equipment Stores and other stakeholders. Results showed that professionals were requesting special chairs when they would facilitate independence (no mention of easing a care assistant's task), and a risk assessment showed a low risk of entrapment. Alternative options had to be considered first. The author's recommendation was for well-defined eligibility criteria to be adopted widely to maximise fairness, and for professionals to be given training in assessment for such chairs.

*Follow-up survey of ten children with spastic diplegia five years after special seating had been prescribed. Videotaped whilst in their usual seat, performing a standardised set of tasks. Sitting Assessment Scale (SAS) used to rate the children from the videos, by three physiotherapists. Two were not using their prescribed seating, and had deteriorated. The others had significant improvement in SAS (p.001). *** [Authors' note: Table III figures are out of alignment.]*

Myhr, U., von Wendt, L., Norrlin, S. and Radell, U. (1995) 'A five-year follow-up of a functional sitting position in children with cerebral palsy.' *Developmental Medicine and Child Neurology 37,* 587–596.

Pountney, T., Cheek, L., Green, E. *et al.* (1999) 'Content and criterion validation of the Chailey Levels of Ability.' *Physiotherapy 85,* 8, 410–416.

*The Chailey Levels of standing, sitting and lying ability were tested for content and criterion validity, the latter against the Alberta Infant Motor Scale and the Gross Motor Function Measure. Results were good for both.****

Chapter 4

Toileting and Continence

Introduction

Before working through this chapter, it is important to do the following:

- Consider your (the user's) requirements, and the requirements of the care assistant and others in the household if applicable (Chapter 1, Stage 1 in Figure 1.3).

- Decide on the priority for tackling the problems.

- Acknowledge the feelings that the problem(s) may have roused.

- Have in mind the environment(s) in which the assistive device(s) will be used (Stage 2 in Figure 1.3).

- Consider whether any alterations to the environment will be necessary.

Problems with toileting can be a particularly sensitive subject. A large proportion of those who have continence problems do not seek help (Asbury and White 2001). In response to this reticence, helplines and organisations have been formed to give advice, such as InContact, the Continence Foundation, ERIC (see Chapter 1, subsection 1.4.1). But many people gain great benefit from seeking advice from specialist services within the Health Service. Ways of solving continence problems often include a combination of medical treatments, assistive devices (ADs) and psychological treatments. This chapter therefore provides an overview of what evidence there is to guide choices, but acknowledges that in many cases these choices will be made collaboratively between yourself and practitioners from a number of allied health professions.

Whether or not you are experiencing continence problems, alterations to the environment may be needed to help make a toilet more accessible. The room may be too small, the doorway too narrow, or you may not be able to get to the room where the toilet is at all.

This chapter guides you through the decisions concerning what types or categories of toileting AD might be suitable, and helps to define what features you would want products to have within your preferred categories. This comprises Stage 4 in the process of choosing a product (see Figure 1.3). Each example will give you an idea of additional things to test or check when trying out the selected two or three products (Stage 5 from the process described in Chapter 1, section 1.3).

In working through Figure 4 *Pinpointing the problem*, note down all the sections that you may need to look at. If you have several needs, more than one solution may be required. Some examples are given to illustrate how the Figures and Tables are used.

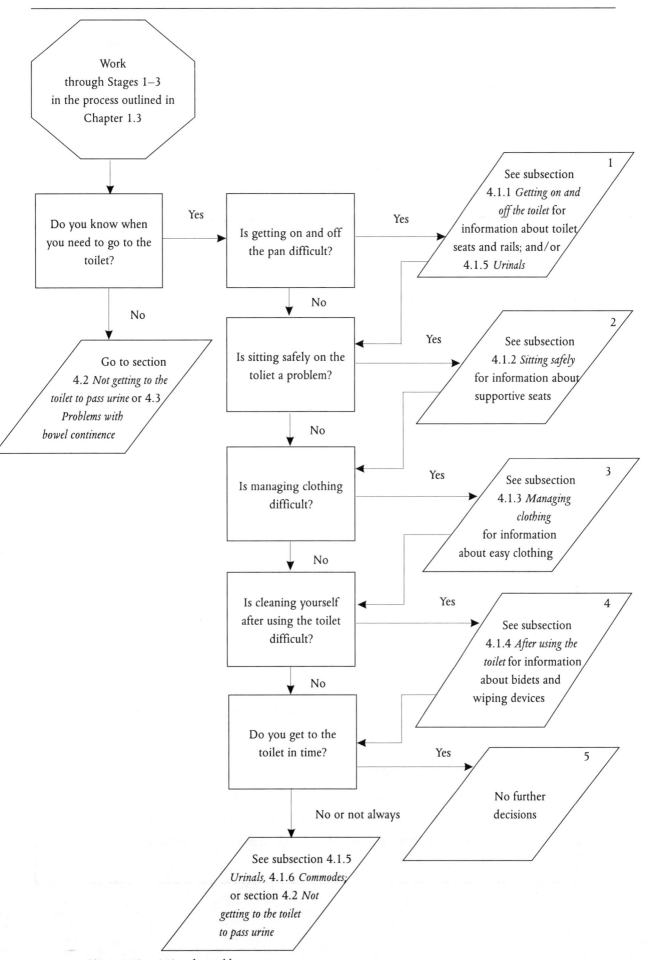

Figure 4 Pinpointing the problem

An example

Harry has multiple sclerosis, lives alone, and gets around at home using a wheelchair. He has a bathboard issued to him from the Red Cross so he can shower himself when the carer comes, but struggles to and from the downstairs toilet. He cannot stand safely at the toilet to urinate and finds getting on and off the toilet pan an increasing effort as the day progresses. He is worried in case he does not get onto the pan and adjust his clothes in time.

- Harry looks at Figure 4 *Pinpointing the problem*. He knows when he needs to go to the toilet; getting on and off it is difficult, but he already has a rail. He notes he could think about a urinal.

- As he continues down Figure 4 he knows he can sit safely enough, but does find his trouser fly opening difficult, so he notes he should look at subsection 4.1.3.

- He sees from Table 4.1.5 that he would want a urinal that was easy to grasp with one hand, as his hands are unreliable when trying to handle things.

- He decides to ask the Red Cross about urinals, rather than asking for advice from the Continence Advisory Service.

- He contacts his local Red Cross office and is invited to visit; he is shown the products they have available.

- He chooses one with a handle and that can stand on its end (as well as on its side) so he can easily reach to pick it up from the floor in the toilet. He buys two, so he can keep one in his bedroom for night-time use.

- In Table 4.1.3 he sees that a longer fly opening would ease the use of the urinal. He takes a pair of trousers to the local sewing shop that does tailoring repairs, and he finds the altered opening such an improvement that he takes two other pairs there soon afterwards.

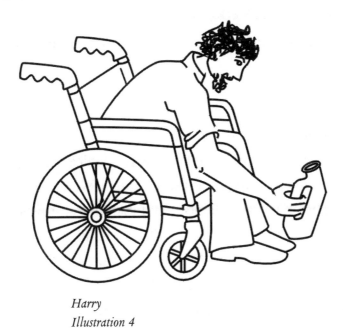

Harry
Illustration 4

Work through
Stages 1–3 in the process
outlined in Chapter 1.3

Do you know when you
need to go to the toilet? — Yes → Is getting on and off
the pan difficult? — Yes → See subsection
4.1.1 *Getting on and
off the toilet* for
information about toilet
seats and rails; and/or
4.1.5 Urinals   **1**

No ↓   No ↓

Go to section 4.2
*Not getting to the
toilet to pass urine*
or 4.3 *Problems
with bowel
continence*

Is sitting safely on the
toilet a problem? — Yes → See subsection
4.1.2 *Sitting safely* for
information about
supportive seats   **2**

No ↓

Is managing clothing
difficult? — Yes → See subsection
4.1.3 *Managing
clothing*
for information
about easy clothing   **3**

No ↓

Is cleaning yourself after
using the toilet difficult? — Yes → See subsection
4.1.4 *After using the
toilet* for information
about bidets and
wiping devices   **4**

No ↓

Do you get to the toilet
in time? — Yes → No further
decisions   **5**

No or not always ↓

See subsection 4.1.5
Urinals, 4.1.6 *Commodes*,
or section 4.2 *Not getting
to the toilet to pass urine*

Harry's route through Figure 4

4.1 Difficulties once at the toilet

From Figure 4 you will have selected the appropriate parts of this section to work through.

4.1.1 Getting on and off the toilet

One of the key reasons people want an assistive device around the toilet is to feel safer and reduce the effort required (Sonn *et al.* 1996).

The main types of assistive device (AD) included in this subsection are rails, rail surrounds (no raised seat), raised toilet seats, lifting toilet seats, and toilet frames (combined seat and rails). Some rail surrounds and toilet frames can be fixed to the floor. Urinals (subsection 4.1.5) and commodes (subsection 4.1.6) may also be useful because these may be used as one way of reducing the number of times it is necessary to struggle to the toilet.

Published literature shows clearly that a good proportion of people over 75 years either need or already use some AD to help them with getting on and off the toilet (George *et al.* 1988; Sonn 1996).

Some people will only need to use products for a short time, for example after an operation such as a hip replacement. Others will be likely to use ADs on a long-term basis, for instance those with rheumatoid arthritis (Clemson and Martin 1996; Meghani 1991).

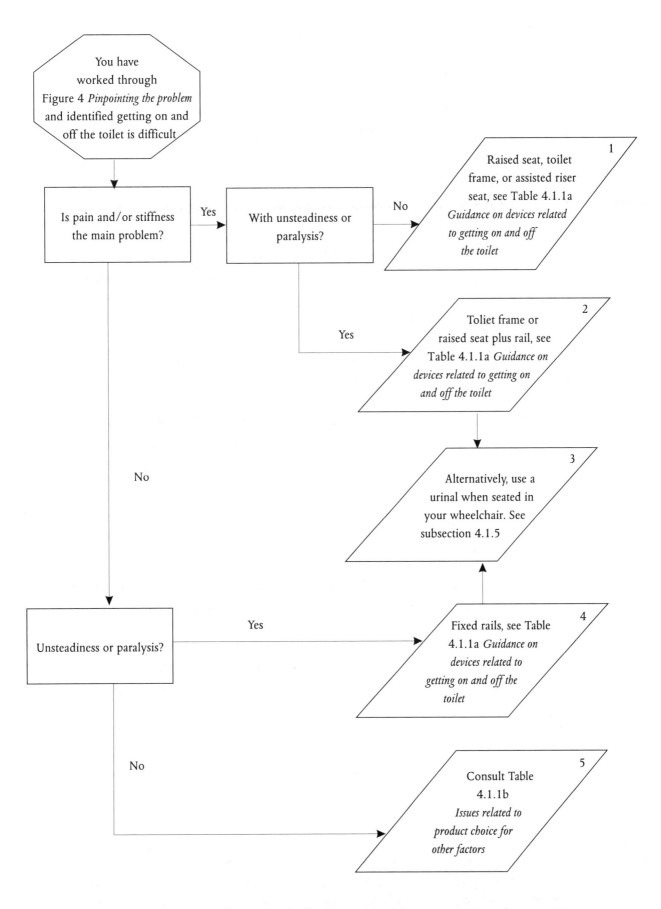

Figure 4.1.1 Getting on and off the toilet. The flowchart is derived from Page, Cooper and Feeney 1981.

An example

John, aged 59, had a stroke and was admitted to hospital. He was soon able to walk again, but his balance was uncertain and his left arm remained weak. He was discharged, with a leaflet about the local Disabled Living Centre (DLC) in case he wanted to ask about devices that might help. He considered he would cope OK, and didn't want gadgets that drew attention to his stroke. He nearly fell in the toilet the other day, and that scared him and his wife, so he now wants to find something that will help him feel safe again. Working through Figure 4, he knows when he needs to go (top left box) but does have difficulty getting on and off the pan.

- Using Figure 4.1.1, he works down it to slanted box 3, noting that fixed rails are recommended.

- In Table 4.1.1a he notes the height at which the rail should go. In Table 4.1.1b John sees the note about others in the household, so he discusses his preference with his wife, and she agrees that a rail is unlikely to inconvenience her.

- He finds the leaflet about the DLC, so goes to get some advice there.

- He is advised to try a raised seat, but decides, together with the staff of the DLC, that he will be fine without, once he has a rail fixed.

- His son gets a hand rail locally and when he comes to fix it, John gets him to hold it where he thinks it should go, and John tests how it is for height, both when standing and seated on the toilet.

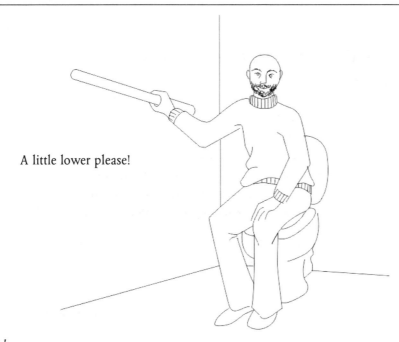

John
Illustration 4.1.1a

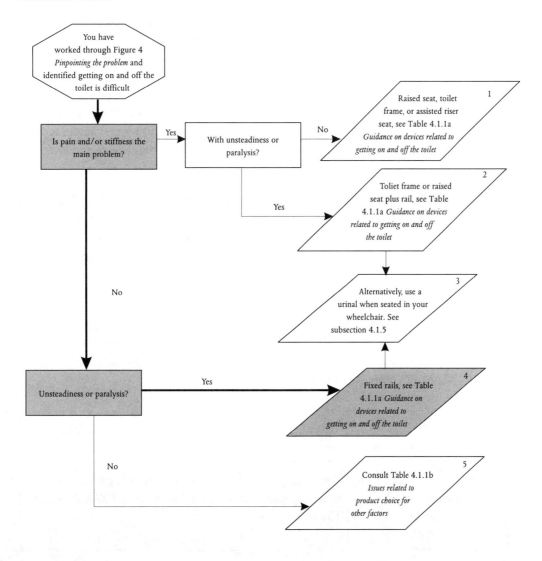

John's route through Figure 4.1.1

Table 4.1.1a Guidance on devices related to getting on and off the toilet

Product type	Factor	Guideline	★
Raised seats, toilet frames, assisted riser seats	Ease of getting on/off	Additional height may be needed when using toilet. Choose lowest satisfactory seat height so that feet can be placed (flat preferably) on the floor .	★
	Comfort	Toilet style seat or avoid sharp edges that might cut into buttocks (MDA 1994; Page *et al* 1981). The seat height affects comfort (see above).	★★
	Hygiene – self	Cut-away contour at front eases access to clean between the legs after using the toilet. No published evidence for cut-away fronts was found, but most raised seats now have them, presumably because of customer demand.	
		Horseshoe seats (seat has a gap at the front) not advised if legs are liable to spasm (MDA 1994).	★★
	Safety	Seat should be adjusted to fit snugly, and all members of household must know how to take it off and refit it correctly. Incorrect fitting leads to instability or damage to the product. The fact that correct fitting remains an issue is supported by several studies (Gitlin, Levine and Geiger 1993; Mann and Tomita 1998).	★★
	Need something to hold on to (with both hands)	Toilet frame, with raised seat incorporated if needed, *only* if pressure will be applied evenly on both rails. Some frames can be bolted to the floor, which would be advisable if there are concerns about unsteadiness or you may not remember to apply even pressure to both rails (Page *et al*. 1981).	★★
	Difficulty in rising even if seat is raised and cannot use hands to help	Assisted riser seat. These are a major expense, so would only be considered when seat and fixed rails are not sufficient. There are both floor-standing and pan-fixed models.	★
	Mild unsteadiness	Toilet frame; seat with handles attached (Gitlin *et al.* 1993).	★★
Seat and fixed rails	Only one hand to hold on to something with	Fixed rail (see below) in conjunction with raised seat if necessary (see above), (Chamberlain *et al*. 1978; Page *et al*. 1981).	★★

	Appreciable unsteadiness or paralysis	Raising the whole pan on a plinth is preferable to a raised seat, as the fixings of a raised seat will break after a time because of the sideways or backwards force on the seat during transfers.	*
	Wheelchair is used	Height of pan plus seat should be equal to the wheelchair seat height when you are on it, using your usual cushion (Clemson and Martin 1996; Page *et al.* 1981).	**
Fixed rails	You walk into the toilet	If there is a suitable wall next to pan place rail horizontally at half the user's standing height. Oblique rail was favoured (Clemson and Martin 1996; Sanford, Arch and Megrew 1995). If there is no suitable wall near toilet, consider a toilet rail surround fixed to the floor; drop-down rail; or rails attached to pan (usually via seat bolt fixing).	**
	Wheelchair is used	Rails should be between 175 and 290 mm higher than wheelchair seat (Page *et al.* 1981; compare Department of Environment 1999) Bilateral drop-down rails were preferred (Sanford *et al.* 1995).	**
		If you pull on rail during sideways transfer, a wall-fixed rail or floor-to-ceiling pole will withstand the forces.	**
		If you transfer onto toilet from one side but only need to *push down* on a rail to do so, consider a wall-fixed drop-down rail, or swing-away rails fixed to toilet seat bolt fixing (Sanford *et al.* 1995).	*
	Ease of movement if you have a rail both sides	Allow 140–200 mm wider than hip width or shoulder width (whichever is larger) (Pheasant undated).	**
	Getting a good grip	Varnish provides a good grip. On other finishes, a very slightly roughened surface is better than very smooth (Pheasant undated).	*
		A good diameter for ease of grip should allow index finger to curl roughly to thumb's top (distal) joint: ergonomic data for handle diameters when using a power grip indicate 40–55 mm diameter is best (Pheasant undated).	***
	Visibility	Contrasting colour advisable, especially for those with sight impairment (Cooper and Stewart 1997).	**

Before rails are secured, try them for position and height both standing and seated.

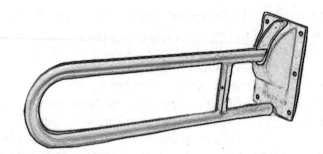

Drop-down rail

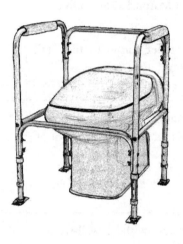

Toilet frame

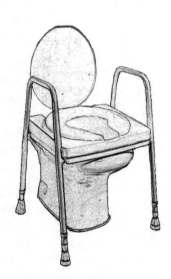

Toilet frame with seat

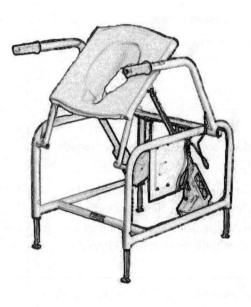

Assisted riser toilet seat

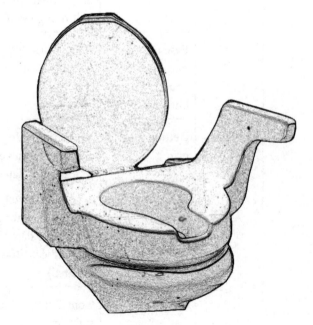

Toilet seat with handles

Illustration 4.1.1b

Table 4.1.1b Issues related to product choice

Factor	Issue	Guideline	★
Others in household not requiring the AD	Children would not be able comfortably to use raised toilet seat or permanently raised pan	Choose raised seat that is easily removed and replaced. If permanently raised pan necessary, provide movable platform in front for children to step onto.	* *
Children (users)	Reduce pan aperture	Products available in high street stores.	
	Support required when seated	See subsection 4.1.2 below.	*
Restricted growth	Pan too high	Platform in front, to step onto (Jepson 1998).	*
	Support required when seated	Rails, see Table 4.1.1a above.	
	Managing clothing	See subsection 4.1.3 below.	
Several users	Cleaning self after using toilet	See subsection 4.1.4 below.	
	Assess height for rails from anthropometric tables (50th percentile)	e.g. for women 65–80 years, fix rail at 785 mm (Pheasant undated). Notes Younger disabled adults may not conform to population norms, especially if disability was congenital (Hobson and Molenbroek 1990).	**** ***
	Removable raised seats and frames not advisable, because uneven pressure is likely to be applied by some users	Permanently raised pedestal preferable. If users will be transferring from wheelchair, the height of 510 mm from the top of the seat to the ground is suggested.	*

4.1.2 Sitting safely

The best position to ease bowel movements is to sit upright or lean slightly forwards, with the bottom well back on the seat, the feet flat on the floor and (for those with a tendency to extend at the hips) a seat-to-footrest height that places the knees a little higher than the hips (PromoCon 2001). The last would not be appropriate if you had recently had a hip replacement. If you need support to achieve this posture in chairs, you will need support for the toilet too. Correct support will enable you to relax, which assists the passing of urine or faeces.

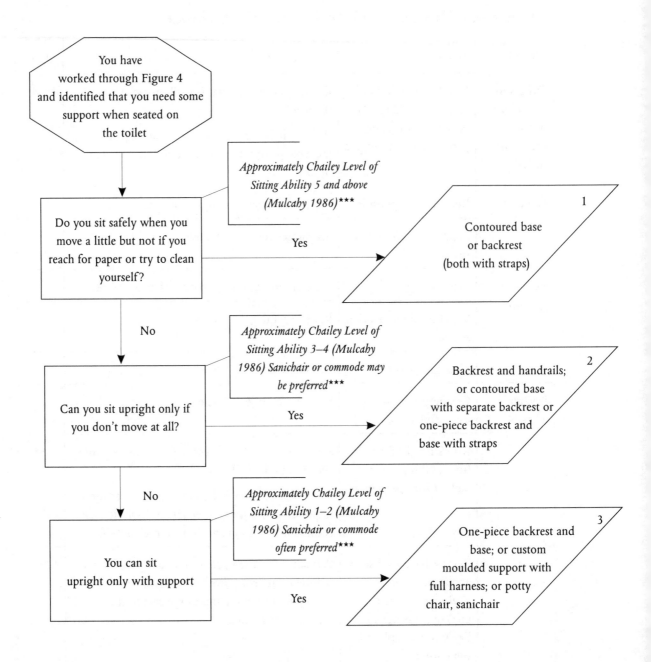

*Figure 4.1.2 Sitting safely. The flowchart is derived from Greenfield and Milne 1985.***

Notes

The decision about the type of product to look for is based on the preferred products for groups of children with similar sitting ability shown in Figure 4.1.2 (Greenfield and Milne 1985).

The scale of Sitting Ability was developed with children who have cerebral palsy (Mulcahy 1986). It is therefore only reliable for that population, but the definitions are used as a basis for the flowchart.

An example

Mary is ten years old and has cerebral palsy and attends a special school. She is trying to get out of nappies, but does not feel safe sitting on a standard toilet.

- Using Figure 4.1.2, Mary knows she does not feel safe unless she stays absolutely still, which is difficult for her anyway. So slanted box 2 indicates a combination of seat, rail and/or backrest.

- Looking at Table 4.1.2, she and her parents decide their preferred option is Octopus rails to give Mary something to hold in front, and a backrest with harness straps, so her parents do not have to take the AD on and off every time Mary wants to use the toilet. A stable seat base is their second option.

- Mary and her parents discuss the possibilities with the occupational therapist (OT) at Mary's school. The school has rails that have handles in front (see Illustration 4.1.2a) on one of their toilets, so the OT invites a representative to come and demonstrate a backrest, using that toilet. Mary finds that, provided she uses the harness strap, she feels safe and comfortable.

- However, the OT also gets her to try a contoured seat base with the rails. She feels there is little difference, so chooses the family's preferred option.

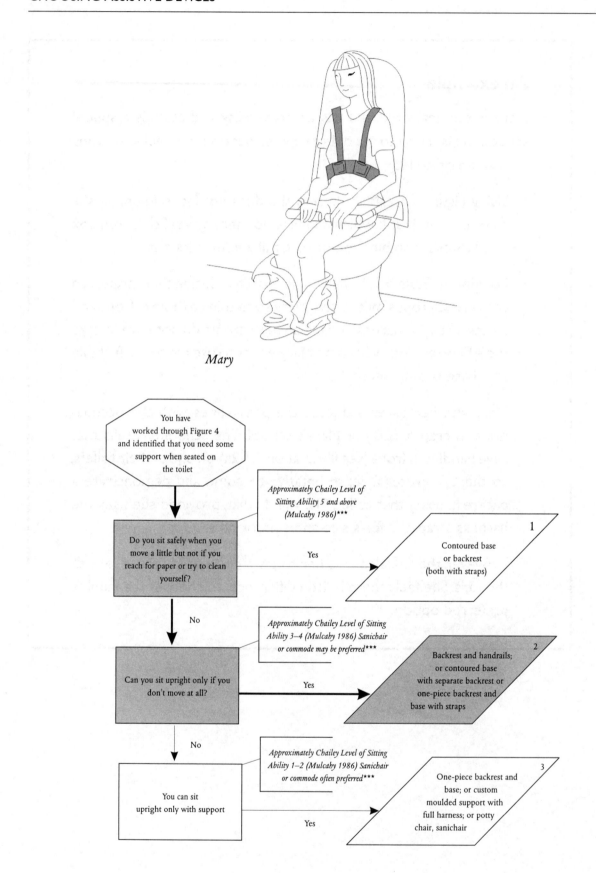

Mary

Mary's route through Figure 4.1.2

Illustration 4.1.2a

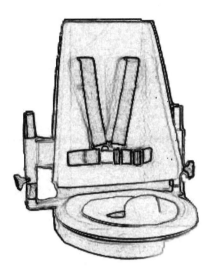

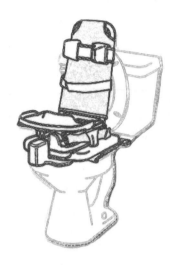

Contoured seat with separate backrest

One-piece support

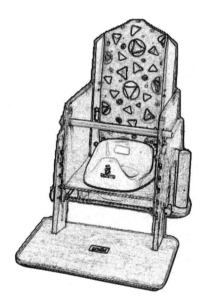

Potty chair

Illustration 4.1.2b

Table 4.1.2 Guidance related to sitting safely on the toilet

Issue	Product type	Guideline	★
You require support Numbers indicate an increasing amount of support	1. Rails each side	Width between 140 and 200 mm wider than hip width or shoulder width (whichever is larger) (Pheasant undated).	★★
	2. Rail that pulls down to give some support at front	Fitted in pairs to toilet seat bolt fixing. Require space at each side to swing them up when getting on or off the toilet; or full frame round toilet, with a movable front rail.	★
	3. Backrest	Usually with contoured edges to keep the trunk upright. Chest or full harness straps. May be used in conjunction with rails and/or seat. May not need to be removed for other toilet users. Some seats may have adjustable lower back support for added stability.	★
	4. Contoured seat base	Usually attached to toilet seat bracket. Lap strap gives added security. May be used in conjunction with rails and/or backrest. Would need to be fitted/removed every time if others wished to use the toilet. Pommel or splashguard at front may hinder independence in getting on and off (Bardsley and Fairgrieve 1981).	★★
	5. One-piece support	Would have to be removed for other toilet users. Storage may be an issue because of its bulkiness. Optional footrests on some products may assist better posture and encourage relaxation, but impede transfers (Greenfield and Milne 1985). Optional headrests are less common.	★
	6. Custom moulded support	This kind of AD would typically double as a commode or shower seat, so would be a sanichair (see Chapter 5).	★

Risk of pressure sores	With padded seat	A cover fitted to standard seat suitable where no shearing (backward or sideways pressure) is involved during transfer on/off. When shearing may occur, choose a padded seat that replaces the standard seat. Seat types 4–6 above reduce the risk of pressure sores because they distribute the weight over a larger surface area than a standard seat does.	*
Alternative approaches	Use sanichair (see Chapter 5, subsection 5.3.5) over toilet. Use commode or potty chair (see Table 4.1.6 below)	A sanichair may double as a shower chair or commode, so reducing number of products required. Sanichairs that offer good postural support are available. Most sanichairs have a commode/potty accessory kit (e.g. Burdon and Craighead 2000).	*

ASSISTIVE DEVICES FOR TOILET VERSUS SANICHAIR

An alternative to putting extra support on or around the toilet is to have a mobile sanichair that you can get on to first, then have someone push you over the toilet. Here are some guidelines to help you judge which might be better for you.

- If you can walk, with or without support, or you are a wheelchair user who can transfer without assistance: try rails and/or an assistive device attached to the toilet.

- If you are a wheelchair user, and also use a shower chair when showering: a sanichair can be used for both functions.

- If you require hoisting: a sanichair may be easier, no matter what arrangement you have for bathing or showering.

4.1.3 Managing clothing

No formal evaluation has been published to indicate how well various approaches to managing clothing work in practice, except for one evaluation of clothes fastenings (Davey 1988). AWEAR (see Reference list) can offer information and advice. Table 4.1.3 provides some suggestions.

Table 4.1.3 Managing clothing

Your difficulty		Guideline	★
Using the toilet	Poor grip	Avoid tight clothing and small buttons; zips can have a tape loop or metal ring attached to their zipper; slightly damp hands give more purchase when pulling tights up.	*
	Only one functional hand	Avoid tight clothing, buttons and zips; trouser fly opening can be fastened with dots of Velcro which press onto a strip, see Illustration 4.1.3 (easier to prise apart than continuous Velcro, Davey 1988).	* **
	Getting trousers and/or pants up and down	Whole gusset area converted into a flap ('drop front') or French knickers (crotch opening). Require good arm movements to reach from front to back, and sufficient dexterity in both hands to pass the flap between legs to refasten.	*
	Handling a skirt	Skirts can be tucked into elasticated waistband to keep the material out of the way (useful if you have only one functional hand); or If you use a wheelchair, a wrapover skirt can be undone and left on the wheelchair.	*
Using a urinal seated	Getting clothing out of the way	Whole gusset area converted into a flap. French knickers (crotch opening). Lengthen trouser fly opening towards crotch. Split gusset with edges overlapped. This would work if you can sit on the edge of your seat (see section 4.1.5).	*
Catheterising yourself	Getting clothing out of the way	Whole gusset area converted into a flap. French knickers (crotch opening). Lengthen trouser fly opening towards crotch.	*
Leg bags	Emptying a leg bag	A zip up the trouser leg makes reaching the bag easier.	*
	Keeping a leg bag comfortably in place	A leg bag sleeve (similar to a stocking) was rated better than holster-type holders (MDA 1995a). An internal pouch in trousers or skirt, or purchase trousers with a side leg pocket and alter this so it opens on the inside too.	*** *

Data from AWEAR, RICAbility (2001) unless cited otherwise

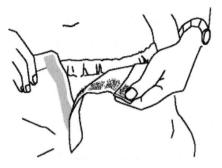

Trouser fly opening with tabs of Velcro one side and a strip on the other

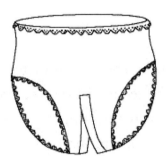

Pants with split gusset

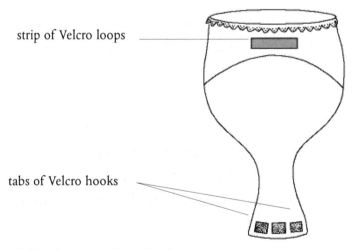

strip of Velcro loops

tabs of Velcro hooks

Pants with drop-down gusset fastened with Velcro
Illustration 4.1.3

4.1.4 After using the toilet

Reaching to clean yourself between the legs is a process which requires good sitting balance, an ability to shift position on the toilet seat, and good control of wrist and hands when at full reach. Poor skill in cleaning yourself would risk both skin problems and odour. Moist disposable wipes may be easier to use than standard toilet paper. Always wipe from front to back to minimise the risk of a urine infection.

Assistive devices (ADs) tackle the problem in one of two ways: ADs can be used to make the wiping easier, by reducing the need to reach and reducing the grip necessary; or a bidet system can be installed.

DEVICES TO EASE CLEANING ONESELF

There are several 'bottom wipers' available. Some are designed for use from the front, some from the back, some for either.

A portable bidet fits between toilet pan and seat. It can be emptied into the pan, but must be filled by hand.

BIDET SYSTEMS

Water regulations have to be checked prior to installation of these systems. A separate water tank may be required for some products.

Plumbed in bidet-toilets are costly, but have the greatest potential for enabling complete independence if your arm and hand function is very limited (Beresford 1999).

Add-on bidet systems have the advantage of not entailing replacement of the existing toilet, but because of the way they are fitted, may have limitations, e.g. sideways transfers may put more strain on the fixing than is advisable.

FLUSHING THE TOILET

Weak or painful grip: Larger levers, either attached to existing lever or replacement.
Poor hand function: Pad on cistern that can be elbow operated.
Remote control: Foot-operated floor-fixed pad: may need special arrangement with water authority (Kelsall and Cochrane 1996). Touch- or movement-sensitive button.

4.1.5 Urinals

The use of a urinal frees you from having to reach a toilet every time you want to relieve yourself. They can therefore be very useful, whether it is to save getting to an upstairs toilet, for convenience when out, or to avoid having to get up at night.

The types may be divided into male urinals (bottles) and female urinals. A few urinals are marketed as 'unisex', but in this subsection are included with the female ones. Bed pans are products designed for bowel movements as well as urine, but brief comments about them are included in Table 4.1.5.

Table 4.1.5 Guidance on choosing a urinal

Product type	Issue	Guideline	★
Male urinals	Ease of holding	If the neck does not provide sufficient grip, select a product with a handle.	★
	Spillage during use	Non-spill products; or non-return adaptors can be purchased to adapt a standard urinal.	★
	Spillage after use	Products with lids are common, but require good function in both hands to use effectively.	★
	Disposable products	Hospital use: require macerating.	★
		Travel use: PVC bag with wire strip round opening and non-return valve (Kelsall and Cochrane 1996).	★
Female urinals	To be used standing or sitting on edge of chair (or sitting back if seat has a cut-away)	A convex curvature to fit around the body reduces splashes and misses; a handle and/or a tube for drainage will make it easier to hold as urine is passed.	★
		Dishes, bottles and cups with drainage tubes could be suitable.	★★
	To be used seated back in chair	A product with a longer neck is recommended. If spillage likely to occur as urinal withdrawn, choose one with a non-return adaptor (McIntosh 1998).	★
	To be used lying down or semi-reclined	Dishes or body-supporting. Often not very successful.	★★
		A handle will make it easier to withdraw. Alternatively, try bed pans.	★
	Disposable products	A shaped cup with bag that has gel crystals in it (gels on contact with urine) (McIntosh 1998).	
Body-supporting female urinals (similar to bed pans but shallower)	Manual handling	Roll the person onto the bedpan if they cannot lift themselves up (Kelsall and Cochrane 1996).	★
	User preference	People prefer to use a commode if at all possible (Kelsall and Cochrane 1996).	★
	Shape	The triangular shape is stable and suitable for use in chair or bed, sitting up, lying or prone (McIntosh 1998).	★
	Lid	Some bed pans have lids; advisable if they have to be carried any distance.	★

Data derived from Fader *et al.* 1999, MDA 1999a unless cited otherwise.

Female urinals may be described as body-supporting, dishes, bottles and cups with drainage tubes (McIntosh 2001). They are used lying, sitting or standing, and with the exception of some dishes, many are designed for use in only one or two postures. McIntosh (2001) lists positions in which specific products can be used, but Table 4.1.5 indicates which type of urinal might meet your requirements in a more general way, because product availability changes over time.

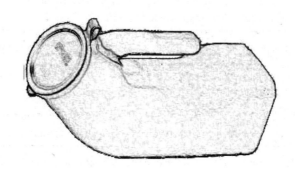

Male urinal with lid

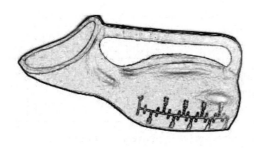

Female urinal with shaped opening

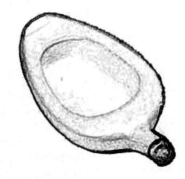

Dish urinal

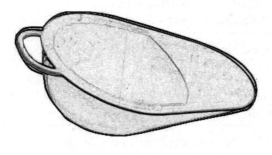

Slipper bed pan

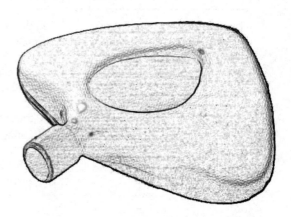

Triangular shaped body-supporting urinal

Illustration 4.1.5

Urinals on the whole are more successful if you can sit on the edge of a chair or stand (MDA 1999b), but if you need to sit back in your chair or lie down, choose from the urinals specifically designed for these positions.

The likelihood of finding a urinal that is suitable is greater if you are fairly independent, compared with if you need personal assistance. This particularly applies to female urinals (Fader *et al.* 1999) because of the greater dexterity needed to position them correctly.

The capacity of a urinal does not indicate the volume of urine that it takes practically. More than half full would be heavy, difficult to keep steady, and raise the risk of spillage. Half capacity is a guide, unless there is a drainage tube and bag attached, when the bag could be nearly filled without repercussions. You therefore need to choose a size according to the volume you typically pass, and if you use one at night and during the day, you may need two, one with a larger capacity (McIntosh 1998).

A trial before deciding on which will suit you best is very important: you need to feel confident when using it. A lending service may be available through the Continence Advisory Service (Vickerman 2001). Although the Continence Advisory Service may not need to be involved with the choice of urinal, they may well be advising on other aspects of continence management, so the responsibility of choosing which urinal would be best can be shared with them.

MULTIPLE USERS

Urinals for use by several people, for example in hospitals or residential homes, should be autoclaved or put in a bedpan washer between users. Not all products can be put through these processes, as it depends on the materials used in their manufacture, so cleaning instructions should be checked prior to purchase.

4.1.6 Commodes

This subsection is bigger than the others for several reasons. First, commodes will usually be chosen without professional advice from the Red Cross, a community loan store or the Continence Advisory Service. Second, there are a number of design types and each has its own advantages and disadvantages. Finally, the issues around residential and community use must be clarified.

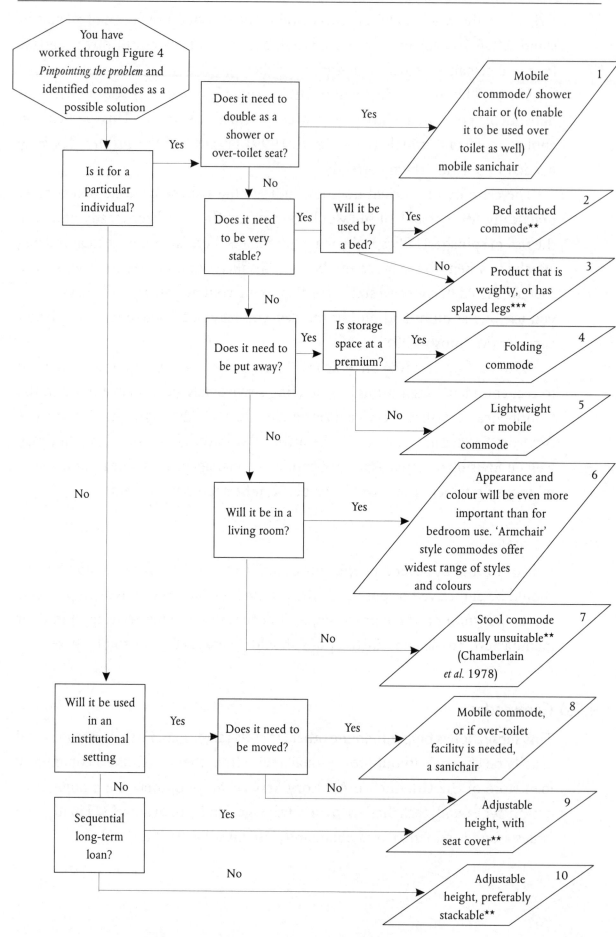

Figure 4.1.6a What type of commode?
Evidence classification derived from MDA 1994, MDD 1993 except box 7.

Notes

Numbers relate to the slanted boxes in Figure 4.1.6a on the facing page.

1. Using a commode for another function as well saves the space and cost of having a second piece of equipment.

2. For people who transfer sideways from bed to commode, a bed-attached commode is the most stable type of equipment, but you have to have good sitting balance because there is only one armrest (MDA 1994).

3. Six out of 18 metal framed commodes failed the BS4875 Part 2 rearwards stability test (MDD 1993). This highlights the need to consider stability when the commode may be used to lean on when unoccupied. Splayed legs increase stability, but also increase the risk of someone tripping over them, or impeding a wheelchair. They do not increase stability if a lateral pull is exerted.

6. Users preferred a commode that looked like an ordinary upright chair, and whose pan was hidden from view (Ballinger *et al.* 1995); colour to fit in with decor was also important (MDA 1994).

8. If a commode/sanichair conforms to BS4751 (BSI 1984) it will fit over a standard-height toilet pan (430 mm (17in.)) provided pan and rack are removed. It will also be maximum width 700 mm (27in.) and at least 2 castors will have brakes. Sanichairs for children often offer good postural support (e.g. Burdon and Craighead 2000).

9. Adjustable-height commodes will enable a range of successive users to gain maximum advantage. Covers are considered an asset with respect to hygiene and appearance (MDA 1994).

An example

Jackie is an elderly lady who likes her home spotless and feels co-ordinated furnishings are important. She lives alone but her son is very supportive. Her neighbour is a good friend and pops in most days to check she's all right. Despite sleeping in a room near the bathroom, Jackie finds she cannot get to the toilet quickly enough at night, owing to general weakness which causes difficulty in getting out of bed. She is shaky on her feet, and uses a walking frame.

*   With her son and the friend she works through Figure 4 and decides to get a commode, and the friend agrees to empty the pan each morning for her.

- Figure 4.1.6a is worked through with the following results: the commode is for a particular individual; it does not need to double as a shower seat; it does need to be stable, because she would pull on it as she manoeuvres off the bed. It therefore is best to look for a bed-attached commode. From Figure 4.1.6b, the seat height, seat depth and seat width are determined for her, but she knows that for a bed-attached commode the seat height has to equal the bed's.

- From Table 4.1.6 Jackie feels that her general weakness, particularly her difficulty getting out of bed, may mean that she also has difficulty rising from a bed-attached commode. This proves to be the case and she is not aware that the bed could be raised using bed blocks (see Chapter 6, Illustration 6.1.5). Figure 4.1.6a is therefore retraced and the next best choice made, namely a commode that is weighty or has splayed legs. The measurement for seat height derived from Figure 4.1.6b is amended to a higher one: an additional 50 mm (2in.) seems sufficient after she has tried different heights to get the right compromise between ease of rising and comfort when sitting.

- The issue relevant from 'pan emptier' section of Table 4.1.6 is that the commode will not be emptied until the neighbour comes in. As the pan will be emptied daily, they decide a large capacity or chemical toilet should not be needed, but choose a commode with a pan lid.

- Jackie's friend accompanies her to the local specialist shop to look at some commodes. Jackie tries sitting on the toilet seat of two or three, checking she can take the seat cover on and off easily.

- Her friend tries putting the pan in and out.

- Jackie chooses the commode that meets their requirements, and orders the colour that fits in with her bedroom.

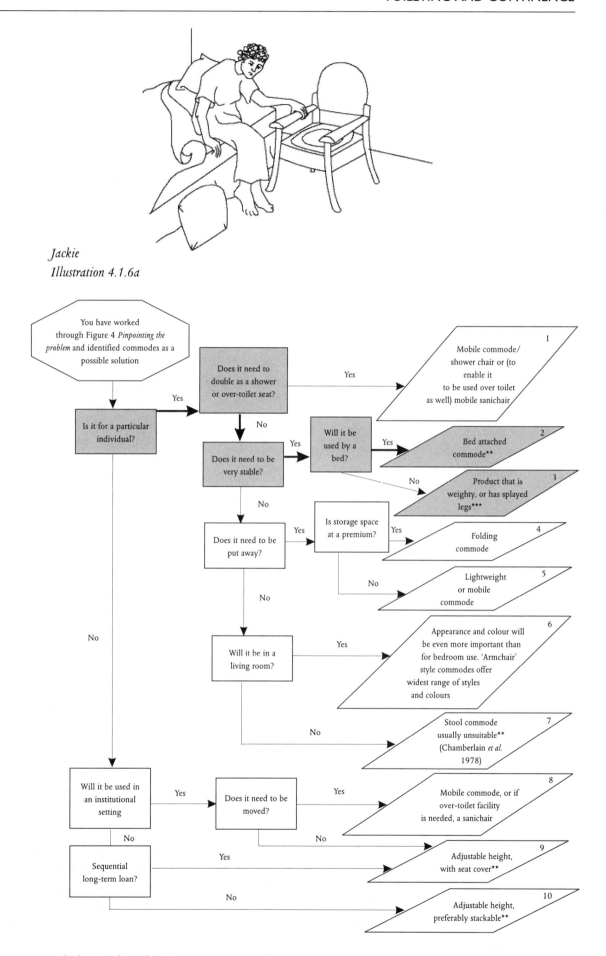

Jackie
Illustration 4.1.6a

You have worked through Figure 4 *Pinpointing the problem* and identified commodes as a possible solution

Is it for a particular individual?

Does it need to double as a shower or over-toilet seat?

Yes → 1
Mobile commode/ shower chair or (to enable it to be used over toilet as well) mobile sanichair

No

Does it need to be very stable?

Will it be used by a bed?

Yes → 2
Bed attached commode**

No → 3
Product that is weighty, or has splayed legs***

Does it need to be put away?

Yes → Is storage space at a premium?

Yes → 4
Folding commode

No → 5
Lightweight or mobile commode

No

Will it be in a living room?

Yes → 6
Appearance and colour will be even more important than for bedroom use. 'Armchair' style commodes offer widest range of styles and colours

No → 7
Stool commode usually unsuitable** (Chamberlain *et al.* 1978)

Will it be used in an institutional setting

Yes → Does it need to be moved?

Yes → 8
Mobile commode, or if over-toilet facility is needed, a sanichair

No → 9
Adjustable height, with seat cover**

No

Sequential long-term loan?

Yes → 9
Adjustable height, with seat cover**

No → 10
Adjustable height, preferably stackable**

Jackie's route through Figure 4.1.6a

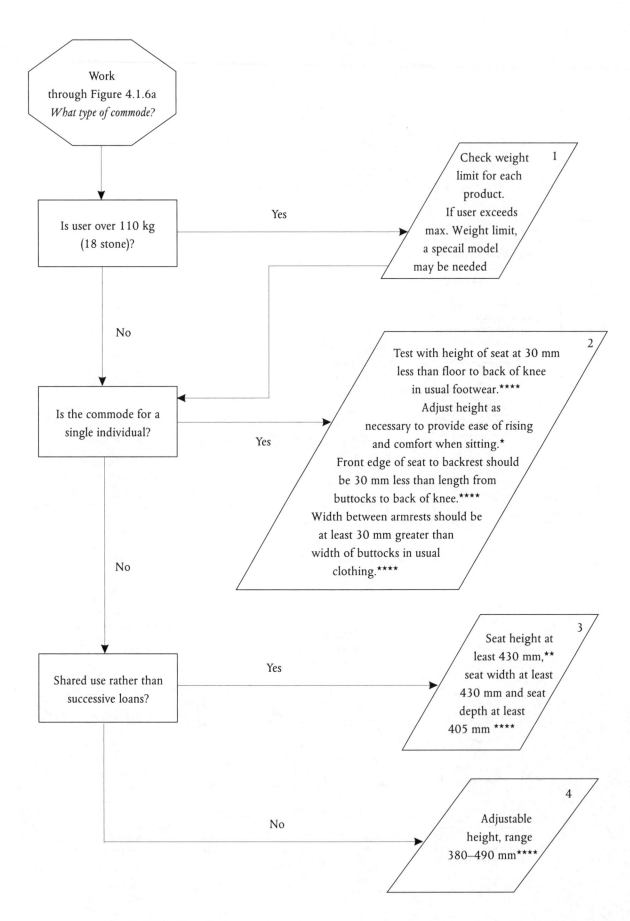

Figure 4.1.6b What dimensions?

Notes

Numbers relate to the slanted boxes in Figure 4.1.6b on the facing page.

1. If difficulty is experienced in rising from the seat height recommended, increase it, bearing in mind that a compromise between ease of rising and comfort of legs whilst seated must be made. If the user is assisted in rising by a care assistant, a minimum height of 480 mm (19in.) is suggested (MDA 1994).

2. Weight limits vary from product to product.

3. The seat height is more than anthropometric tables would suggest, but the majority of commode users were found to prefer this height (or greater) because of arthritis or general leg weakness (MDD 1993; MDA 1994).

    Seat width of 430mm (17in.) is the 95th percentile for 65–80-year-old women and seat depth of 405 mm (16in.) is the 5th percentile for elderly women (Pheasant undated). These dimensions are chosen to accommodate 90–95 per cent of the anticipated user population.

4. These measurements enable optimal adjustment for nearly 90 per cent of the population (Pheasant undated).

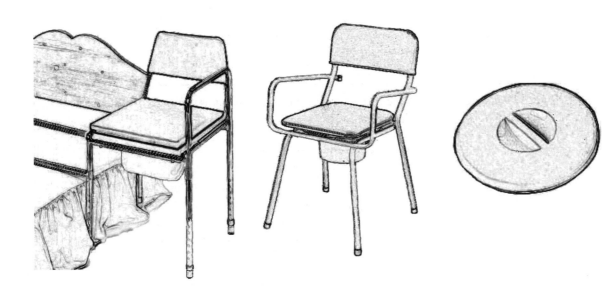

Bed-attached commode   Stackable commode   Recessed bar handle or pan lid

Illustration 4.1.6b

Table 4.1.6 Guidance on issues related to commode features

Factor		Issue	Guideline	★
User: any age	General weakness	Difficulty in rising	Higher seat than that recommended in Figure 4.1.6b *What dimensions?* (Finlay *et al.* 1983).	★
		Difficulty in removing commode seat cover	Lightweight cover that is easy to grasp.	★★
	Poor grip	Removal of lid	Knob may be easier to grasp than recessed bar (see Illustration 4.1.6b).	★★
	Liable to extensor spasm	Legs getting caught in opening	Horseshoe seat (see Illustration 5.3.4 in Chapter 5) *not* advised.	★★
		Risk of commode tipping backwards	Select mobile commode with footrests, *or* stable commode.	★★
			Footrests keep the ankle bent which lessens the risk of extensor spasm, and also means that the commode is not tipped if some downwards pressure is applied on the footrests by the user (MDA 1998a).	★★
	Unsteadiness	Use commode to steady oneself when standing	Select stable commode (see Figure 4.1.6a).	
	Poor function in hands	Need help with cleaning perineum	Commode pan that is removable whilst user is seated.	★★
	Comfort	Thinness	Comfort is an issue, especially in some residential homes where the user may be on the commode for some time. Choose commode seat with contours similar to standard toilet seat or padded seat.	★★
			Padded backrest.	★★
		Narrow pelvis	Some apertures do not fit the bony prominences comfortably.	★★
User: child	Able to walk	Enable child to get on and off independently	Low potty chair (Greenfield and Milne 1985).	★★
	Needs to be lifted or hoisted	Ease for the care assistant	High seat height (min. 435 mm) or adjustable in height.	★★

Pan emptier	General weakness	Emptying pan	Small pan (half capacity 1.7 litre) unless volume passed exceeds this.	**
	Unsteadiness	Emptying pan	Pan that removes upwards, rather than on runners.	**
			Pan with lid to reduce risk of spillage when carrying. This is preferred even without unsteadiness.	**
	Not always available	Commode not always emptied between uses: odour	Pan with lid to reduce odour, especially if used for faeces (Naylor and Mulley 1993).	*
			Pan with large capacity.	*
			Consider a chemical toilet, especially if used for faeces (Naylor and Mulley 1993).	*
Commode features	Dual purpose	Choose a product that is described as a sanichair	Ensure it fits over toilet once pan and rack removed; conformance to BS 4751 (BSI 1984) should ensure this.	*
	Manoeuvrability	Space to turn	Overall length rather than wheelbase length affects turning circle.	*
		Ease of moving	Thresholds and loose mats are difficult to negotiate because mobile commodes do not have *tip* bars.	*
	Brakes	Ease of applying	Test with care assistant's usual footwear.	*
Commode features	Brakes	Number	For greatest stability when the user is transferring, all four castors should be braked, but in practice, some carers found this too time consuming, and preferred two only.	**
			These comments derive from six mobile commodes being put through a laboratory circuit which simulated a range of environmental factors (unpublished).	
	Removable armrests	Ease of removal	Often difficult for user (MDD 1993): test before choosing.	**
	Pans	Compatibility with pan washers; or (for disposables) macerators	Check prior to purchase.	*
		For people with learning disabilities	Pans that lift upwards or backwards are the most tamperproof designs (Greenfield and Milne 1985).	**

Data drawn from MDA 1994, MDD 1993 unless otherwise stated.

4.2 Not getting to the toilet to pass urine

Introduction

This section provides a brief description of the types of urinary incontinence (see section 4.3 for bowel incontinence) and their treatment and management.

It is quite common for there to be a problem with leaking some urine before you want to: up to 5 per cent of the population may have continence problems (Vickerman and Whitehead 2001). It is even more common amongst those over 65 years (1 in 10 for women, 1 in 14 for men, Department of Health 2000) and higher still amongst those in nursing homes (2 in 3, Department of Health 2000).

Incontinence problems of people in residential homes are high because they are more likely to have physical conditions that cause them, but the environment may contribute as well, for instance by making the toilets less available in practice (Riley and Tobin 1986). Toilets being further than 10 metres from sitting and dining rooms, lack of clearly visible signs, and lack of timely help are all cited by these authors. Sadly, 15 years later, these obstacles are still to be found in some residential homes.

In the community, these principles of availability can also be applied, even though the context will be rather different. Thus a confused person may benefit from clear labelling of the toilet (ADS 1997), and if you use a walking aid a cluttered room may make getting to a toilet seem like a walk of more than 10 metres. A chair that is difficult to get up from, doorways that are difficult to negotiate, or internal steps, may act as barriers to successfully reaching the toilet without mishap.

These things must all be considered at Stage 3 in the process described in Chapter 1, section 1.3, either before or in conjunction with choice of assistive devices (ADs). In some instances, an AD will itself be the way of increasing the availability, e.g. a commode by the bed reduces the distance that must be travelled, or a rail by the toilet reduces anxiety and effort required to use the toilet effectively.

Your diet, fluid intake pattern and how much you move around can all affect continence. It is important not to cut down too much on your fluid intake. Drinking less than 1.5 litres a day may make matters worse. A good fluid intake makes the urine more dilute, which may increase the bladder's tolerance to storing it, and decrease the risk of getting an infection. Some food and drinks, though, do encourage the body to make more urine, so these could be avoided. Examples are coffee, Coca-Cola and alcohol (Engberg *et al.* 1998; Incontact 1999; Multiple Sclerosis Council 1999). If night time is the main worry, avoiding a late night drink of any sort may help, combined with having one's legs up during the afternoon. If you have diabetes, maintaining good glucose control will help (Engberg *et al.* 1998). Long periods of inactivity can make you more liable to have problems.

A bladder or bowel problem can have a great impact on your quality of life, and some people stop going out or lose their self-confidence because of it (Asbury and White 2001). This can be overcome by getting treatment, learning how to manage the leaks, and tackling any negative feelings you may have. Asbury and White (2001) address the latter in a humorous and practical way.

You may find it possible to manage minor problems by attention to your diet and by using the helplines and information services (see Chapter 1, subsection 1.4.1). It is wise to seek advice if the problem persists. You can contact your local Continence Advisory Service direct, or ask your family doctor or another health professional. The key fact is that there are a number of treatment approaches, all of which have good reported rates of improvement for those for whom they are appropriate. The National Institute for Clinical Excellence (NICE) is currently auditing continence treatments and should report in 2002.

Continence Advisory Services (CAS) in the UK are free. You would be checked for any medical reasons for the continence problem, and products and treatment suggested after assessment (Department of Health 2000). Products that the CAS can provide may be limited because special contracts are usually negotiated for their purchase in bulk.

SEXUAL ACTIVITY

You may be anxious about having sexual intercourse when there is a bladder problem. SPOD's (2001) information leaflet advises emptying your bladder immediately before, and putting an absorbent sheet under you so you do not need to worry about any leakage.

TYPES OF INCONTINENCE

- Problems only at night time.

- Stress incontinence. This occurs when the muscles that hold the urine in the bladder are weak, and it is particularly common in women, for example following childbirth. Men may also experience stress incontinence, for instance after a prostate operation. Leaking will occur when coughing, sneezing, laughing or other activity that raises the pressure within the abdomen.

- Urge incontinence. This may occur if you have difficulty in getting to the toilet in time because you do not have much warning that you need to go (urgency). It is common for people who have urgency to want to pass urine frequently, sometimes every half-hour. Urgency may be the result of damage to the nervous system, e.g. multiple sclerosis or stroke, but may occur with no apparent cause.

- Continence problems are often a mixture of stress, urgency and frequency.

- Overflow incontinence. This is caused by the bladder being unable to empty properly. This may be due to an obstruction to the flow of urine, such as an enlarged prostate in men, or because the bladder muscle is unable to contract properly because of nerve damage.

- When the nerves that control the bladder are not working properly, your bladder may either empty without you knowing (reflex bladder), or not fill at all (spastic bladder).

Fuller descriptions can be found elsewhere (e.g. Asbury and White 2001; RICAbility 2001).

Figure 4.2 is designed to guide you to appropriate subsections to look at regarding products, but as these are only part of the picture of managing continence problems, an indication of the range of possible treatments is given on the facing page

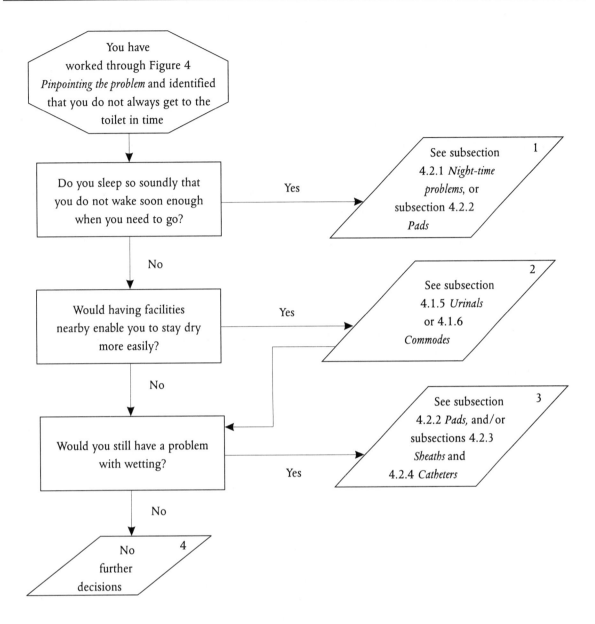

Figure 4.2 What type of product?

TREATMENTS THAT MAY BE RECOMMENDED

Because there are many types of incontinence, and each has a number of possible causes, it is sensible to have a full assessment of your difficulties by the Continence Advisory Service. Quite often the problem is tackled in several ways, and so advice from more than one person from the team of health professionals will be offered.

EVIDENCE FOR THE EFFECTIVENESS OF WAYS OF MANAGING CONTINENCE PROBLEMS

A high proportion of people who have treatment for their continence problems find that they improve or are resolved completely.

Pelvic floor muscle exercises, sometimes with biofeedback or electrical stimulation, and the use of vaginal cones for women, are all effective (e.g. Elser *et al.* 1999; Holtedahl, Verelst and Schiefloe 1998; Laycock *et al.* 2001) and there is no evidence that one (or any particular combination) is better.

Behavioural approaches and bladder training are effective (Anders 1999; Burgio *et al.* 1998) but those younger than 80 years are more likely to benefit (Weinberger, Goodman and Carnes 1999).

Vaginal and urethral devices can be helpful for some people; studies have only been on single devices.

For information on pads, sheaths and catheter, see subsections 4.2.2, 4.2.3 and 4.2.4 respectively.

Table 4.2 Some treatments for continence problems

Incontinence type	Treatment approach	Comments
Stress	Pelvic floor muscle exercises	A physiotherapist will teach you how to do these effectively and give you an individualised programme aimed at strengthening the muscles sufficiently to reduce or stop the unwanted leaks.
	Biofeedback	A way of showing on a screen how well you are contracting the right muscles, and it is useful because people may find it difficult to do the exercises correctly.
	Electrical stimulation	Helps the muscles to contract.
	Pads	Used in conjunction with treatments. Reduction in the need for pads provides an indication of improvement. See subsection 4.2.2.
	Vaginal devices	Help to reposition and put pressure on the urethra; help the pelvic floor muscles to contract more effectively; may feel uncomfortable, especially at first.
	Female urethral devices	To block the flow of urine. Can be uncomfortable and increase risk of infection.
Urge with frequency	Behavioural approach; bladder retraining	A combination of things to help you reduce the need to go, including practical and psychological elements. 'Treatment of choice' for women, but they must be highly motivated (Anders 1999). The first step is a diary to record when you go and when accidents occur.
	Biofeedback; pelvic floor muscle exercises	May be used alone or as part of the behavioural approach.

Urge with frequency (continued)	Medication	Helps to reduce the 'urge' to pass urine.
	Urinals	See subsection 4.1.5.
	Pads	See subsection 4.2.2.
Overflow	Catheter	Indwelling or intermittent as appropriate.
Nerve control of bladder impaired	Penile sheath	Used with leg bag or a valve. See subsection 4.2.3. For men, a sheath could be used as an alternative to pads.
	Intermittent catheterisation	More difficult for women; requires good dexterity.
	Indwelling catheter	Used with a leg bag or a valve. See subsection 4.2.4.
	Medication	For example, to reduce spasticity in the muscles.
	Penile clamp	Only if sensation is present and other ways have proved unsuitable.
Reduced awareness of need to go or does not know what to do owing to dementia	Toilet regime, so person is prompted to go at times that coincide with usual habit. Pads would be used in conjunction with or instead of such a regime.	Often difficult to effect in residential settings because responsibility for a person is shared, and staff are busy.
Night-time problems	Urinal Commode by bed Pads	See subsection 4.1.5. See subsection 4.1.6. See subsection 4.2.2.

4.2.1 Night-time problems

For those who have difficulty at night in waking before beginning to pass urine, there is a number of ways of approaching the problem. First, the adjustment of diet and fluid intake, as suggested at the beginning of section 4.2, should be experimented with. If problems persist, your local doctor should be consulted.

Elderly people who have accidents at night may benefit from being woken at night to use a toilet or commode, but it is by no means clear whether this outweighs the sleep disruption (Engberg *et al.* 1998). Pads may be the better option.

An estimated 15 per cent of children aged 5 years, decreasing to 1 per cent of 15-year-olds, have at least one episode per month of incontinence at night (Ryan-Woolley 1987). A proportion of these will benefit from formal intervention.

Enuresis alarms are either body-worn, or a pad in the bed. The jury is out concerning which might be better, but those who have tried body-worn devices tended to achieve dryness more quickly – in 5 weeks compared with 8 weeks (MDA 1998b).

The device features that affect how easily a child can accept using one, and how effective it will be are first, the comfort of the device, and second, the volume of the alarm (MDA 1998b). The volume of the alarm seemed to be a more subjective preference, with some reporting it too soft and others that it made them jump. The family would need to hear it in their home to give their preference, because disturbing other members of the household is also an issue.

4.2.2 Pads

Pads are either body-worn or for use on bed or chair. The major division within those categories is whether they are disposable or reusable.

Pads are available with different levels of absorbency, chosen according to the typical amount lost. If you need pads on a regular basis, it is recommended that you consult your doctor or the Continence Advisory Service.

The absorbent layer in disposables is usually a fluff pulp often with a superabsorber; the latter takes longer to absorb the urine, but then gels, so leakage on applying pressure is less. The combination of these materials gives better performance than either on their own. There are guidelines for testing the absorbency of a product (BSI 1999).

Washable pads usually have a thick felt layer to absorb the urine, enclosed between a fabric layer next to the skin and a waterproof backing. The fabric is either cotton, which is comfortable when dry, or a synthetic fibre that repels water, which is comfortable especially when wet. The pattern of leakage will therefore indicate which fabric might be more suitable for an individual.

Minimising leakage from the pad when wet is the most important goal. Leakage can be minimised by selecting pads that fit snugly to the body contours; by using the most appropriate pad absorbency; and by regular pad changes. Ease of changing pads should always be assessed, and a product type selected to make the process as easy as possible, whether for yourself or a care assistant.

Those with sensitive skin may find some products cause a skin rash, but this is rare except where there is bowel leakage too.

DISPOSABLE PADS

There are different designs: to apply to regular underwear by adhesive strips, to insert into a pouch in specially designed washable pants, to use with mesh pants, or all-in-one diapers.

REUSABLE PANTS WITH INTEGRAL PADS

These tend to be used more for those with light incontinence, and most users want the pad to be as discreet as possible (MDA 2001). A good fit around the crotch reduces risk of leakage.

DISPOSABLE BED PADS

These are best used in conjunction with a body-worn pad as they are not very effective on their own.

REUSABLE BED PADS

No studies have indicated that any specific features of bed pads are favoured for particular requirements. Choice of features such as flaps to tuck under the mattress, and whether the waterproof layer is integral or separate, is a matter of personal preference (Cottenden in press).

Table 4.2.2 Guidance on pad choice

Incontinence	Issue	Guidelines	★
Light Pads of approx. 170–700 ml absorbency	Cost	Reusable more cost effective, but not acceptable to some. Some people continue to use sanitary pads when they actually need greater absorbency (Mann and Tomita 1998).	★★★
	Appearance	Minimal bulk is wanted to reduce visibility. This must be balanced against the absorbency performance required.	★★★
Moderate Pads of approx. 700–1300 ml absorbency	Pad type	Disposable more commonly used than reusable; pads with adhesive tapes or pads for use with mesh pants.	★★★ ★
	Absorbency	Choose products with superabsorber. Some users felt their pads were insufficiently absorbent (Mann and Tomita 1998), demonstrating the need for careful selection.	★★★
	Comfort	Shaped pads are more comfortable than rectangular ones.	★★
	Noise	Products which rustle may be disliked (Mann and Tomita 1998).	★★★
Heavy Pads or pants with 1300+ ml absorbency	Pad type	Disposable more commonly used than reusable; either pad with mesh pants or all-in-one (diaper style).	★★
	Cost	Prices vary widely and are not a reliable indication of performance (MDA 1998c).	★★★
	Leakage	If leakage still occurs after careful selection of appropriate pad (for absorbency and fit), a pad on chair or bed may be needed.	★★★
	Skin irritation	Skin may show sign of irritation after exposure to urine over many days, i.e. wet most of the time. But most products' top layer keeps the skin relatively dry, so skin problems are unlikely unless both bowel fluid and urine are present.	★★★

THE CHOICE BETWEEN DISPOSABLE OR REUSABLE

In addition to the guidance given in Table 4.2.2, the issue of laundering is a key factor. For those with light incontinence, laundering may not be a problem. If reusable pads are used by more than one person it is essential that they are cleaned according to the guidelines of 71°C for a minimum of 3 minutes (MDA 1996) to ensure harmful micro-organisms are destroyed. More details on cleaning can be found in Chapter 6.

Environmental costs are considered about equal for either type of product (MDA 2001) as costs of laundering reusables balance the materials and waste management costs of the disposables.

Financially, the cost of reusables is lower than that of disposables provided they last at least 100 washes (MDA 2001) but the initial cost is higher.

In practice, use of each type of product for differing situations gives a flexibility that many appreciate.

4.2.3 Sheaths and other body-worn devices

A penile sheath with a tube connecting it to a drainage bag is a commonly adopted option for men whose bladder empties without leaving a residue in it. The sheath is usually made of silicone rubber. Some sheaths are made of latex, which produces an adverse reaction in a small number of people. The sheath may have an integral adhesive strip on it, or a separate strip which has to be applied before the sheath. A formal comparative trial found that one-piece products were preferred (MDA 1995b; MDA 2000). Some products have applicators. A formal comparative trial has shown those without are often preferred (MDA 2001).

A sheath is not suitable for a number of elderly men because the sheath cannot be securely applied to the penis. A common problem with these devices is that they loosen or slip off.

When choosing a penile sheath, it is therefore important to try several to ensure ease of application and secure fitting.

Studies indicate that urinary infection rates are lower with penile sheath use than with indwelling catheters (Warren 1990) but higher than for those who had no need for such devices (Cottenden in press). There is some debate about whether tugging a sheath increases the risk of infection, but kinking of the tube will encourage pooling of urine which will increase the risk of skin problems and infection.

Other-body worn devices have not been evaluated, but female devices tend to leak and no design has been particularly successful.

LEG BAGS

Bags to collect the urine are used with penile sheaths and catheters. They are obtainable in two main sizes, a smaller one for day use and a larger one for night. The latter may be attached to the sheath or catheter tube, or to the open drainage tap of the day bag.

Studies have shown that the ease of operating the valve to empty the bag is a key factor (MDA 1996), so trial of several is recommended to ensure you can operate it easily and without wetting your fingers.

The acceptability of day bags was affected by the comfort of the straps and how discreet the bag was (MDA 1999a). The elastic straps were considered uncomfortable by some of the study's participants; alternative ways of supporting the bag could be tried such as a holster, a pouch in the trousers or skirt, stretch shorts or a leg bag sleeve (see subsection 4.1.3).

A secure fixing is particularly important for those who are able to walk. A bag designed for wheelchair users proved more comfortable for that user group (MDA 1999a).

4.2.4 Catheters

For some people a catheter may be an effective option. Your local Continence Advisory Service will assist you in the choice of the most appropriate product. When nerve damage causes inability to empty the bladder, or incomplete emptying of it, catheters are often used. If the bladder allows the urine to seep out constantly, pads may be a preferred alternative, see subsection 4.2.2 above.

There are two types of catheter use, namely indwelling catheters and intermittent catheterisation. The former have an inflatable balloon that rests in the bladder with a tube that either passes through the urethra (the passage the urine normally takes) or through the abdomen wall above the pubic bone (a suprapubic catheter). Intermittent catheterisation is the term for the insertion of a catheter into the bladder simply to drain the urine; the catheter is removed immediately afterwards.

Indwelling catheters are connected to a leg bag or catheter valve (see below) to allow for emptying. Indwelling catheters may seem preferable to bulky pads for people with long-term incontinence, but risk of urine infection is higher than with other devices (Warren 1990) and it is quite common for catheters to leak or become blocked. Some people need to have a catheter because they have overflow incontinence owing to an obstruction which cannot be removed surgically.

In view of the higher risk of infection and other problems, catheterisation is often used for short-term needs such as when a person has a pressure sore or is terminally ill. Long-term use requires vigilance and good hygiene practice to minimise the risk of complications such as urine infections originating from sources outside the bladder, and mechanical damage to the urethra. More information can be drawn from books such as Norton (1996), RCP (1995) and Roe (1992).

CATHETER VALVES

Instead of uncontrolled drainage into a bag, indwelling catheters can be drained through periodic opening of a valve.

The ability to use catheter valves successfully is dependent on a number of factors. A formal user evaluation (MDA 1997) showed that the following affect acceptability and ease of use:

- mental ability

- ease of turning the valve tap: bigger taps are easier but more visible beneath clothing

- likelihood of getting fingers wet

- ability to see whether valve is open or closed

- whether a night drainage bag (when desired) can be attached.

When valves can be used, they are usually more acceptable than bags (Lewington *et al.* 1989); a small study suggested that combining day use of a valve with night-time drainage was the ideal (German *et al.* 1997).

4.3 Problems with bowel continence

This section briefly describes the types of bowel incontinence, and approaches to the treatment and management of bowel incontinence. The prevalence of faecal or bowel incontinence is less well documented than urinary incontinence: it is estimated at 1 per cent in the community and 1 in 4 (25 per cent) in nursing homes (Department of Health 2000).

Table 4.3 Guidance on ways that bowel incontinence may be managed

Issue	*Guideline*	★
Secondary incontinence due to constipation	Plenty of liquid helps, and additional roughage in the diet, if necessary supplemented with bulking agents. Laxatives. Suppository or enema to clear the bowel (Edwards and Bentley 2001).	★★
Reduced awareness of need to go	Biofeedback, Manual stimulation, electrical stimulation (Glia *et al.* 1998). Anal plug.	★★★
Nerve damage	Enema or manual evacuation.	★
Anal sphincter muscle damaged or misshapen	Anal plug. Surgery may be suggested (Glia *et al.* 1998).	★
Disease of lower bowel	Cause must be treated first.	★

The purpose of this section is to give an overview of how the problem with continence may be tackled by your local Continence Advisory Service or the medical profession, rather than by providing great detail. Professionals will explain the advantages and disadvantages of the preferred approach for your particular case.

The most common reason for bowel incontinence is constipation. The bowel motions become hard and block the bowel. Bowel fluids seep round the blockage, and come out looking like diarrhoea. A nurse or your family doctor needs to confirm the cause of the problem, and the bowel will usually require suppositories or an enema to clear it (Edwards and Bentley 2001). Preventing the situation from recurring is key, and diet and fluid intake are the first steps. Laxatives, suppositories and enemas are progressively more aggressive so would be used as necessary.

Other causes of bowel incontinence may be treated in a number of ways, depending on their cause. Possibilities include diet, habit training, biofeedback, stimulating the lining just inside the bowel manually or electrically, or surgery if the sphincter muscle at the bowel entrance is damaged.

Disposable pads are commonly used (see subsection 4.2.2), and for some people an anal plug may be suggested, although not everyone finds these comfortable (RICAbility 2001).

Key points

This chapter has reviewed evidence concerning assistive devices (ADs) for the toilet, and alternatives to using a toilet.

The first decision is whether you have difficulty getting to or onto the toilet (section 4.1), difficulty controlling your bladder (section 4.2), or difficulty controlling your bowel (section 4.3).

Difficulty getting to or onto the toilet

- Choose assistive devices (ADs) that make you feel safe.

- There is evidence to guide your choice of rails, seats, urinals and commodes, but suggestions for choosing other ADs are based on expert opinion.

Bladder or bowel problems

- Consult your local Continence Advisory Service or family doctor.

- Treatments will be proposed that are tailored to your particular problems.

- There is evidence for the efficacy of many of the treatments.

- There is some evidence to guide choice of pads, penile sheaths, catheter valves and leg bags but you need to try out a few products to find the best one for you.

References

ADS (1997) *Incontinence.* Advice Sheet 3. London: Alzheimer's Disease Society.
Information on causes, ways of dealing with problems and products that might be helpful. *

Anders, K. (1999) 'Bladder retraining.' *Professional Nurse 14*, 5, 334–336.
Reviewed the literature for frequency and urge incontinence and found cure rates between 44 and 90 per cent with bladder retraining. **

Asbury, N. and White, H. (2001) *Don't make me laugh.* North Shields: Northumbria Healthcare NHS Trust.
A self-help book for users to address the psychological and practical problems of incontinence.

AWEAR. Tel: 0115 9530439.
An umbrella organisation that offers information about clothing suitable for people with disabilities or special needs.

Ballinger, C., Pickering, R., Bannister, S., Gore, S. and McLellan D.L. (1995) 'Evaluating equipment for people with disabilities: user and technical perspectives on basic commodes.' *Clinical Rehabilitation 9*, 157–166.
Additional analysis on MDD 1993 data.

Bardsley, G. and Fairgrieve, E. (1981) 'An evaluation of a children's toilet aid developed in Memphis, USA.' *British Journal of Occupational Therapy 44*, 9, 280–282.
A single product evaluation of a contoured toilet seat with hip strap and some lumbar support. It was tested for a week by nine children with 'appropriate' needs, at school and home. The comfort and 'fit' of the child when seated was good for all nine. **

Beresford, S. (1999) 'The Clos-o-mat shower toilet.' *British Journal of Therapy and Rehabilitation 6*, 7, 343–6.
A professional's review of a bidet-toilet. *

BSI (1984) BS 4751 *Mobile sanitary chairs.* Milton Keynes: British Standards Institution.

BSI (1999) BS ISO 15621 *Urine absorbing aids – general guidance on evaluation.* Milton Keynes: British Standards Institution.

Burdon, D. and Craighead, S. (2000) 'Seahorse sanichair for use by children and adolescents.' *British Journal of Therapy and Rehabilitation 7*, 7, 310–313.
An informal evaluation of a single product with an unspecified number of disabled children. *

Burgio, K., Locher, J., Goode, P. *et al.* (1998) 'Behavioral v. drug treatment for urge urinary incontinence in older women.' *Journal of American Medical Association* 16 Dec., 280, 23, 1995–2000.

Randomised controlled trial of people with urge incontinence; 197 randomised to one of three groups: a) pelvic floor muscle exercises, behaviour therapy and biofeedback, b) drug treatment, c) placebo pill. The proportion who felt they were much better were 74 per cent, 51 per cent and 27 per cent for the respective groups.***

Chamberlain, M.A., Thornley, G. and Wright, V. (1978) 'Evaluation of aids and equipment for the bath and toilet.' *Rheumatology and Rehabilitation* 17, 187–194.

Survey by interview of 150 people 6–24 months post discharge, of whom more had neurological than arthritic conditions. Thirty-two had raised toilet seats and 12 had a free-standing toilet frame. Only half of the users of the rails felt confident in using the rails because of their instability. Additionally, 41 were commode users, an undisclosed proportion of whom used stool commodes which 'afforded no support' (p.191).** *[Note that floor fixings for toilet frames were not as common in 1978 as now.]*

Clemson, L. and Martin, R. (1996) 'Usage and effectiveness of rails, bathing and toileting aids.' *Occupational Therapy in Healthcare* 10, 1, 41–59.

Survey follow-up of 144 people at up to two years post-discharge: 56 per cent non-use of raised toilet seats. In contrast, rails by the toilet had only a 17 per cent disuse rate. Oblique rail was favoured by 26 of the 28 people who had rails.**

Cooper, B. and Stewart, D. (1997) 'The effect of a transfer device in the homes of elderly women.' *Physical and Occupational Therapy in Geriatrics* 15, 2, 61–77.

Single product evaluation of a floor-to-ceiling pole which was fitted in 30 women's flats (mean age 77 years). Significant changes in the Canadian Occupational Performance Measure showed the positive impact of having the pole. ** *All chose to keep the pole. A contrast colour provided a visual reminder of the rail (16 chose to keep the contrast).*

Cottenden, A. (in press) 'Pads and appliances.' In P. Abrams, L. Cardozo and A. Wein (eds) *Incontinence. Proceedings of the 2nd International Consultation on Incontinence*. Paris, 1–3 July 2001. UK: Health Publications Ltd. To be published 2002.

Literature review.

Davey (1988) *Assessment of clothes fastenings*. DH Disability Equipment Assessment Programme. Heywood: HMSO.

A selection of fastenings (buttons, zips, button hooks, Velcro and poppers) were tested on a specially designed garment by 48 people, aged 33–78 years, with a range of disabilities. Although no one fastening was easiest for all, the larger items or Velcro were generally easier, and the Velcro dot-on-strip was the easiest Velcro configuration.**

Department of the Environment (1999) Approved document 'Part M: access and facilities for disabled people'. Building Regulations (Amendment) 1998. London: The Stationery Office.

This document applies to buildings 'other than dwellings' excepting level thresholds and access to a toilet on entrance storey for all new dwellings. Recommended grabrails by a toilet for a wheelchair user are a wall fixed horizontal one at 700mm with a matching drop-down one at the accessible side of the pan. With a toilet seat height of 450-475mm this falls within the height recommended by Page et al 1981.

Department of Health (2000) *Good practice in continence services*, Ref. 211133 1p 5k.Mar00. London: Department of Health. Or accessed on www.doh.gov.uk/ continenceservices.htm

Literature review, position statement and targets set.

Edwards, M. and Bentley, A. (2001) 'Nursing management of constipation in housebound older people.' *British Journal of Community Nursing 6, 5,* 245–252.

*Literature review and synthesis of two flow charts, one for acute and one for chronic constipation.** Some but not all of the decisions are supported by evidence. The charts are not designed for those with neurological damage.*

Elser, D., Wyman, J., McClish, D. *et al.* (1999) 'The effect of bladder training, pelvic floor muscle training or combination training on urodynamic parameters in women with urinary incontinence.' *Neurology and Urodynamics 18,* 427–436.

*Randomised trial with 204 people with stress incontinence. They were assigned to bladder training, pelvic floor muscle training or combination training, for 12 weeks. 181 had post-treatment evaluations. No significant difference between the groups' response, but all were 'effective'.****

Engberg, S., Organist, L., Lafayette-Lucey, A., and McDowell, B. (1998) 'Treatment of urinary incontinence among caregiver-dependent adults.' *Urologic Nursing 18, 2,* 131–136, 155.

*Expert opinion and literature review.**

Fader, M., Pettersson, L., Dean, G. *et al.* (1999) 'The selection of female urinals: results of a multicentre evaluation.' *British Journal of Nursing 8, 14,* 918–925.

Thirteen urinals were tested by between 28 and 32 people; an article based on MDA 1999.

Finlay, O., Bayles, T., Rosen, C. and Milling, J. (1983) 'Effects of chair design, age and cognitive status on mobility.' *Age and Ageing 12,* 329–335.

*All except four residents of three homes (n = 92) were included in one of two studies: 1. A survey of 61 residents who were assessed as able or unable to rise from 3 chairs. More could rise from the highest chair (seat height 445mm) p. 0.002. 2. Formal trial with 31 residents which compared ease of rising from 2 chairs. Whole sample showed those who could rise without difficulty were younger (p. 0.05) and those who did not benefit from higher seat tended to have greater cognitive deficit (p. 0.02). ****

George, J., Binns, V., Clayden, A. and Mulley, G. (1988) 'Aids and adaptations for the elderly at home: underprovided, underused and undermaintained.' *British Medical Journal 296,* 1365–1366.

*A random sample of people aged 75 years and over was surveyed; 11% needed at least a rail by the toilet.***

German, K., Rowley, P., Stone, D. *et al.* (1997) 'A randomised cross-over study comparing the use of a catheter valve and a leg bag in urethrally catheterised male patients.' *British Journal of Urology 79,* 96–98.

*Randomised trial with 18 males who tried a drainage bag and a valve, for 3 weeks each. Seventy-two per cent preferred the valve as it was more comfortable during the day.*** However, at night more episodes of frequency and urge incontinence were found with the valves, so the authors advised a night-time drainage bag.**

Gitlin, L., Levine, R. and Geiger, C. (1993) 'Adaptive device use by older adults with mixed disabilities.' *Archives of Physical Medicine and Rehabilitation 74,* 149–152.

*Survey of 8 AD users after discharge from hospital. A second survey of 31 therapists about their perceptions of AD use and reasons for non-use was undertaken. Reported that therapists deemed lack of knowledge in correct use was a major cause of discontinued use of ADs.***

Glia, A., Gylin, M., Åkerlund, J. *et al.* (1998) 'Biofeedback training in patients with fecal incontinence.' *Diseases of the Colon and Rectum 41,* 359–364.

Reviewed the literature and reported improvement rates between 50 and 92 per cent of patients for conservative therapies. Biofeedback was the 'preferred' conservative therapy for those with faecal incontinence, but actually only 18 of the study's 26 subjects showed improvement with this approach. Highlighted anal asymmetry as one* *factor that indicated conservative treatment may not be successful, and surgery might be suggested instead.*

Greenfield, E. and Milne, J. (1985) *Summary report of an assessment of toilet aids for handicapped children.* DHSS Aids Assessment Programme. Lancashire: HMSO.

*Formal comparative trial with 40 children who tested up to 10 toilet assistive devices (ADs) for 10 weeks each, mainly in school or hospital environment but a few at home. Products were tested between 7 and 36 times, depending on the number of participants for whom the given product was suitable. Trainer seats were only useful with children with minimal disabilities.** Other recommendations used in Figure 4.1.2.*

Hobson, D. and Molenbroek, J. (1990) 'Anthropometry and design for the disabled: experiences with seating design for the cerebral palsy population.' *Applied Ergonomics 21,* 1, 43–54.

*Anthropometric measurements of 25 adults with cerebral palsy.****

Holtedahl, K., Verelst, M., Schiefloe, A. (1998) 'A population based, randomised controlled trial of conservative treatment for urinary continence in women.' *Acta Obstetrica Gynecologica Scandinavia 77,* 671–677.

*Ninety women were randomly allocated to a treatment group or control. On follow-up at six months, treatment group mean severity score for symptoms dropped from 3.9 to 1.9 (max. 8) compared with no change for controls.*****

INCONTACT (1999) *Bladder and Bowel Problems.* London: Incontact.

Leaflet written for the public about causes, medical investigations and treatments available.

Jepson, J. (1998) 'Study into the equipment needs of people with restricted growth.' *British Journal of Occupational Therapy 61,* 1, 22–26.

*A postal survey to people with restricted growth (31 respondents) asked about ADs and suggestions for new devices. Eight suggested a folding lightweight step (which could be used by a toilet, and would also be appropriate for children.)***

Kelsall, A. and Cochrane, G. (eds) (1996) 7th edition. *Personal care.* Oxford: Disability Information Trust.

Disabled people and professionals informally evaluate assistive devices, but no description of their needs, numbers or method of evaluating ADs is given. The book contains helpful 'Points to consider' at the beginning of each section.*

Laycock, J., Brown, J., Cusack, C. *et al.* (2001) 'Pelvic floor re-education for stress incontinence: comparing three methods.' *British Journal of Community Nursing 6,* 5, 230–237.

*Multinational trial of 101 women aged 20–64 years. Randomised at ratio of 2:2:1 to exercises with vaginal cone, with biofeedback device, exercises alone. After three months, n=68 reassessed. No significant difference between the groups, but all groups showed significant improvement in quality of life, reduction in wet episodes, increase in muscle contractility.*****

Lewington, C., Morgan, M., Noone, P. and Kairsary, A. (1989) 'The value of catheter valve use in long-term bladder drainage.' *British Association of Urological Surgeons* (BAUS), *Conference Proceedings.*

*One hundred elderly people were randomly assigned to either catheter valve or drainage bag, and the valves were highly acceptable to users.****

McIntosh, J. (1998) 'Realising the potential of urinals for women.' *Journal of Community Nursing 12,* 8, 14–17.

*Expert opinion. Female urinals are classified and guidance concerning choice and correct use given.**

McIntosh, J. (2001) 'A guide to female urinals.' *NT Plus, Nursing Times 97,* 6, VII–X.

A guide to female urinals, for which positions they were designed, and guidelines for selection. *

Mann, W. and Tomita, M. (1998) 'Perspectives on assistive devices among elderly persons with disabilities.' *Technology and Disability 9*, 119–148.

Interviewed 508 current users of assistive devices as part of a ten-year longitudinal study. They do not state how many of the sample used raised toilet seats, but a comment is recorded that a splatter guard is necessary. Rather than a front cut-away, one respondent suggested a cut-away at the side. Several requested more comfortable seat design. **

218 people had continence problems. Three of these people were using sanitary pads knowing they were not absorbent enough; a further ten with undefined level of continence complained of pads insufficiently absorbent. Five comments related to poor fit; three found the pads too 'flimsy', one citing turning in bed caused it to tear; one disliked the rustling sound of the material. **

MDA (1994) *Mobile, armchair, folding and bed-attached commodes: a comparative evaluation*, DEA A9. Medical Devices Agency. Norwich: HMSO.

Formal comparative user trial in which 55 people were allocated to test one of four groups of commodes. Fifteen users tested mobile commodes and some of them and their carers commented favourably on the dual use of mobile commodes either as a shower chair or as a sanichair. Two commodes with a split seat caused discomfort when a leg in spasm caught in it. ** *With regard to comfort, comments from the participants showed that it was usually the sharpness of the inside edge that caused discomfort.* ** *Pans smaller than 1.7 litre half capacity were considered too small by some users.*

MDA (1995a) *Suspension systems for urine leg bags: a comparative evaluation* DEA A11. London: Medical Devices Agency.

Formal comparative user trial in which three holster-style and one mesh leg sleeve were tested by 52 leg bag users, 22 of whom were ambulant. The mesh sleeve was higher on overall performance (p. 0.001) and better than at least one of the others for comfort, ease of emptying and being discreet under clothing.

MDA (1995b) *Penile sheaths: a comparative evaluation* DEA A15. London: Medical Devices Agency.

Formal comparative user trial in which 36 men tested 2 one-piece and 2 two-piece sheaths. No statistically significant difference was cited between the product types but on overall performance, one-piece sheaths were preferred whichever type had been used prior to the study. Two-piece sheaths were 'unpopular'. **

MDA (1996) *Sterile 500ml leg bags for urine drainage: an evaluation* DEA A20. London: Medical Devices Agency.

Formal comparative user trial of 14 leg bags by 83 people who tested 7 bags each for one week. Results indicated the main concerns related to tap, straps and leakage. **

MDA (1997) *Catheter valves: a multi-centre comparative evaluation*, DEA A22. London: Medical Devices Agency.

Formal comparative user trial with 46 people who tested either 4 or 7 catheter valves for one week per product, in the community. A further 30 (mostly catheter users) conducted ergonomic assessment of the 7 valves. Substantial differences were found between valves and it was concluded that, to be successful, a valve needs to be easy to use, leak-free, comfortable, and inconspicuous beneath clothing. **

MDA (1998a) *Seating for young children with disabilities: a comparative evaluation*, DEA A23. London: Medical Devices Agency.

Formal comparative user trial with 40 children under 5 years who tested up to 4 seats each. Further details in Chapter 3.

MDA (1998b) *Enuresis alarms: an evaluation*, DEA A24. London: Medical Devices Agency.

Formal comparative user trial with 129 children who tried 1 of 4 alarms, i.e. each alarm was tested by 29–34 children. For each device, about one-third were reporting discomfort with the device, regardless of whether it was body-worn or pad.

There were many more false alarms with the pad than the body-worn devices (65 per cent compared with 14–39 per cent), possibly due to sweating triggering the alarm.** The literature review cited a study that compared body-worn and pad alarms: 20 children in each group. There was no significant difference in effectiveness, but those in the body-worn device group tended to achieve dryness more quickly – in five weeks compared with eight weeks.

MDA (1998c) *Disposable, shaped body-worn pads with pants for heavy incontinence: an evaluation*, IN1. London: Medical Devices Agency.

Formal comparative user trial with 228 users who tested 4–8 products from the 20 ranges on the market at the time of the study. The results showed that individual products' performance varied considerably, and higher cost did not necessarily indicate better performance.**

MDA (1999a) *Non-sterile 500–700 ml leg bags for urine drainage: an evaluation*, IN2. London: Medical Devices Agency.

Formal comparative user trial of 5 leg bags by 29–31 men. One was less liked than the other four. The one designed for wheelchair users was found more comfortable for this group of users.**

MDA (1999b) *Reusable female urinals: an evaluation*, IN3. London: Medical Devices Agency.

Formal comparative user trial of 13 urinals. Between 28 and 32 people tested each product.

MDA (1999c) *All-in-one disposable bodyworn pads for heavy incontinence: an evaluation*, IN4. London: Medical Devices Agency.

Formal comparative user trial with 192 users, who tested 6–8 of the 36 pads then on the market. (All 36 products were evaluated.) Results showed that individual products' performance varied considerably, and higher cost did not necessarily indicate better performance.**

MDA (2000) *Self-adhesive sheaths for men using sheath systems: an evaluation*, IN6. London: Medical Devices Agency.

Formal comparative user trial with 58 men, who tested 6 one-piece sheaths, some with applicators. Those with applicators were significantly less acceptable than those without (p. 0.0001).

MDA (2001) *Reusable review: a guide to washable absorbent incontinence pads*, IN8. Medical Devices Agency's website: www.medical-devices.gov.uk. Accessed on 9/11/01.
A review of the literature.

MDD (1993) *Basic commodes: a comparative evaluation*, DEA A5. Medical Devices Directorate. Norwich: HMSO.

Formal comparative user trial of 18 commodes which were divided into 3 groups; 40 users tested one group of 6 commodes. Eighty-three per cent (range 50–100%) of those testing adjustable-height commodes reported ease in rising when adjusted according to the guidelines (Pheasant undated).** Of those subjects who tested the 8 commodes with removable armrests, 52 per cent found difficulty in removing, 64 per cent in replacing, them when seated on the commode.**

Meghani, Z. (1991) Study of selfcare and mobility aids and appliances by the elderly. M.Sc. Gerontology, Kings College, University of London.
Surveyed 29 people 4–8 months post-discharge and found 33 of 36 toilet devices in use.**

Mulcahy, C. (1986) 'An approach to the assessment of sitting ability for the prescription of seating.' *British Journal of Occupational Therapy* 49, 367–368.
A sitting ability scale developed for use with children with cerebral palsy.**

Multiple Sclerosis Council (1999) *Urinary dysfunction and multiple sclerosis.* Washington: Paralyzed Veterans of America.

Flow charts for treatment decisions based on published evidence plus an expert panel.** to **** Intermittent catheterisation is the preferred management for difficulty in voiding urine if medical and behavioural interventions have failed.

Naylor, J., and Mulley, G. (1993) 'Commodes: inconvenient conveniences.' *British Medical Journal 307*, 1258–1260.

Survey of 150 randomly selected current users of commodes: 115 were interviewed, with 105 of their carers. Emptying commodes was particularly disliked by carers,** so a chemical toilet was recommended for those who use a commode for defaecation. Seventeen per cent of commodes were too low to rise from comfortably. Appearance was important (77 were kept in living room).

Norton, C. (1996) 2nd edition. *Nursing for continence.* Beaconsfield: Beaconsfield Publishers.

Page, M., Cooper, S. and Feeney, R. (1981) *The selection of toilet aids for disabled people.* Loughborough: Institute of Consumer Ergonomics.

Interviewed 500 users of ADs, of whom 20 per cent had toilet devices. Recommended basing choice of toilet device on pain and stiffness versus unsteadiness.*** Only recommended free-standing frames when there are no problems with balance or co-ordination. Recommended a convex rather than a concave seat. [However, ergonomically designed, slightly contoured seats that are rounded on the inside edge are comfortable. In 1981 such shapes were not yet thought of!]

Pheasant, S. (undated; c.1997) 2nd edition *Bodyspace.* London: Taylor & Francis.

Recommendations for seat height, depth and width based on data from a large sample representative of the general population.*** to ****

PromoCon (2001) Children's continence products. Manchester: PromoCon.

An information leaflet for users about products.*

RCP (1995) *Incontinence: causes, management and provision of services.* London: Royal College of Physicians.

RICAbility (2001) Choosing products for bladder and bowel control. London: RICAbility.

A user guide to the causes, treatment and products available for continence.*

Riley, M. and Tobin, G. (1986) 'The ten metre hurdle.' *Community Care 4 Sept.* 18–19.

One hundred and seventy-four residents in 30 homes were interviewed.

Roe, B. (ed) (1992) *Clinical nursing practice: the promotion and management of continence.* New York: Prentice Hall.

Contributions by different clinical experts. Includes a chapter on assistive devices (Cottenden; pp.129–156).

Ryan-Woolley, B. (1987) *Aids for the management of incontinence: a critical review.* London: Kings Fund Centre.

Reviews the literature. Good results with those willing and able to self-catheterise to drain the urine from the bladder were reported.

Sanford, J., Arch, M. and Megrew, M. (1995) 'An evaluation of grab bars to meet the needs of elderly people.' *Assistive Technology 7*, 36–47.

Formal comparative user trial of four configurations of rails around a toilet, by 116 people who were over 60 years old, independent in transfers, predominantly male; 66 ambulant, 50 wheelchair users. Bilateral drop-down rails were favoured most highly (62%), especially by wheelchair users. Oblique rail almost equally utilised by both groups, but ambulant users voted this as best.***

Sonn, U. (1996) 'Longitudinal studies of dependence in daily life activities among elderly persons.' *Scandinavian Journal of Rehabilitation Medicine Supplement 34*, 1–35.

*A longitudinal study of 659 elders reported an increase in difficulty with toileting from 0 per cent at 70 years to 3.6 per cent at 76 years.****

Sonn, U., Davegårdh, H., Lindskog, A-C. and Steen, B. (1996) 'The use and effectiveness of assistive devices in an elderly urban population.' *Aging Clinical and Experimental Research 8*, 3, 176–183.

*Survey of 150 who were visited by an occupational therapist as part of a larger population study of people over 70 years old (see reference above). The most frequent reason for needing ADs was to feel safer.***

SPOD (2001) Resource and Information leaflet No.14 *Incontinence and sex.* London: The Association to aid the Sexual and Personal Relationships of People with a Disability.

Vickerman, J. (2001) 'Developing a specialist continence occupational therapy service.' *Occupational Therapy News 6*, 11, 31.

Vickerman, J. and Whitehead, J. (2001) 'Continence management: an occupational therapist and physiotherapist perspective.' *Nurse 2 Nurse 1*, 11, 34–37.

An overview of the incidence of incontinence, the multi-disciplinary team required to provide a service to people with continence problems and the role of the occupational and physiotherapist. Quotes Thomas 1980 who stated that up to 5 per cent of the population may have continence problems.

Warren, J. (1990) 'Urine collection devices for use in adults with urinary incontinence.' *Journal of the American Geriatrics Society 38*, 364–367.

*Reviewed the literature and concluded that, 'external urine collection devices appear to be the most attractive' because they incurred the lowest incidence of urinary infections. Rates of new bacteria per 100 days of use were: indwelling devices 8; intermittent catheterisation 3; external collection device (male) 3; external collection device (female) 1.****

Weinberger, M., Goodman, B. and Carnes, M. (1999) 'Long-term efficacy of nonsurgical urinary incontinence treatment in elderly women.' *Journal of Gerontology 54A*, 3, M117–M121.

*Survey to follow up 81 elderly women 13–29 months after completion of non-surgical treatment. Of the 53 who responded, 43 per cent reported their incontinence was now mild or absent.****

Bibliography

BSI (1985) BS 4875 *Strength and stability of furniture, Part 1 Strength, Part 2 Stability.* Milton Keynes: British Standards Institution.

This standard wwas used to test commodes technically for strength and stability, see MDA 1994 and MDD 1993.

Forsythe, W. and Butler, R. (1989) 'Fifty years of enuresis alarms.' *Archives of Disease in Childhood 64*, 870–885.

*Literature review: authors' opinion was that body-worn alarms were preferred by children to pad alarms.**

Korpela, R., Seppänen, R-L. and Koivikko, M. (1992) 'Technical aids for daily activities: a regional survey of 204 disabled children.' *Developmental Medicine and Child Neurology 34*, 985–998.

Survey of 752 children with neurological disorders in a region in Finland; 209 used assistive devices (ADs). Forty-eight had toileting ADs but 11 did not use them: 5 had faults, 2 were too small. ** An additional 38 children were assessed as needing ADs but did not have them.

MDA (2000a) *Hydrophilic coated catheters for intermittent self-catheterisation: an evaluation,* IN5. London: Medical Devices Agency.

Formal comparative user trial with 61 men, who tested 4 hydrophilic coated catheters and the results showed that the performance varied considerably, with 2 performing better than the others.*** The literature review cited 4 studies that have shown inflammation and strictures to be less frequent with hydrophilic coated catheters.

A SELECTION OF SINGLE PRODUCT EVALUATION OF CONTINENCE DEVICES

Bellin, P., Smith, J., Poll, W. *et al.* (1998) 'Results of a multi-center trial of the CapSure (ReStor) continence shield on women with stress urinary incontinence.' *Urology 51,* 5, 697–706.

Single product evaluation with 100 women who tested a single product for up to 12 weeks (84 for the full period); 91 per cent had reduction in number of accidents.

Eckford, S., Jackson, S., Lewis, P. and Abrams, P. (1996) 'The continence control pad – a new external urethral occlusion device in the management of stress incontinence.' *British Journal of Urology 77,* 538–540.

Single product evaluation with 19 subjects who used a single device for two weeks. Reduction in leakage (p. 0.002) and the number of leaks (p. 0.001).

Gallo, M., Hancoch, R. and Davila, G.(1997) 'Clinical experience with a balloon-tipped urethral insert for stress urinary incontinence.' *Journal of Wound, Ostomy and Continence Nurses 24,* 1, 51–57.

Clinical experience with a single device; expert opinion.

Hahn, I. and Milsom, I. (1996) 'Treatment of female stress incontinence with a new anatomically shaped vaginal device (Conveen continence guard).' *British Journal of Urology 77,* 711–715.

Single product evaluation in which 90 of 115 women completed a four-week trial of a single device. Leakage significantly less (p. 0.001); 46 per cent had no leakage; 62 per cent had some vaginal discomfort, however 60 per cent wished to continue with the device.

Thyssen, H. and Lose, G. (1996) 'New disposable vaginal device (continence guard) in the treatment of female stress incontinence.' *Acta Obstetrica & Gynecologica Scandinavia 75,* 170–173.

Single product evaluation. Of 26 women who tested a single device, 4 discontinued, 9 were subjectively cured, 12 did not notice the device after a few days.

Versi, E., Griffiths, D. and Harvey, M-A. (1998) 'A new external urethral occlusive device for female urinary incontinence.' *Obstetrics and Gynaecology 92,* 2, 286–291.

Single product evaluation in which 96 of 155 women completed the trial. Symptoms improved (p.001) at the expense of increased irritation (p. 0.001); 39 per cent wanted to continue with the product but no rationale for this choice could be detected from baseline data.

Chapter 5

Bathing and Showering

Introduction

This chapter considers devices which assist people with washing, bathing and showering.

Before working through this section, it is important to do the following:

- Consider your (the user's) requirements, and the requirements of the care assistant and others in the household if applicable (Chapter 1, Stage 1 in Figure 1.3).

- Have in mind the environment(s) in which the assistive device(s) will be used (Stage 2 in Figure 1.3). Include decisions and arrangements for any necessary alterations to it.

In the case of bathing and showering, Stages 3 and 4 must often be taken together instead of one after the other. The decision-making process may require holding the environmental alterations and the quest for an assistive device (AD) in parallel because they impact on one another. Possible options can be narrowed down until the advantages of two or three particular devices and/or a bath/shower facility outweigh others.

This chapter guides you through the decisions on what types or categories of AD to choose, starting with the choice between bath and shower. It helps to define what features you would want products to possess, which is Stage 4 of the process of choosing a product (see Figure 1.3). In the examples you may find hints about additional things to test or check when trying out the selected two or three products (Stage 5 from Figure 1.3).

This chapter does not provide guidance on getting undressed before bathing or showering or getting dressed afterwards.

It is important to consider what your future needs may be, and to plan for those that are likely to arise. This may be hard to do, as we do not really know what the future holds and also perhaps because none of us finds it easy to admit we may not be able to do in the future what we can today.

Practitioners can help in this regard because they have the experience of others in similar situations to yourself to draw upon. Forward planning is particularly necessary in the sphere of bathing and showering, because some decisions may entail major expense and disruption to the home, and it would be better for this to be done only once. But smaller items will repay forward planning too. For example, seek products for children that are adjustable to allow for growth (Korpela, Seppänen and Koivikko 1992). Regular review of whether ADs continue to meet your requirements will also be needed.

5.1 Keeping ourselves clean

5.1.1 Background

Difficulty with bathing or showering, especially bathing, is widespread amongst the older population (George et al. 1988, Sonn et al. 1996). The most common stated objective for assistive devices (ADs), particularly for bathing, was to feel safer. Rails in bathrooms should be fitted as standard (CAE; Sonn et al. 1996). This seems a sensible strategy particularly for accommodation designated for elderly people or those with physical impairments.

Before ideas are put into common practice they should be well piloted, otherwise designs may incur disabling results which prove expensive to rectify. An example was the low-level baths fitted in retirement flats in the UK in the 1970s–1980s with a vertical pole positioned halfway along the bath edge from ceiling to floor. This pole was ideal for those who could stand to step in, but impossible if a bath board and seat were needed to lift the legs over the bath rim from a seated position. Pesola (1999) approached bathroom design more thoroughly by producing a mock-up of a bathroom design which elderly people were asked to test out.

In the UK, bathing used to be the preferred method for achieving all-over cleanliness. In recent years showering has become more popular, especially amongst younger people. The housing stock predominantly offers bath only; having a shower unit too is less common. Very few dwellings have a shower with no bath. In many of those that do it is because an adaptation has been made for a person with disabilities, who required a shower facility in a house where there was insufficient room for both.

Space is frequently an issue, because bathrooms tend to be minimal in size, and often have a narrower door to enter them (Chamberlain, Thornley and Wright 1978). However, some aspects of the situation are set to change. Since 1999, new buildings must have doorways with a minimum 775 mm clearance to make passing through easier for wheelchair users (Department of the Environment 1999).

Taking a bath or shower is considered the appropriate way for cleanliness, at a social level. It is also for many a physically enjoyable and relaxing experience. However, all-over washing ('strip washing') is adequate to maintain personal hygiene. In the light of increased numbers of people for whom bathing or showering is difficult, local authorities in the UK have to make policies to enable them to cope with demand, and consequently their duty to enable people to manage in their own homes (Chronically Sick and Disabled Persons Act 1970) is interpreted accordingly. Thus the extreme is to define the need as achieving personal cleanliness rather than being able to bath or shower. Whilst those with disabilities and the majority of older people have difficulty bathing, few are unable to wash, with care assistant help if necessary (Parker and Thorslund 1991). So the provision of ADs for people experiencing difficulty bathing may in some areas be low priority unless there are additional factors such as incontinence, or a quickly deteriorating condition. In addition to social services provision, the demand for bathing ADs in many areas of the UK is currently addressed through provision of basic equipment by the Red Cross, and by people purchasing products for themselves.

Occupational therapists and assistants are the people who usually recommend ADs for provision through the social services departments. Their assessment will be comprehensive, and include your wishes and preferences. The home is your domain, and you must feel comfortable about what is proposed, otherwise you may reject the device or adaptation (Steward 2000). The local authority will have criteria that guide what may or may not be offered (LBOTM 2000), and it is useful to ask what these are if you are not entirely satisfied with what is being recommended for you.

Careful consideration of what you and others in the household want is essential when considering possible solutions, especially if structural adaptation to the home will be involved.

Sometimes providing assistance to people who are physically less able proves difficult, especially if the physical impairment is accompanied by cognitive impairments such as dementia or brain damage. Sometimes the difficulty may be lack of co-operation or outright refusal to do anything whilst the care assistant is present. Such reactions may arise from the fact that the person cannot accept that help is needed, and washing is a personal matter (Gitlin and Corocan 1993). ADs can ease the task for care assistants, as Gitlin and Corocan's study showed. It is probable that the positive role that ADs can play in caring for a person with dementia can be underestimated (Mann, Hurren and Tomita 1993).

People are more likely to use bathing devices if given adequate training in their use, than if not given such training (Meghani 1991; Schemm and Gitlin 1998; Stowe *et al.* 1982). A short demonstration and try-out should be sufficient for simple devices, but when requirements are complex, a trial period is strongly recommended to supplement the initial demonstration. In either case, written instructions should accompany any product, new or loaned (MDA 1998c), so that you can refer to them if necessary.

If you need support in the bath to prevent the risk of injury or to prevent your head slipping under the water, bathing devices are a necessity rather than a luxury. However, a survey in Finland found a high proportion of children without suitable devices, or their parents struggling with inadequate products, or none at all (Korpela *et al.* 1992). An assessment of the risks (see Chapter 6, section 6.2) involved with your current way of washing will contribute to the decision about how to solve your problem.

Very little has been published about the effectiveness of shower installations. Although problems of a technical nature occur, such as leaks or poor drainage, the finished facility seems to restore or improve independence for most people (Adams and Grisbrooke 1998; Rhodes 1989).

5.1.2 The decision whether to bath or shower

The preference for a bath or shower is largely a personal matter, but social and cultural norms and expectations also play a part. As mentioned above, people increasingly prefer a shower, or at least the option of a shower. By contrast, when 60 older people were surveyed, roughly 62–71 per cent preferred to bath (Parkes 1993). Parkes's respondents gave several reasons for not bathing or showering, which are shown in Table 5.1.2a.

Table 5.1.2a Reasons elderly people gave for *not* taking a bath or shower

Factor	*Bath*	*Shower*
Fear of slipping	11%	19%
Difficulty getting in, out or both	55%	0%
Water spillage	0%	16%
Difficulty getting water temperature correct	0%	23%
Difficulty washing self	0%	6%

Data from Parkes 1993.

This study's respondents were mainly frail elderly. In contrast, Table 5.1.2b draws on information from younger people with severe disabilities (MDA 1999), endorsed through professional experience (Harpin 2000).

Comparison of the two Tables illustrates that people with greater needs for body support and personal care assistance may have particular additional concerns compared with elderly people. There are common concerns, however, about safety, ease of washing and the need for confidence that the water will be at the desired temperature.

Tables 5.1.2a and 5.1.2b should be used to list factors relevant to your situation, so helping to see whether the advantages of bathing or of showering outweigh those of the other.

The ideal solution to the dilemma between choosing bathing or showering is to provide facilities for both. Although most residential homes now do so, few private dwellings will have the space except when a shower is installed over the bath.

Table 5.1.2b Factors affecting choice between bath and shower, with particular reference to those who require assistance and supportive seating

Factors to consider		Bath	Shower
Yourself (the user)	Incontinence	Skin gets well soaked but water soiling is a risk.	Commode aperture in seat provides easy access around the bottom.
	Warmth	Immersion in warm water is relaxing and provides buoyancy that improves movement if you have muscle weakness.	You can get cold unless the room is well heated.
	Stimulation	A 'spa' facility is invigorating and provides buoyancy.	The spray pressure is invigorating but causes a startle reaction in some people with cerebral palsy.
	Degree of freedom of movement	Support within the bath is often needed.	A shower chair will often mean straps are required. Shower trolleys can usually be used without straps.
	Those with cerebral palsy	Immersion can help to reduce muscle spasm. Jerky movements can cause bruising when arms are knocked against the bath.	May cause startle reaction.
	Those with muscular dystrophy	Once reclined, help may be needed to sit back up.	Showering often maintains independence longer.
	Those with neurological conditions, e.g. multiple sclerosis; cardiac conditions; respiratory conditions[1]	The heat of a bath may make you feel exhausted, or cause some breathing distress.	Shower may be preferred.
	Those with spina bifida or spinal deformities	A mesh seat or moulded cushion may be needed.	A mesh shower cradle may be preferred.

Care assistant or family	Handling	Mechanical assistance in lowering and raising you is recommended.	Lateral or *horizontal* transfers are possible alternatives to hoisting.
	Washing	More bending is required, the lower you sit in the bath.	Shower chairs entail bending. Trolleys can be used at optimal height for care assistant.
	Splashing	Only from your movements.	Protective screen or curtain necessary to avoid appreciable splashing on care assistant's legs.
	Drying	A place for you to get dried and dressed is needed at a height which reduces bending.	Shower chair users are often dried whilst seated, necessitating bending. Trolleys can double as a drying and dressing area.
	Shared use of bathroom	Assistive device must be lightweight and easy to store.	Shower stretcher can be wall mounted, over a bath if necessary, and folded away when not in use.
The environment	Space	Bath size, hoist and a place for you to get dry must all be considered. Access to both sides of the bath may be needed.	Level access shower area maximises use of space. A trolley requires a great deal of space to manoeuvre.
	Time	You may want to linger in the bath.	A shower is usually quicker than a bath.
	Water	When using a bath chair, a good depth of water is needed.	Less water is usually used compared with bathing.
	Heating: a smaller room is more economical to heat but there will be less space to manoeuvre.	You may want the room warmer if you have a bath that must be filled after you enter rather than a standard bath.	Showering normally means the room has to be warmer than for bathing.

Data from Medical Devices Agency (1999) EL3, used with permission.

1. Additional information from Hill 1996; Kimbell 1999.

Table 5.1.3 Guidance on some washing and drying devices

Your difficulty	Product type	Advantages	Disadvantages	★
Poor grip	Soap on a rope	You do not have to pick up and retain hold of a slippery bar of soap.	It has to be hooked over something, or the user must be able to pass the cord over his or her head.	★
	Liquid soap	Pressing the dispenser is easier than using a bar of soap.	The bottle has to stand on a flat surface.	★
	Flannel mitt	Less grip required.	Some practice needed to prevent it falling off during use.	★
	Sponge washing-up mop; long handled sponges	Increases reach; handle can be bent if desired, but reaching some parts of the body is still difficult for some people (Mann and Tomita 1998).	Handle may be difficult to grip – the longer the handle the firmer the grip needs to be to get pressure on the other end (Mann and Tomita 1998).	★★
Poor grip	Lambswool pad (short or long handle)	Soft to the skin.	Quite heavy when wet.	★
Reaching your feet	Toe washer (flannel-covered wire on long handle)	Can be passed between toes.		★
Reaching your back	Sponge on suction pads	Can be used in shower, to rub your back against.	More effort to move your whole body across the sponge.	★
	Towelling strap with plastic ring each end; may have sponge one side	Can be used to dry your back, or to wash back or feet using the sponge side.	Some practice needed to flick it over your head, especially when wet.	★
Drying yourself	Wall-mounted air blower	Push button or touch pad to start.	Vent must be altered to direct air flow; difficult to reach feet.	★
	Full-length vertical tube air blower	Pressure pad on floor can be activated by foot or wheel.	If you are seated, some areas will not dry well.	★

Some data from Kelsall and Cochrane 1996.

5.1.3 Difficulty with washing, drying and hair washing

Little is written about these activities in the literature, and no formal evaluations have been published. The following guidelines are based on the available data, and include some advantages and disadvantages of product types (see Table 5.1.3).

Personal assistance is more commonly used when upper limb tasks are difficult, and assistive devices (ADs) when lower limbs are affected (Verbrugge, Rennert and Madans 1997). Tasks people feel *unable* to do are more likely to need personal assistance than those they feel are *difficult*, for which an AD may be used (Agree 1999). The AD is useful either if it reduces the time and effort taken to complete the task, or if the advantage of greater independence in the task is felt to outweigh the time and effort taken.

How well you think washing and drying will be done using an AD is another factor. Using an AD may mean some compromise between how you would ideally like the task done, and how it actually may be achieved. We therefore suggest the following approach:

- If you can manage the task without increasing pain or getting frustrated, continue without an AD.

- If the task risks joint damage, gives you pain or is really difficult, try out a few devices (after looking at Table 5.1.3).

- If the task is impossible or still frustrating even if you use an AD, get personal assistance.

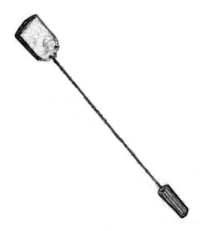

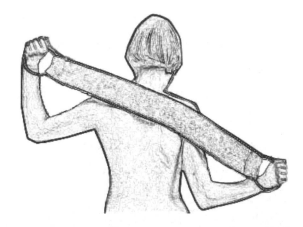

Toe washer

Towelling strap

Illustration 5.1.3

An example

Stephen is a wheelchair user, and has muscular dystrophy. He and his partner Sharon, who has cerebral palsy and is also a wheelchair user, are looking for a house.

- They consider subsection 5.1.2 *The decision whether to bath or shower.* As he can transfer sideways, Stephen feels he could be independent if he showers. Sharon needs to be hoisted in and out of her chair, so requires assistance anyway, and feels a bath full of warm water would be relaxing for her.

- Stephen is not able to sit back up if he bends to wash his feet, so he looks at subsection 5.1.3 *Difficulty with washing, drying and hair washing.* This subsection indicates that Stephen could try a toe washer and confirms to Sharon that personal assistance is her best option for washing and drying.

HAIR WASHING

Hair washing is more of an issue for some people than others, depending on culture, sex and age. Each person has his or her preferred way of dealing with hair washing.

For some, showering provides an easy solution (Adams and Grisbrooke 1998), but head support may be required if it is difficult or painful to hold your head tipped back slightly. A reclined mobile shower chair with a drop-down head section could be used for washing the hair whilst clothed, for example positioning the chair so the head section is over a bath or against a half-height shower screen.

If you bath and require head support, the issue is whether the seat design allows your head to be tilted back slightly, and allows the water to run away easily. A mesh bath seat (see section 5.2.6) has been reported useful or a product with a head section that drops down to facilitate hair washing (MDA 1999).

5.2 Bathing

There is a great variety of devices to assist with bathing, but many do not enable you to get right to the bottom of the bath. You may therefore have to accept a change in how you take a bath. For clarity, each subsection addresses a separate type of bathing device, but combinations of them are frequently advisable, and an indication of the commonest combinations will be given in each subsection.

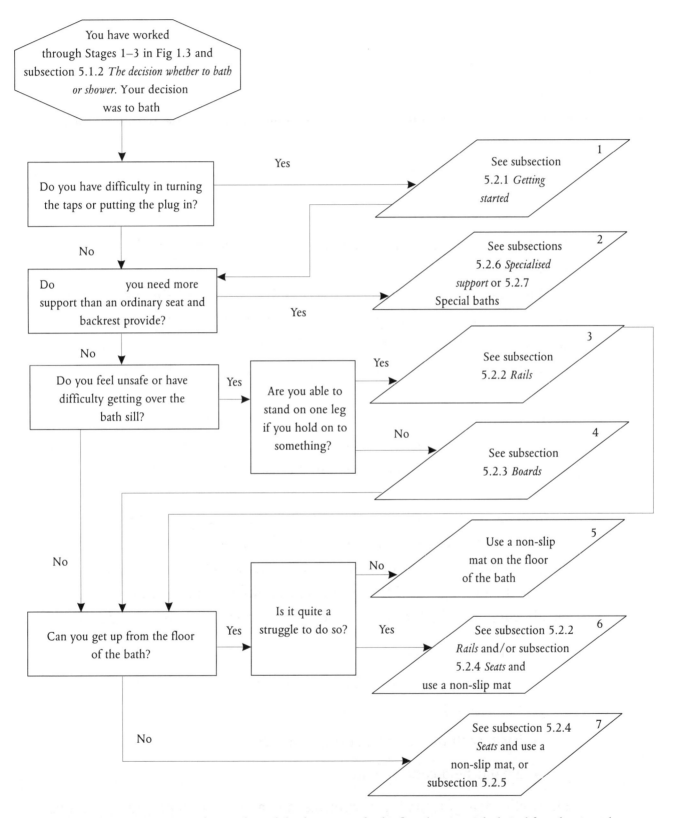

*Figure 5.2 Pinpointing what may be needed. The structure for this flow chart is mainly derived from data in ; Edwards and Jones 1998. Mann et al. 1996***

A combination of non-slip mat, rails, board and seat (or rails and lifting seat) is satisfactory for most people (Edwards and Jones 1998; Galer and Feeney 1979; Mann *et al.* 1996). Assistive devices reduce the need for personal assistance (Gitlin *et al.* 1999).

5.2.1 Getting started

Safety in bathing is a key concern for people. This encompasses all components of bathing, including filling, entering and getting out of the bath, sitting safely whilst washing, and being able to empty the bath. The impact of having an assistive device (AD) on each of these must be considered. If any of these remain unsafe or difficult after considering ADs or techniques, it would be sensible to bath only when someone else is at hand to help if necessary. The risks to any care assistant in providing help must also be assessed and minimised (see Chapter 6, section 6.2).

Taps should be easy to operate (see Table 5.2.1) and the water run to the correct temperature before getting in. If you want to add water after getting in, a thermostatic control on a mixer unit is imperative if your sensation is impaired, but advisable for anyone. The plug should also be easily pulled if you bath alone in case of an emergency; those liable to have a fit should always have someone to keep a check on them.

A non-slip bath mat on the bottom of the bath is recommended whenever you stand or move in the bath, as this gives greater grip against the skin as well as making you feel safer.

Water gives buoyancy, so getting up from the bottom of the bath whilst water is still round you is less of an effort. For safety, though, it is sensible to pull the plug out just before you stand up or move onto a bath board or seat.

If standard plugs are difficult to manage, differing designs can be found but mostly entail new bath or basin units. The following may be considered:

- pop-up plug with control at top of basin or bath
- bath with the controls along the side of the bath for easy reach when the user is seated in the bath
- basin with the controls at the front edge
- a hand-held control unit.

Electronic detectors and tap controls are already installed in some public washrooms and toilets, so should be available for ordinary homes as alternative means of controlling plug and taps.

Table 5.2.1 Guidance on choice of taps and tap turners

Your difficulty	*Type of product*	*Guideline*	★
Poor grip that is expected to improve	Tap turners avoid having to have new taps fitted	Choose a product according to the style of tap.	
	Tap turner for crystal style taps	The devices can be fiddly to fit (MDD 1993a). To be practical, the tap should be sufficiently far from wall for the device to be left on the tap once fitted.	**
	Tap turners for cross-head taps	Although these are easier to get on and off than the crystal style tap turners, the products vary, with some requiring a technique that poses difficulty to users (MDD 1993a).	**
Poor grip that is likely to persist, but able to reach across basin	Short lever taps (61–71 mm)	Off positions at right angles to the spout create less obstruction than those parallel to the spout. These taps can be up to three times more effective than crystal style taps (Rogers *et al.* 1996).	* ***
No useful grip or poor grip, but able to reach across basin	Long lever taps	Suitable if you have little hand function but can reach and move your arm out from midline. Considered obtrusive (MDD 1993b).	* **
No useful grip or poor grip, but able to reach upwards	Vertical lever taps	Most who tested them found them 'awkward' to use (MDD 1993b).	**
No useful grip or poor grip, and not able to reach far	Tap control at front of basin or at centre of bath side	Suitable if you have limited reach. Test control option: knob, pad, lever.	*
	Remote tap control	Operated by hand-held control unit.	*
	Automatic tap control	Sensor detects when your hands are under tap, or the sensor can be placed elsewhere so you can move a part of your body in front of it.	*

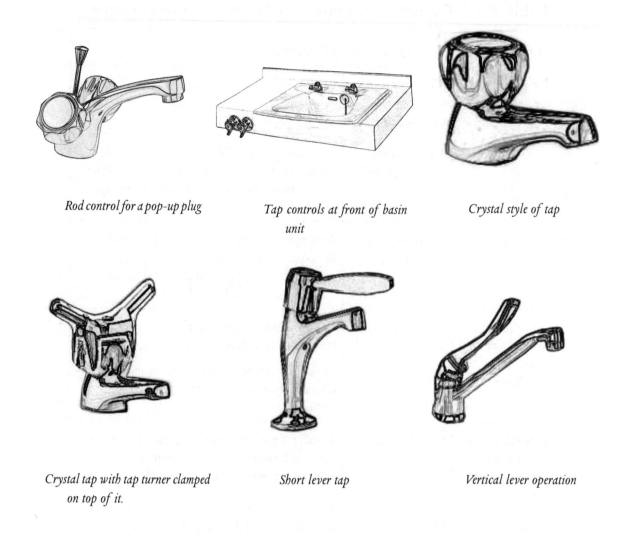

Rod control for a pop-up plug

Tap controls at front of basin unit

Crystal style of tap

Crystal tap with tap turner clamped on top of it.

Short lever tap

Vertical lever operation

Illustration 5.2.1

5.2.2 Rails

Rails in the bathroom will be used for steadying, pulling or pushing. Given the confidence that feeling safe confers, rails will be of benefit to a large proportion of the population, and to all who are elderly. They are particularly helpful because wet skin and wet surfaces are more slippery than dry ones.

If you have difficulty in grasping, or find it painful, rails will be of less benefit. Sometimes a horizontal rail to push or *lean* on proves useful.

The diameter of rails suggested is 40 mm (1.6in.)(Pheasant undated), but with no supporting evidence. However, other handle diameters Pheasant recommended are similar, as cited in Chapter 4 (Table 4.1.1a *Guidance on devices related to getting on and off the toilet*).

The finished surface should be slightly roughened to reduce the likelihood of the hand slipping when wet, but not so much that it chafes the skin (Pheasant undated). Metal rails may need to be earthed in case they give an electric shock (Disability North 1998), and will tend to be slippery when wet.

If the height of the bath rim makes lifting the legs over it an effort, a small platform to step onto first may help. Such a platform must be stable even if you step on its edge, and the edges could be highlighted with warning tape or a colour contrast to reduce the risk of tripping over it.

MULTIPLE USERS

Residential homes for those who are disabled or elderly should have 'a good number of grab rails' (Parkes 1993, p.60) in the bathroom. A colour contrast will give maximum visibility to encourage their use. Unfortunately there has been no study to determine their optimum configuration and heights; Clemson and Martin (1996) pointed out that 'further research is essential to establish optimum rail placement for confidence and safety' (p.56). Their study findings tentatively indicated that people with lower limb impairments preferred oblique and horizontal rails to vertical rails.

The new British standard 8300:2001 provides recommendations for en suite bathrooms in residential establishments (BS1 2001). This comes into force in 2004, and is based on wide consultation and user input. Taking the 50th percentile of a 65–80-year-old woman (Pheasant undated) as the average resident of a rest home, with mainly lower limb and balance problems, the following configuration could be helpful:

Horizontal wall-fixed rail (towards the tap end)	705 mm (28in.) from the *bottom of the bath*
Oblique rail (in the middle third of the bath's length)	535 mm (21in.) at lower end, from the *bottom of the bath*

Continuous horizontal/oblique rails may have to compromise between these heights. *System rails* are worth considering if you want to customise lengths, angles and combinations of rails. System rails have components from which you select, according to the configuration you require. Examples can be seen in Figure 5.2.2 and Illustration 5.2.2.

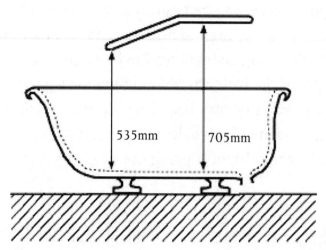

Figure 5.2.2 Optimum position for a bath rail for use by several people, e.g. in a residential home.

INDIVIDUAL USERS

Guidelines for rail heights are appropriate for residential homes, but each individual is proportioned differently, so when the rails are for an individual in his or her own home, rail heights and positions must be judged on site. You can tell where they should be by acting out the tasks.

If a rail is needed to lean on as you get in and out of the bath, one fixed across the bath may be of help, provided it does not impede other aspects of the bathing process. It is suggested that it is placed a little beyond halfway towards the tap end, i.e. between 900 and 1100 mm (36–43in.) from the sloped end of a 1.7 m (5ft 6in.) bath. An alternative is a rail attached to the edge of the bath and the floor (see Illustration 5.2.2).

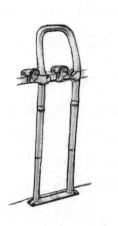

Rail attached to edge of bath and the floor

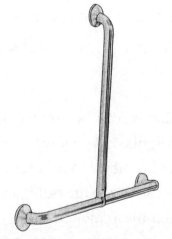

An example of a rail system where a vertical and horizontal rail are combined, instead of using two separate rails

Illustration 5.2.2

Table 5.2.2 Steadying and pulling

Activity	Your needs	Type of rail	Guideline	★
Getting over the bath rim	Bending forward is difficult or painful	Vertical pole, floor-to-ceiling (Cooper and Stewart 1997**) or horizontal rail next to bath	Fix by bath so it can be reached when seated in the bath too. If you may need to use a bath board to get into the bath in the future, a spring-loaded pole is more expensive but easier to remove and relocate. A horizontal rail that is attached to the bath and not the floor may only by used for steadying, not pulling.	★ ★
	Leaning over the bath to a rail in the wall would feel unsafe	Rails attached to taps, or rail system (see text)	Rails attached to taps may only have downwards pressure applied, so the weight is taken by the bath rim not the tap fitment. A design that is higher than the bath rim is available.	★
	Leaning over the bath is OK	Horizontal rail in wall	Fix at knuckle height (Pheasant undated) when *standing in* the bath. A rail both sides may be helpful: leading edge of bath side rail should be nearer the taps than the wall-fixed rail.	★ ★
Getting up from the bottom of the bath	Rail on one side should be sufficient	Integral handle in bath	'Not generally helpful' for getting up from the bottom of the bath, possibly because they are usually horizontal (Chamberlain *et al.* 1978).	★
		Oblique wall-fixed rail	Lower end at shoulder height when *seated in* the bath.	★
	Need rail for both hands	If rail in wall plus integral handle not satisfactory, a rail fixed at edge of bath may be suitable (as in Illustration 5.2.2)	Alternatively, a rail system to provide rail over the bath width. Fix at shoulder height or slightly above if you can lift your arms above shoulder level.	★
Both getting in bath and up from bottom of the bath	Need rail for both activities	Combination of rails, or a rail that has a horizontal and oblique section	Alternatively, a combination of rail and bath seat.	★

5.2.3 Boards

A bath board rests on the bath rim, with brackets that brace it against the inner sides of the bath to steady it. You sit on it outside the bath, then lift your legs over into the bath. You then move your hips along the board to position them centrally across the bath, usually in 'steps' by bracing your arms on the board to lift your bottom and move sideways a little at a time. This is easy when clothed, but bare skin, especially when wet, will not slide so easily. A small piece of dry towelling between you and the board often helps. Trying out a bath board in an actual bath is therefore recommended before finally deciding whether you can manage.

The board must not be longer than the width of the bath, otherwise sitting on the overhang will cause the board to tip up (Disability North 1998; MDA 1998a). The bath rim must be wide enough (MDA 1998a recommended a minimum of 25mm (1in), but Disability North 1998 considered 37 mm (1.5in.) to be the minimum) to support the board adequately. Baths set into the tiles often result in the bath rim being too narrow to fit a bath board safely.

A board is usually used in conjunction with a bath seat (see subsection 5.2.4) so you have to move from the board to the seat rather than sit directly on the bath floor.

Using a bath board requires the ability to swing the legs both outwards and inwards at hip level, as you lift the legs over into the bath. This means that those who have had hip replacements should *not* attempt to use a board for some months after the operation, because the joint is at risk of dislocating.

Notes

Numbers relate to slanted boxes in Figure 5.2.3a.

1. Using a shelf at the head end of a bath is helpful only if you can then get onto and up from the bottom of the bath. This is because a seat would have to be fitted some distance from the shelf, making it unsafe to transfer on and off.

3. If it is difficult to lift your legs over the rim, a manual leg lifter may enable you to do this independently (see Chapter 6, Illustration 6.1.6). A manual leg lifter is a stiffened strap with a loop both ends. One loop is passed over the foot, the other used as a handle. To use it effectively, good arm strength is needed. If a leg lifter is not suitable, a special lifting seat that has an elevating leg board, a hoist, or a special bath may be considered. Personal assistance is another option.

4. An extended bath board is continuous from the wall across the bath and projecting into the bathroom sufficiently for you to sit down on it with hips and legs aligned to the length of the bath. The projecting board is supported on legs. This type of board eliminates the need to swivel the hips; they will only have to be moved sideways along the board.

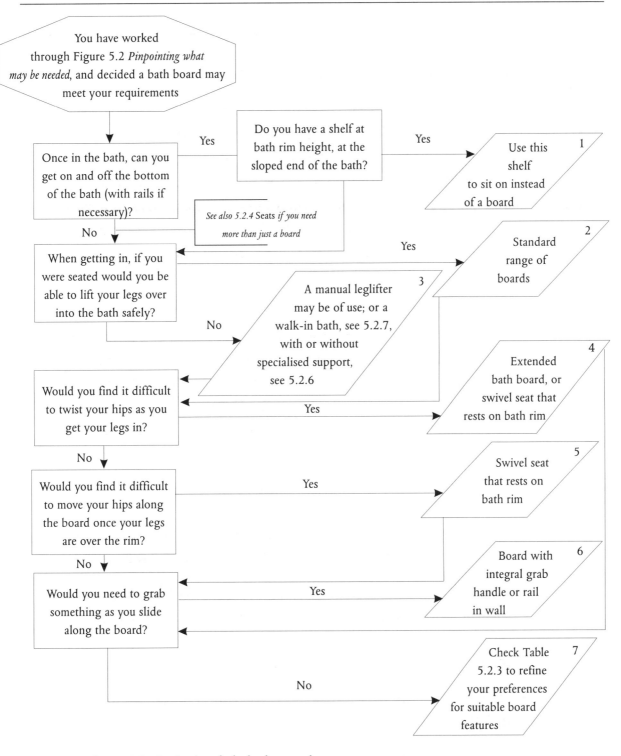

Figure 5.2.3a Getting into the bath when seated

5.   A swivel seat rests on the bath rim, and rotates through 90° so that you can sit on it when standing at the edge of the bath, then swivel it as the legs are lifted over the rim until you are aligned with the bath length. This type of seat would be particularly useful for over-bath showering, because of the drainage holes in the plastic seat.

6.   Many people find a wall-fixed rail helpful to pull on when using a board. From the comments in subsection 5.2.2 above, a horizontal or oblique rail is suggested, fixed at approximately 150 mm (6in.) higher than the bath rim.

An example

Primrose has rheumatoid arthritis, and has seen an occupational therapist because of her difficulty getting up from a chair. She is generally weaker than she used to be, has painful wrists, and cannot lift her arms above her shoulders. She is wary of her knees buckling under her as they did last week when she was stepping over the bath rim. She was lucky to get away with bruises, and does not want to risk stepping into the bath again. She has looked at Figure 5.2 *Pinpointing what may be needed* and feels a bath board is worth trying.

- She sees in Figure 5.2.3a that she could look at subsection 5.2.4 *Seats* too. She has been getting up from the bottom of the bath, but it has become such a struggle she answers 'No' and continues down the flow chart. She feels she should be able to lift her legs over the rim and move her hips along a board, and decides she would not use rails unless she had to because they would increase the pain in her wrists.

- In Table 5.2.3 *Guidance on issues related to bath boards* she notes that for comfort she should try plastic rather than wood or metal boards, and that drainage holes would be an advantage as she has an over-bath shower, so she could shower when she wanted.

- When she asks her social services occupational therapist, she is offered only a metal board with holes, or a padded plastic board. Primrose tries both, and decides she would prefer the greater comfort of the padded board above the need for drainage holes.

- They then discuss the possibility of a bath seat (see subsection 5.2.4).

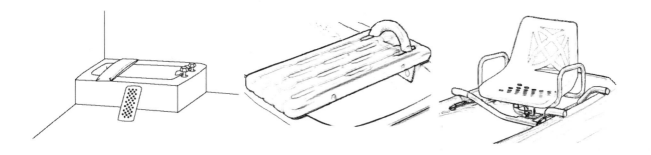

Primrose's bath boards

Bath board with handle

Swivel bath seat. Note that the holes may need to be covered for male users. See Table 5.2.4

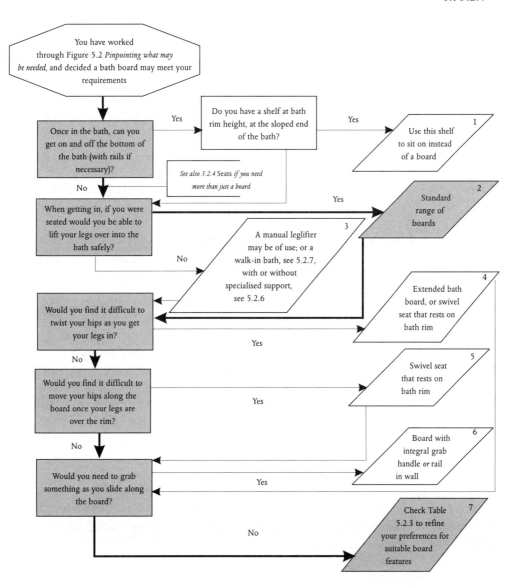

route through Figure 5.2.3a

Primrose's

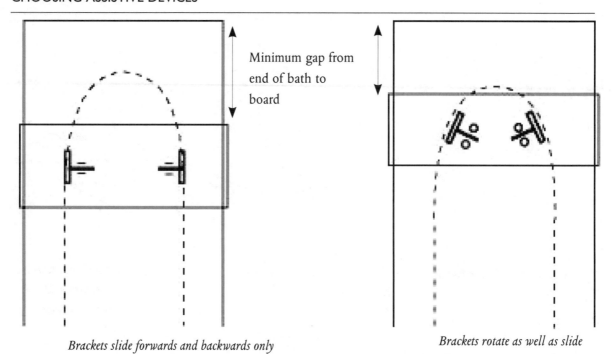

Brackets slide forwards and backwards only

Brackets rotate as well as slide

Bath board brackets
Illustration 5.2.3a

Table 5.2.3 Guidance on issues related to bath boards

Factor	Issue	Guideline	★
Safety	Your weight	Ensure the board will safely take your weight by checking the instructions about maximum load.	★★★★
	Slipping	Seldom a problem, but if you are concerned, do not choose painted metal or padded PVC (MDA 1998a). A damp towel between skin and board would reduce slippage.	★★
Comfort	Different surface finishes	The wood and metal boards were rated less comfortable than plastic and padded ones (MDA 1998a).	★★★
Skin care	Shearing when getting in and out	Brace your arms to lift weight off buttocks and move to the centre of the board in several small moves. If sliding is necessary, place something between skin and board to reduce friction.	★
Space for you to sit in the bath	Some brackets do not accommodate the curvature of the bath	Boards that have to be fitted in front of the curvature at the end of the bath will limit space further.	★★
Use with over-bath shower	Drainage	To reduce spillage over bath side, the board should have drainage holes.	★

5.2.4 Seats

Bath seats are designed to provide a seat higher than the bottom of the bath. They are used when getting up from the bottom of the bath is too difficult or risky to attempt. They rest on the bath floor, hang on the bath rim edges, or are braced against the bath sides. A few seats may retain some water in crevices, so would need to be removed and dried after each use; others are designed to drain spontaneously and may be lifted and cleaned less frequently.

You may be able to step into the bath, with or without a rail to steady yourself.

It may be safer or easier to use a bath board (see subsection 5.2.3 above) in conjunction with a seat. Having sat on the board and lifted your legs over, you then rest your hands on the bath rim and swing your buttocks off the board and down on to the seat. To get out, the hands must be placed on the edge of the board. The buttocks are then lifted up and back on to the board. If unable to use your arms in this way, you will probably find a board and seat difficult to use.

An alternative to a bath board and seat is a shallow bath insert, which rests on the bath rim. You would need to be comfortable with your knees out straight, and probably live on your own, as moving and storing it makes this option impractical in a shared bathroom unless there is ample space. Another possibility is a lifting bath seat (subsection 5.2.5).

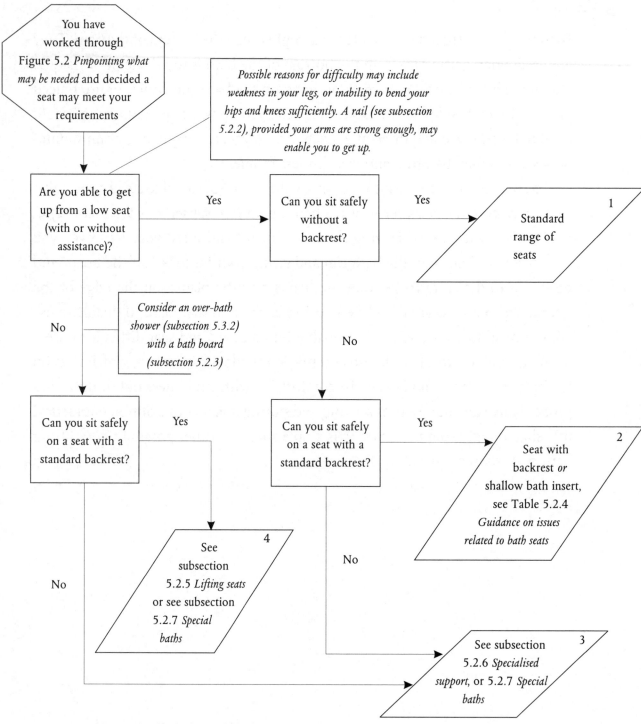

Figure 5.2.4 Sitting higher in the bath

Note

Number relates to slanted box in Figure 5.2.4.

2. Some seats have backrests, either at fixed height or adjustable. Combined bath board and seat sets, where they are fixed together, may also have a small backrest incorporated. The backrest will provide additional security for those who are unsteady when sitting, and may be more comfortable for those with back pain.

An example

Primrose has rheumatoid arthritis and has difficulty in getting up from the bottom of the bath. She has already decided what bath board to have (see subsection 5.2.3).

- She works her way down Figure 5.2.4, and she feels she should be able to get up from a seat, and can sit safely without a backrest, so a standard seat should be suitable.

- Looking at Table 5.2.4 *Guidance on issues related to bath seats*, she notes that her bath is acrylic, so she cannot have a seat that braces against the bath sides. She also feels comfort will be important.

- Her occupational therapist from the social services department lets her try a seat suspended from the bath rim, and also a contoured plastic seat that rests on the bottom of the bath. She cannot use handrails because of her painful wrists, so although she prefers the contoured seat, it is too difficult to get up from, so she chooses the suspended seat which is higher. She can get up from this more easily, leaning her elbows on the bath rim.

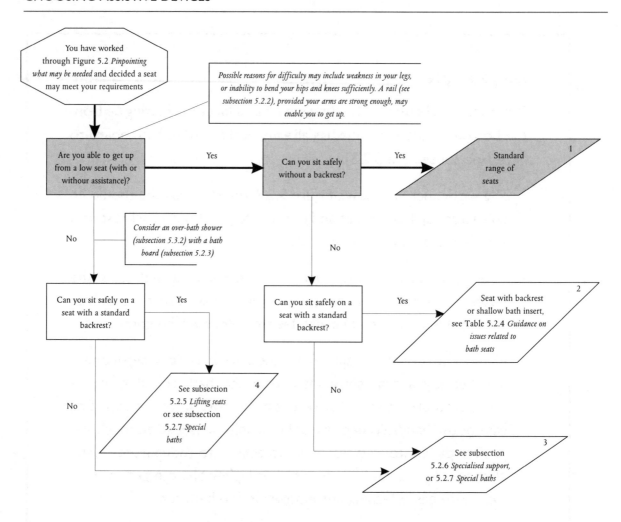

You have worked through Figure 5.2 *Pinpointing what may be needed* and decided a seat may meet your requirements

Possible reasons for difficulty may include weakness in your legs, or inability to bend your hips and knees sufficiently. A rail (see subsection 5.2.2), provided your arms are strong enough, may enable you to get up.

Are you able to get up from a low seat (with or withour assistance)?

Yes → Can you sit safely without a backrest?

Yes → Standard range of seats   1

No

Consider an over-bath shower (subsection 5.3.2) with a bath board (subsection 5.2.3)

Can you sit safely on a seat with a standard backrest?

Yes

No

Can you sit safely on a seat with a standard backrest?

Yes → Seat with backrest or shallow bath insert, see Table 5.2.4 *Guidance on issues related to bath seats*   2

No

See subsection 5.2.5 *Lifting seats* or see subsection 5.2.7 *Special baths*   4

See subsection 5.2.6 *Specialised support*, or 5.2.7 *Special baths*   3

Primrose's route through Figure 5.2.4

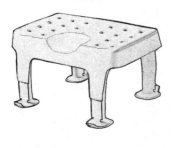

Bath seat with cut-away at the front

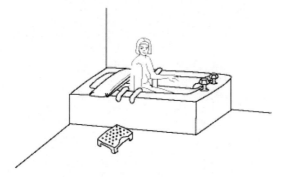

Primrose tries a bath board and seat

Illustration 5.2.4

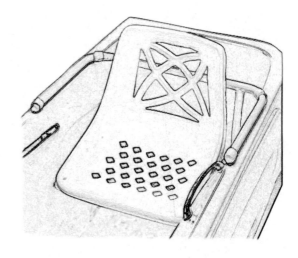

Seat with holes that may be an entrapment hazard

Table 5.2.4 Guidance on issues related to bath seats.

Factor	Issue	Guideline	★
Your safety	Support for back	Some seats have a backrest; combined seat and board units have a small integral backrest. Choosing a seat without a backrest when you need one will increase the likelihood of your not using it (Shipman 1986).	* ★★★
	Risk of entrapment of testicles	If the seat has holes for drainage (as in Illustrations 5.2.3 and 5.2.4) they must be covered with a flannel unless the holes are small (MDA 1997).	★★
Comfort	Depth of seat	Acceptability dropped rapidly for seats deeper than 280 mm, unless they had a cut-away front (MDA 1998a).	★★
Personal hygiene	Washing	Cut-away at front of seat makes washing your bottom easier (MDA 1998a).	*
Safety for others	Risk of injury to any who assist you	Physical assistance on and off the seat should be confined to steadying you, because the care assistant has to bend and twist the spine (Aitchison 1999).	★★
	Risk of injury when removing and replacing the seat	Place one foot in the bath to reduce twisting of the spine. Suction pads must be released individually unless they are linked with a quick release band.	*

5.2.5 Lifting seats

Lifting seats are those that do all or part of the work of getting you up from the bottom of the bath, to level with the bath rim. Some products also have a turntable in the seat to help you pivot through 90° once up. Alternatively, the seat itself pivots. This is either a powered movement which is an integral part of the lifting sequence, or has to be done manually. In the latter, there is a locking mechanism so that pivoting does not occur except when the seat is up.

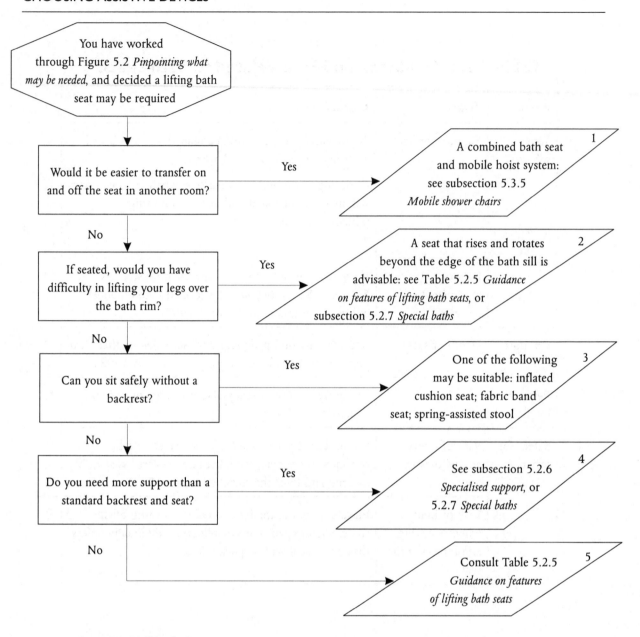

Figure 5.2.5 Lifting bath seats

Note: There is increased risk of injury to the spine when it is bent and rotated.

Notes

Numbers refer to slanted boxes in Figure 5.2.5

1. If you require hoisting you may find getting onto a bath seat easier in a larger room than the bathroom. The seat is part of a hoist system that then lifts the seat into the bath. An alternative is being hoisted directly into the bath. For more information, see Chapter 6. Systems that can be used for bath, shower or over the toilet are included in subsection 5.3.5 under 'Multiple functions', and Chapter 6, Table 6.3.4.

2. For some users, getting their legs over the bath rim is difficult because they cannot straighten their knees or bend their hips sufficiently. The seats that go higher than the rim will be helpful if this is the case for you, as your legs do not then have to be lifted so high, relative to the body. The extra height also makes it easier for a care assistant

to guide your legs over the rim. Products that rise this extra height are floor fixed, integral to a special bath, or part of a hoist system.

3. The fabric band seat is contained within a wall-fixed unit. For bathing, it is pulled out, stretched over the bath rim and attached to a7 fixing at floor level.

An example

James lives with his wife in a bungalow. He has Parkinson's disease with some dementia, which means that sometimes when he cannot do things his wife is not sure whether he is unable, or just unwilling. James has always enjoyed a bath, but recently coaxing him to get into the bath even with a rail is becoming impossible. Also, his wife is anxious about him being able to get up again, because she could not lift him if he got stuck.

- James agrees with his wife that something to help would be a good idea, but firmly states he wants to continue to bath if at all possible. They have a leaflet about their local Disabled Living Centre, so make a visit. Together with the occupational therapist there, they discuss James's needs, the bathroom facilities, and what his wife's requirements are.

- They work through Figure 5.2 and decide they would prefer a lifting seat so that James could get nearer to the bottom of the bath.

- In Figure 5.2.5 they feel James would be able to get on and off a seat in the bathroom for the foreseeable future, that he should be able to lift his legs over the rim, perhaps with a little help from his wife, and that a backrest is sensible but a standard one should be sufficient.

- From Table 5.2.5 *Guidance on features of lifting bath seats* his wife decides against seats operated by compressed air because these have trailing tubes, and James might trip on them. However, she is concerned about lifting the electrically powered ones in and out of the bath, as they are heavy.

- They try two or three. They all fit in the bath, but one does not rise high enough to be level with the bath rim. James is much happier with the one which has a reclined backrest, and his wife feels she could manage to get it out of the bath, once the backrest is detached. They check his weight, 15 stone (94 kg) to ensure he is under the maximum load for the seat.

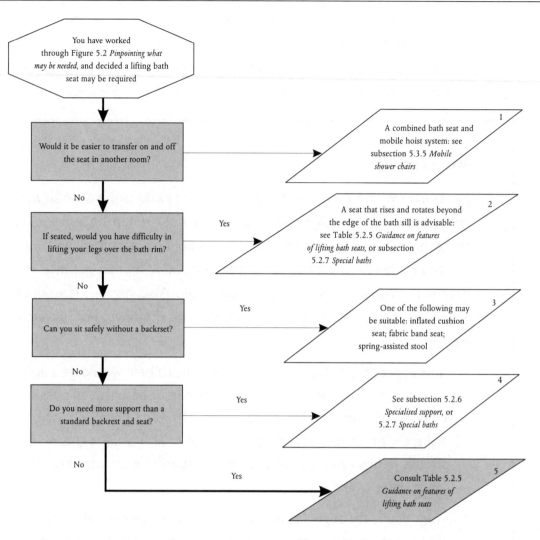

You have worked through Figure 5.2 *Pinpointing what may be needed*, and decided a lifting bath seat may be required

Would it be easier to transfer on and off the seat in another room?

A combined bath seat and mobile hoist system: see subsection 5.3.5 *Mobile shower chairs*   1

No

If seated, would you have difficulty in lifting your legs over the bath rim?

Yes

A seat that rises and rotates beyond the edge of the bath sill is advisable: see Table 5.2.5 *Guidance on features of lifting bath seats*, or subsection 5.2.7 *Special baths*   2

No

Can you sit safely without a backrset?

Yes

One of the following may be suitable: inflated cushion seat; fabric band seat; spring-assisted stool   3

No

Do you need more support than a standard backrest and seat?

Yes

See subsection 5.2.6 *Specialised support*, or 5.2.7 *Special baths*   4

No

Yes

Consult Table 5.2.5 *Guidance on features of lifting bath seats*   5

James' route through Figure 5.2.5

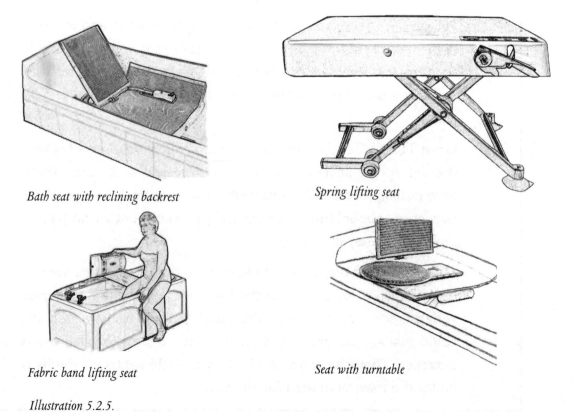

Bath seat with reclining backrest

Spring lifting seat

Fabric band lifting seat

Seat with turntable

Illustration 5.2.5.

5.2.6 Specialised support

Requiring special support means that you cannot sit safely and/or comfortably on standard seats. The two main types of product that will provide specialised support in the bath are cushions, and chairs or cradles. Products from this subsection may be needed in conjunction with special baths, as not all special baths offer specialised support.

For this level of need, it is assumed that mechanical assistance with raising and lowering you into the bath will be necessary. There is a spring-assisted platform on which some chairs can be fixed (but you would sit quite high in the bath), which would be suitable for children and smaller adults (see Illustration 5.2.6). For young children there is a mesh seat that rests on the bath rim, with a bar that is swung up and over to lower the child into the water, see Illustration 5.2.6. With all other products, a hoist will usually be needed (see Chapter 6, section 6.3). If a mobile hoist is to be used, there has to be sufficient clearance under the bath for its legs, and holes cut in the bath panel.

A place to be dried is also needed. Many put towels on their wheelchair, but a shelf or trolley (mobile or wall-fixed and hinged so it can be folded against the wall when not in use) at a good working height for the care assistant would provide an ideal place to be dried.

The ability to raise you *during* a bath is useful for soaping, then to lower you again to rinse.

Table 5.2.5 Guidance on features of lifting bath seats

Factor	Issue		Guideline	★
Your (the user's) requirements	Able to sit upright	Backrest or not	To manage without a backrest you either need to be able to sit without support for the length of time you bathe, or choose a product that sinks to the bottom of the bath so you can lean on the bath slope; most are on a platform so this is not possible.	★
	Able to adjust hip position as seat rises and lowers	Some types of lifting seat require you to shift your hips as they rise and lower	Compressed air operated seats are only stable when you are right in the centre: in practice this means that the hips may have to be shifted if the seat seems uneven. The fabric band seat may require constant hip adjustment as it rises and lowers.	★
	Able to use arms to assist rising and lowering	Spring-assisted seats require a light push or pull to effect the movement	You must be able to raise your arms at least as far as shoulder height. Ensure the springs are set at the appropriate weight for you.	★
	Able to swing legs over bath rim	Side flaps	If you sit on the seat then swing your legs over the bath rim, side flaps make this safer and easier. You need good balance for transferring.	★
	Difficulty in turning your hips when seated	Some products have a turntable to make this easy	The alternative is a seat on a floor-fixed post that swings through 90°, or a special bath (subsection 5.2.7).	★
	Limited hip flexion	Ease of getting in and comfort when seated	A product with a backrest that is raked back, or that can be reclined is recommended.	★
	Comfort	Padded surface	Some products are padded, but these did not score higher for comfort than unpadded seats (MDA 1998b). If the seat and backrest are smooth plastic a cushion can be used (see subsection 5.2.6).	★★
	Ease of washing your bottom	Cut-away on seat	If you cannot transfer weight on to one buttock, a cut-away may prove helpful.	★
Safety in the bathroom		Trailing pipes or leads	If you are liable to trip on pipes that carry air into the seat, a battery operated seat may be advisable.	★

Safety when handling the seat		Lifting it in and out	All potentially pose a risk of injury to the person who lifts the seat in and out because of the weight and the difficulty of keeping the spine in a good position (Aitchison 1999). Spring-assisted seats are heavy. Battery packs can be removed and stored separately. Some products have detachable backrests.	★★★
Product	Maintenance	Some products require more attention than others	Battery packs need to be removed and recharged frequently: some manufacturers recommend doing so after each use (Disability North 1998).	★★★
	Robustness	Has it been designed for a person of your weight?	Ensure you choose a product that has a maximum weight limit (frequently 127 kg) greater than your weight. More robust products are available.	★★★
	Compatibility with bath	Deep baths	Ensure the seat rises level with, or just above, the bath rim.	★★★
		Side flaps	Ensure the flaps are not obstructed as the seat rises and lowers (MDA 1998b).	★★★
	Multi-purpose	As sanichair and shower seat	One seat can be lowered into a bath by attachment to a hoist, or placed on a mobile base for use over the toilet or in a shower.	★
	Damage to some types of plastic	Use of bath oils (not bubble bath)	Check with manufacturer if you have to use bath oils regularly.	★

An example

Sharon, who has cerebral palsy, and is a wheelchair user, has decided she wants to bath, and has seen from Figure 5.2 that she needs specialised support.

- Sharon looks at Figure 5.2.6; she does like water round her, so looks at Table 5.2.6 *Guidance on bath chairs, cradles and cushions*.

- From this Table, she notes that, although a mouldable cushion would meet her needs, it may be more difficult for her assistant to help her wash, so decides to try a mesh seat with adjustable legs.

- Sharon knows that she must check the size of every chair to make sure it is big enough; she is quite prepared to ask manufacturers if she finds nothing standard that meets her requirements, as many firms do accommodate such requests. However, she finds one that is large enough and has adjustable legs.

- Sharon tries this, and checks that the bath is wide enough for the legs to sit on the bottom of the bath correctly, and that her sacrum does not rest on the bath surface when the mesh gives with her weight.

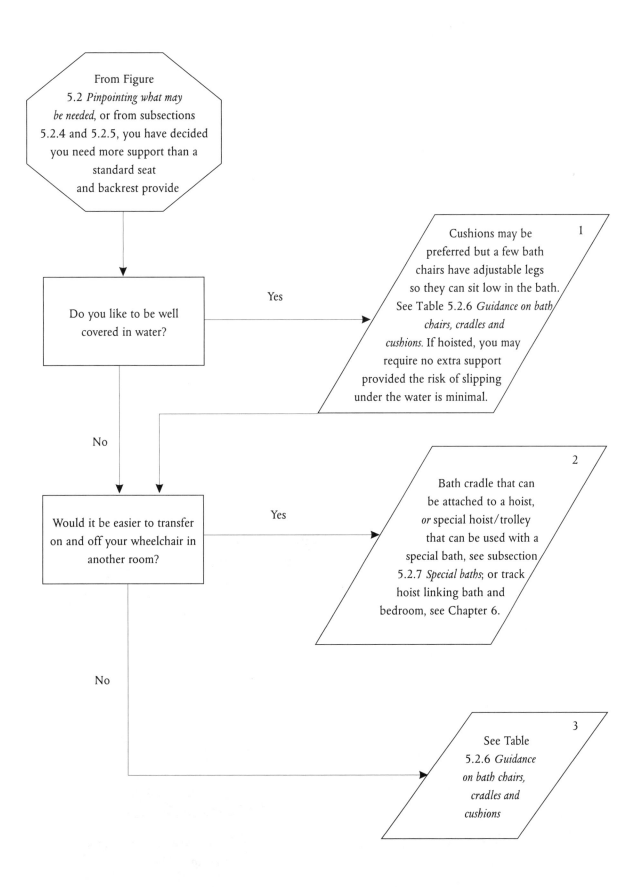

From Figure
5.2 *Pinpointing what may
be needed*, or from subsections
5.2.4 and 5.2.5, you have decided
you need more support than a
standard seat
and backrest provide

Do you like to be well
covered in water?

Yes

1
Cushions may be
preferred but a few bath
chairs have adjustable legs
so they can sit low in the bath.
See Table 5.2.6 *Guidance on bath
chairs, cradles and
cushions.* If hoisted, you may
require no extra support
provided the risk of slipping
under the water is minimal.

No

Would it be easier to transfer
on and off your wheelchair in
another room?

Yes

2
Bath cradle that can
be attached to a hoist,
or special hoist/trolley
that can be used with a
special bath, see subsection
5.2.7 *Special baths*; or track
hoist linking bath and
bedroom, see Chapter 6.

No

3
See Table
5.2.6 *Guidance
on bath chairs,
cradles and
cushions*

Figure 5.2.6 Specialised support in the bath

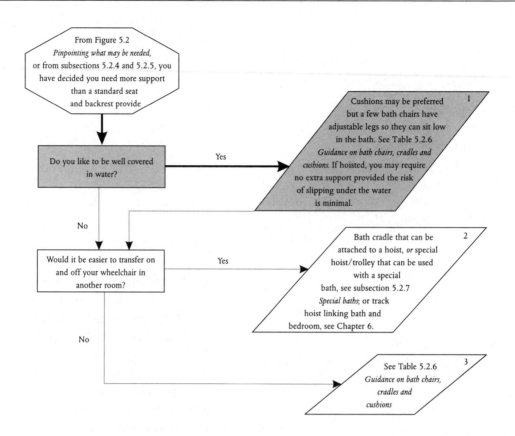

From Figure 5.2
Pinpointing what may be needed,
or from subsections 5.2.4 and 5.2.5, you
have decided you need more support
than a standard seat
and backrest provide

Do you like to be well covered
in water?

Yes

Cushions may be preferred
but a few bath chairs have
adjustable legs so they can sit low
in the bath. See Table 5.2.6
*Guidance on bath chairs, cradles and
cushions.* If hoisted, you may require
no extra support provided the risk
of slipping under the water
is minimal. 1

No

Would it be easier to transfer on
and off your wheelchair in
another room?

Yes

Bath cradle that can be
attached to a hoist, *or* special
hoist/trolley that can be used
with a special
bath, see subsection 5.2.7
Special baths; or track
hoist linking bath and
bedroom, see Chapter 6. 2

No

See Table 5.2.6
*Guidance on bath chairs,
cradles and
cushions* 3

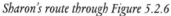

Sharon's route through Figure 5.2.6

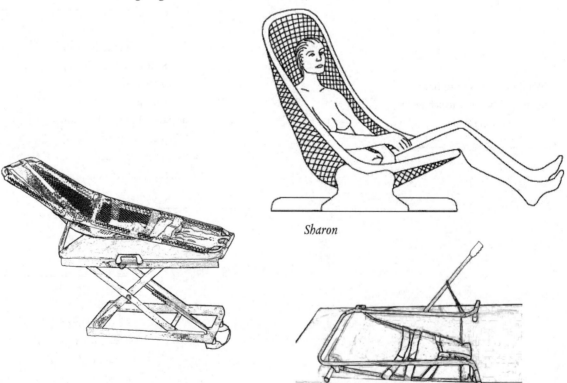

Sharon

Bath cradle on spring-assisted lifting platform

*Bath cradle with lifting mechanism operated by a bar
that swings up and over.*

Illustration 5.2.6

BATH CUSHIONS

These have waterproof covers and are usually fixed to the bath by suction pads. If the cushion is to be attached to a lifting bath seat or platform, a manufacturer may be able to put eyelets on the cushion so it can be tied on. This is an advantage because many seats and platforms have a stippled surface which reduces suction pad adhesion. Cushions are made in a range of sizes, but if a special size is required, it is worth asking the manufacturer if they can produce a custom-made size for you. Cushions are of four main types (MDA 2001):

1. Comfort cushions: foam or air filled. These come in many sizes, from head pads to full bath linings. *Advantages* include ease of use and the feasibility of using them for more than one user in a residential setting. *Disadvantages* include the limited support they provide.

2. Self-moulding cushions: bead filled, enclosed in the cover with sufficient air so that they allow body contours to settle into them. *Advantages* include ease of use and the feasibility of using them for more than one user in a residential setting. *Disadvantages* include instability if the user moves, and a tendency to float.

3. Vacuum moulded: bead filled, with a pump to extract air. The cushion is moulded round you whilst the beads are mobile. As air is extracted from the cushion it becomes firm. *Advantages* include provision of customised support. *Disadvantages* include the bulkiness of some, which sits you higher in the bath; the firmness makes washing the back and bottom more difficult; and these cushions are only practical to use for one individual. This is due to the moulding process requiring time and care. (The cushion is stored in its moulded shape.)

4. Pressure relieving: gel filled. This softens in the warm water. *Advantages* include comfort. *Disadvantages* include their weight, limited support and risk of the gel 'bottoming out' under thin people's bony prominences.

BATH CHAIRS AND CRADLES

These support you in a semi-reclining position. They usually comprise a metal frame with a mesh cover, but some products for children are moulded plastic. MDA 1999 highlights the following:

Straps: many chairs and cradles have straps as standard, but several manufacturers will supply additional straps if required. *Advantages* include being safely able to use a product that otherwise may not seem to offer quite enough support.

Disadvantages include reduced freedom of movement and a mild hindrance when washing.

Size: many products are primarily for children, but the largest sizes may be satisfactory for smaller adults. It is therefore worth looking at the children's range even for adults.

Table 5.2.6 Guidance on bath chairs, cradles and cushions

	Factor	Bath chair / cradle	Bath cushion	★
Your (the user's) requirements	A little side support for trunk	Most chairs and cradles should be satisfactory	Comfort cushion to line the bath, *or* non-bulky mouldable cushion.	★★
	Full trunk support	Chest strap may be required	Comfort cushion lining whole bath may be satisfactory especially in narrower baths, *or* mouldable cushion long enough to reach mid-thigh to shoulder.	★★
	Head support	Head positioning pads available on most products	Comfort cushion lining whole bath may be satisfactory, *or* mouldable cushion long enough to reach mid-thigh to top of head, *or* head cushion alone (mouldable most effective).	★★★
	Support or padding for misshapen spine	Material mesh (not welded) accommodates bony prominences, provided the spine does not press against the bath surface; mesh *laced* on allows greater customised shaping than covers attached by sewing or poppers	Comfort cushion may be satisfactory, but bulky, mouldable cushion more likely to be needed.	★★★
	Protection from bath surface because of jerky movements	Straps are advisable; bath pads on inside wall of bath will cushion your flailing limbs	Comfort cushion lining whole bath may be satisfactory; other cushions usually shift with your movements so posing a risk to your safety.	★★★
	Tendency for hips and knees to straighten in spasm: you should have hips and knees bent	Most products enable this; straps are advisable as well	Bulkier vacuum moulded cushions will enable this.	★★

Your (the user's) requirements (continued)	Concerns about pressure points, shearing or sensitive skin	Moulded plastic seats not advisable; if mesh is uncomfortable, a towel can be placed between you and the mesh Crotch strap is often uncomfortable	Comfort cushions usually satisfactory; ensure a gel cushion does not 'bottom out' as the gel gets warm, so leaving you unprotected from the bath surface. Moulded cushions: extract air until beads stay in place, so cushion still yields a little.	★★
Care assistant	Lifting you on and off	A hoist will normally be used. See Chapter 6, subsection 6.3.4.		
		A mobile hoist with a stretcher style seat is available for use with a special bath range (see Table 5.2.7 and Illustration 5.2.7)		
	Assisting with washing	Good water circulation around mesh seats; mesh yields to allow soaping; commode aperture available on some products	Vacuum moulded cushions make back and bottom more difficult to reach.	★★★
	Placing and removing the product	Most do not have suction pads, but weight varies a lot from product to product	All except gel cushions are light, but suction pads have to be disengaged carefully.	★★★
	Adjustments	None needed after initial fitting of pads, straps etc	Vacuum moulded cushions are best if fine tuned each bath.	★★
Product	Maintenance	Products should be dried after use; mesh and straps should be laundered occasionally	Products should be removed and dried after use; thorough cleaning round suction pads recommended weekly to retain their effectiveness.	★★★
		Bath oils may cause damage to product: check with manufacturer	Bath oils will coat the suction pads, so careful cleaning necessary; they may also damage the cover: check with manufacturer.	★
	Replacement parts	Covers can usually be replaced; Velcro on straps can be renewed once effectiveness declines	Two types of cushion have detachable suction pads: replacement pads can be obtained.	★★

Source: MDA 1999, 2001

5.2.7 Special baths

The number of special baths has greatly increased in recent years, and new models continue to come onto the market regularly. The description of types may not therefore remain comprehensive as time passes.

Special baths are on the whole well designed, and the range offers features that equal or exceed all the benefits that assistive devices used in a standard bath provide. It is suggested that you familiarise yourself with the features you may wish to have, and the amount of support required in the bath, by reading through previous subsections in this Chapter (5.2.3 – 5.2.6).

The cost of purchasing and installing special baths is high. Also, many of them require more space than a conventional bath.

If you require assistance with bathing, the adjustable height facility is the most important feature, combining ease of getting in (with or without a hoist) and ease for the care assistant when washing you. The other key option is thermostatic control, which gives confidence that no risk is taken when water is added once you are in the bath. A shower spray is popular to enable hair to be washed during the bath, and is standard on several of these baths.

A 'spa' or whirlpool facility is available on several of these baths. Many people find this stimulating and relaxing. If you need cushioning you should not choose a spa bath that has jets situated under the body, because there are currently no cushions with holes that coincide with the jets. However, some products have the jets only in the side walls of the bath, so a cushion could be used. A whirlpool mat can be purchased for use in baths without the spa facility, but no cushioning could be used with this. Manufacturer guidelines for keeping the jets clean should be followed to minimise infection risks.

If you seek to achieve or preserve independence, the range can offer features to suit most needs, as can be seen from Table 5.2.7. Some suppliers may bring a mock-up of the bath for you to see. Alternatively, it may be possible to go and visit a place that has one installed.

Objective evidence is sparse for these baths.

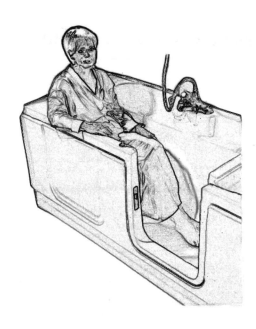

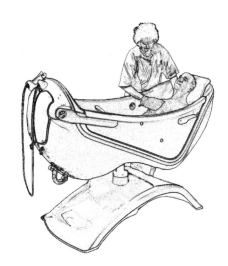

Tilting bath with upward lifting side door

Bath with side door (step-in; not suitable for lateral transfers)

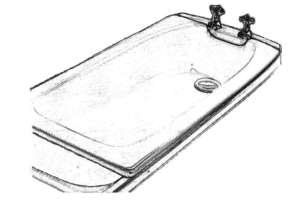

Shallow bath insert

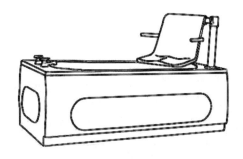

Bath with integral lifting seat

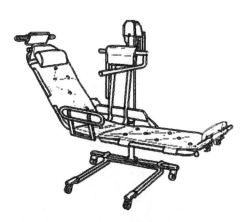

Mobile hoist with stretcher style chair that is designed to be used in a special bath

Illustration 5.2.7

Table 5.2.7 Advantages and disadvantages of special baths

Bath type	Advantages of the design over standard bath with appropriate assistive device	Disadvantages	Comments
Moulded with shelves that function as a bath board and seat (subsections 5.2.3, 5.2.4)	No need to position and remove separate devices.	You cannot lie down as in a standard bath.	
Walk in (seat faces you)	You bath seated with hips and knees bent at approximately right angles; rim to step over is low; reduced floor area required compared with a standard bath.	Water had to be run after you are in: some people do not like the feel of this; coldness of seat can be reduced by running hot spray over seat area before entering. You cannot recline.	Some products have a seat that slides forward, so you do not have to step over the rim, and a transfer from a wheelchair may be possible.
Side entry (more like a car door) with seat area	Provided the door opening is adjacent to the seat area as well as foot area, ideal for lateral transfer from a wheelchair; reduced floor area required compared with a standard bath.	Need to be able to turn hips once seated and lift legs over low rim, and shift hips to centre of bath; water has to be run after you are in, which some people do not like; coldness of seat can be reduced by running hot spray over seat area before entering.	Ensure bath is installed so seat height is correct.
Side entry with drop-down side	Ideal for lateral transfer from a wheelchair.	Water has to be run after you are in – some people do not like the feel of this; coldness of seat can be reduced by running hot spray over seat area before entering. Most models are longer than standard traditional bath. A deep drop-down side could impede a mobile hoist once lowered, so care would have to be taken when installing the bath to provide sufficient clearance for hoist base to pass under it.	Ensure bath is installed so seat height is correct. One product is fully cushioned, and has adjustable height, spa facility and a knee rest as options. It is therefore suitable for those needing high levels of support.
Side entry with tilt mechanism	Height suitable for most adult users transferring sideways or from standing. Tilt option means that those who need support to sit safely may feel safe once reclined. Some water can be run into the foot well prior to entry, so a 'top up' is all that is required.	Requires more space than standard bath, and is usually positioned so a care assistant can approach from either side.	Tilt mechanism can be manually or electrically operated. Bath cushions can be used in conjunction with the bath provided a spa facility is not used and the cushion is not bulky. Suitable for use with a mobile hoist. Adjustable height option; spa facility option.
Integral lifting seats: with lowering fabric band seat	Lowers from both sides so no need to shift your hips as you may with the add-on products (see Table 5.2.5).		You need good sitting balance.

manual swivel:		Seat would impede others using the bath. You need to be able to sit on the seat from a standing position because the height would be too great for a lateral transfer from a wheelchair.	
seat lowers outside the bath after rotating	Seat can be lowered to the optimum height for transfers.		Check with manufacturer re suitability for use with hoist. Cushioning or soft seats available on some products.
bath has moulded knee rest as well	Seat reclines slightly once down in the bath; if you need some support to sit upright you may feel safe once fully lowered. Knee rest contour is comfortable if you cannot straighten your knees.	Other bath users cannot slide down to immerse their shoulders.	Suitable for use with mobile hoist. Adjustable bath height option.
Integral platform: bath rises around it	Bath can be lowered for ease of soaping. Suitable for lateral or standing transfers. Contoured platform option for those who need support when reclining. Spa facility option.	Single working height not suitable for all care assistants.	If cushioning is required for support or comfort, choose a manufacturer that can put eyelets on instead of suction pads, so that the cushion can be tied onto the platform. Suitable for use with mobile hoist.
Adjustable-height tub suspended at foot end only	Free access around head and both sides. Small head cushion standard.	Requires more space than a traditional bath. Because of the wider head end, you may need a supportive cushion to keep you upright.	A mobile hoist with stretcher style chair is available from the same manufacturer, for use in conjunction with the bath. Spa facility option.
Shallow bath insert	Standard bath does not have to be replaced. Provides better working height for care assistant than if you were on the bottom of the bath.	Bulky to store if others use the bath. Depth of water is limited.	

Source: MDA 1999

Notes

With side entry baths, check the speed of emptying as well as the speed of filling, especially if you tend to feel cold when you are wet.

All guidelines have ** classification and arise from MDA 1999. Twenty respondents of a postal survey (111 responses in total) were current users of special baths. Site visits were also made to 12 residential homes where such baths were in use.

- *Side entry, drop-down side*: ten baths (Kingkraft Easibath) were reported on: five in the community and five in residential settings. The level of support provided was considered satisfactory by all except one user, and it was liked by users. The standard width (520 mm; 20.5in.) may not be sufficient for larger people, but an extra-wide model is available.

- *Side entry with tilt*: nine baths (Parker 400) were reported on: four in the community and five in residential settings. The bath encourages independence, and the recline enables many of those with support needs to feel safe, but some still required a cushion for comfort or support.

- *With lifting seat and moulded knee rest*: six baths (Parker 300) were in use in the community. All users found the support good, and the bath comfortable.

- *Platform and rising bath*: five baths (Aquanova and Parker 500) were reported on: two in the community and three in residential settings. Comfort was satisfactory, but the fixed height of the platform was not optimal for all care assistants, and users for whom additional support was required complained that the cushion or moulding tended to float during bathing.

- *Adjustable height baths*: eight baths (Arjo) were reported on: two in the community and six in residential settings. All users were reasonably satisfied with the comfort and support, but two sites found the bath did not lower sufficiently to get users' feet over the rim when they were hoisted in.

5.3 Showering

Each of the following subsections deals with a different type of showering device. In practice, whichever type of shower (subsections 5.3.1 – 5.3.3) is selected, some sort of seat or supportive product (subsections 5.3.4 – 5.3.6) will usually be needed with it. The need for rails (subsection 5.2.2) must also be considered.

As stated in subsection 5.1.2 *The decision whether to bath or shower*, the ideal is to provide facilities for both. If the bathroom is not large enough, and an over-bath shower is not appropriate, a shower cubicle may be sited in another room.

If an extension is being considered, a well-designed shower room need not be large. Pesola (1999) demonstrated that a 1.95 m x 2.1 m design could satisfactorily provide toilet, basin and level-access shower area. Harpin (2000) suggests a minimum of 1.8 m x 2.2 m; this could be reduced marginally if the toilet and shower area are combined.

BS8300 (BS12001) recommends different minimum sizes depending on intended use, varying from 2.0 x 2.2m for those who can walk, to 2.5 x 3.1m for those requiring an overhead track hoist.

As with all decisions concerning assistive devices (ADs), but particularly with major installations such as showers, your future needs must be taken into account, so that you will be able to get full use from the facility for a good length of time.

For short-term needs, options need to be considered that are speedy to install and easy to remove.

If you have difficulty in washing, subsection 5.1.3 *Difficulties with washing, drying and hair washing* should be looked at. Hair washing may be easier in a shower than in a bath, provided you can tilt your head back slightly, and lift your arms up and apply some pressure. If you cannot tilt your head back, a care assistant's hand can shield your face from the shampoo during rinsing.

When choosing a shower, it is important to consider the position and type of controls. You are advised to shower seated, because the risk of slipping is higher if you are standing whilst concentrating on washing and rinsing yourself (Kimbell 1999); so the controls should be easily reached from the seated position. The continuous spray of a shower is culturally disliked by some people, so if a tap is to be installed in the shower area to provide bowls of water, it should be sited within easy reach for yourself and the care assistant as appropriate.

The use of shower gel or emollients will make surfaces more slippery, so extra care is needed. If a care assistant is to operate the controls, these should be sited within reach for a person standing outside the shower area.

A thermostatic shower will prevent changes in water temperature during a shower. However, this requires a minimum head of water, so advice must be taken before choosing one. An alternative is an instant heater shower which runs off the mains cold water supply (DLF 1998). For either, it is worth asking for a safety cut-out facility to avoid risk of scalding.

Power showers may be invigorating but could be too forceful for children and frail adults (Kimbell 1999). Shower tray drainage may not cope with the rate of flow from power showers, so the rate of flow that the drain can take would need to be compared with the rate of flow from the shower: a higher flow from the latter will result in flooding!

The range of controls available includes touch panels, buttons, levers, dials with raised central flange, and rocker switches (DLF 1998). Testing the controls is recommended to ensure you can use the shower independently. Consider what you might need once in the shower, such as shower gel, shampoo or sponge, and plan where you can put them so they are easily reached. Over-reaching would increase the risk of your slipping and falling.

Ensure the hose is long enough to spray under the bottom when you are seated (Kimbell 1999).

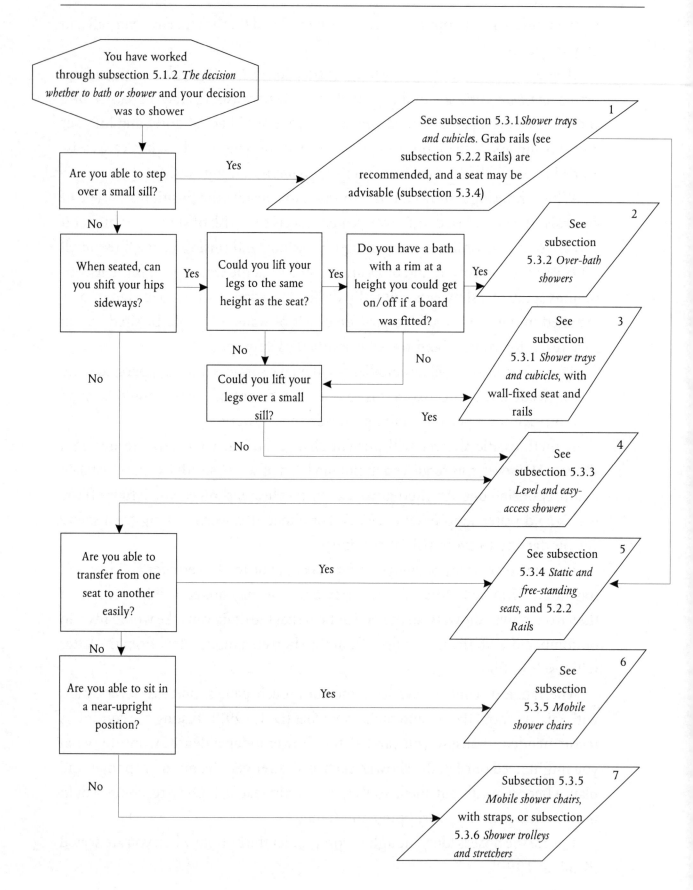

Figure 5.3 Pinpointing the type of shower

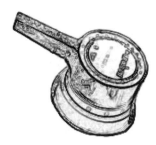
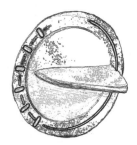
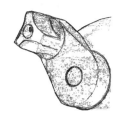

Some shower controls
Illustration 5.3a

An example

Stephen has muscular dystrophy, uses a wheelchair and can transfer sideways without help. He and his partner Sharon are looking for a new home.

- He has decided he prefers to shower, so looks at Figure 5.3, and notes that he cannot step over a rim, but can transfer sideways. He feels lifting his legs as high as the seat is tiring and difficult, so answers 'no' to that box. Although he can lift his legs over a small rim, he may not be able to do this in the longer term, so looks at subsection 5.3.3. Continuing down Figure 5.3 he again feels he should not assume he will continue to be able to transfer easily so goes to subsection 5.3.5 *Mobile shower chairs* instead of 5.3.4 *Static and free-standing seats*.

- From Table 5.3.3 *Advantages and disadvantages of level-access and easy-access showers* he feels a graded floor area would be ideal.

- From Table 5.3.5 *Guidance on mobile shower chair features* he notes he will need a self-propelling shower chair.

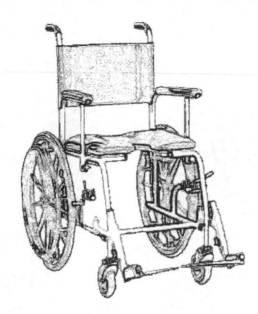

Self-propelled shower chair with padded horseshoe shaped seat

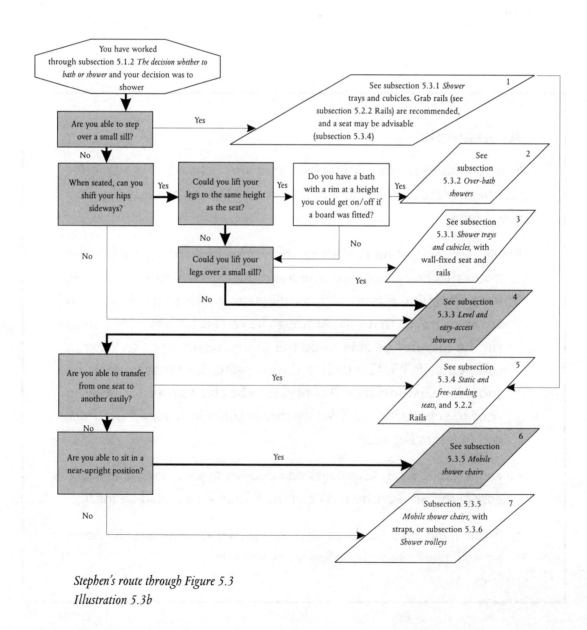

Stephen's route through Figure 5.3
Illustration 5.3b

5.3.1 Shower trays and step-in cubicles

Shower trays are usually plastic with reinforcement in the base, but non-slip stainless steel ones are also available. They may have panel screens that are full height or half height, fixed, sliding or swing-away, but these are usually assembled around the tray on site. The way that the panels move to allow you to get in and out should be easy to manage: some can require considerable dexterity (Kelsall and Cochrane 1996). The trays may have a lip to retain the water, in which case lips of 70-100 mm (3-4in.) should be relatively easy to step over (Kimbell 1999). However, it may be that you find steps more difficult when you are tired, or may do so in the future, so a level or easy-access (rim less than 15 mm (0.5in. or a ramp edge) shower might be a better choice. If you need a shower area with little or no lip, go to subsection 5.3.3 below.

Table 5.3.1 Guidance on shower trays and cubicles to step into

Factor	Issue	Guideline	★
Feeling safe	Steadying yourself as you step in	Vertical or oblique rail. Bear in mind that it will be used both entering and exiting the shower area: ensure it is within reach for both, or fix two.	★
	Steadying yourself as you shower	A combination of horizontal and vertical may be needed, or vertical and oblique if you use a seat in the shower (Kelsall and Cochrane 1996).	★
		If a vertical rail is used, ensure it is within easy reach (Clemson and Martin 1996).	★★
Warmth	Preference for a soak	A unit with seat area that allows some pooling of water around buttocks and footwell to soak feet is available, but it may be more difficult to get in and out (Hill 1996).	★
	Tendency to feel the cold	Heat is retained better in more enclosed shower areas.	★
Limited space in bathroom	Bath has to be removed to fit shower	Trays that fit within the space freed up by bath removal are available.	★
		Allow enough elbow room (min.800mm width recommended, Harpin 2000)	★★
Siting of shower elsewhere in house	You wish to retain bath, but no room for shower as well; or you cannot get to the bathroom	Free-standing cubicle will minimise the alterations needed. Some products have a toilet too.	★

219

In contrast to trays with panel screens, a cubicle is a free-standing unit with sides and doors, although it may look similar once fitted. A cubicle is easy to place in a corner of any room, and relatively simple to remove if no longer required. It may have a toilet and hand basin, or a drop-down or swing-out seat. If you use a mobile shower chair, see subsection 5.3.5 below.

Rails by showers to assist you when getting in or out have been studied very little. More than one rail is usually required because steadying is needed both as you get into the shower area and when actually using the shower, see Table 5.3.1.

It is recommended that you are seated during showering, so look also at one of the subsections 5.3.4 – 5.3.6. Ensure there is enough elbow room when seated in the shower area, and for a care assistant to reach where necessary.

5.3.2 Over-bath showers

The main advantage of an over-bath shower is that it entails no major upheaval in the bathroom.

The main disadvantage of this type of shower is that you have to lift your legs over the bath rim, and if the ability to do this is lost, the facility will no longer be suitable for you.

Always use a non-slip mat inside the bath. If the bottom of the bath is moulded, use strategically placed self-adhesive non-slip shapes.

It is assumed that stepping over into the bath will not be possible (see subsection 5.2.2 *Rails* if this assumption is wrong) so you should select a bath board with drainage holes for use when showering (subsection 5.2.3), or try a swivel seat that rests on the bath rim.

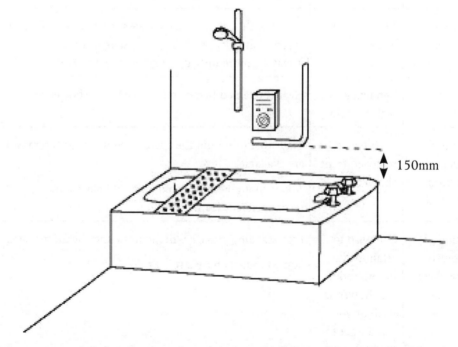

150mm

Figure 5.3.2 A suggested configuration for rails and over-bath shower for use with a bath board

Table 5.3.2 Guidance on over-bath showers

Factor	Issue	Guideline	★
Getting in	Sliding along the bath board	A horizontal rail in the wall about 150 mm higher than the rim.	*
Your safety	Steadying yourself if you stand when showering	The rail should have a horizontal section above the bath board with a vertical (or oblique then vertical) section in front of the board extending to a height suitable to hold when standing. Or fix a second rail.	*
You require a backrest	You cannot sit with your back unsupported for duration of shower	Swivel seat with backrest is available that rests on the bath rim, see Illustration 5.2.3.	*
Safety	Good water temperature control	Thermostatic control shower recommended. Use of hose spray fixed on the taps is generally unsatisfactory, and not advisable as temperature more difficult to control (Mann and Tomita 1998).	*
Able to reach the controls	Independence in controlling the shower	Site the control box within reach when seated on bath board.	*
Use of a bath board means a screen cannot be fitted to retain the spray	Water spillage	Ensure the curtain is draped with fold inwards across the bath board.	*

5.3.3 Level-access and easy-access showers and cubicles

If you cannot step over a low rim into a shower tray, then you need to consider a shower that has ramped access or is flush with the rest of the floor. An installation like this can either be a tray with level or ramped access, a cubicle with ramped access, a sunken tray with grille to provide level access, or a waterproofed area with a slight gradient to the drain. There is now a wide range of such products.

It is important to have sufficient room to shower safely, and for yourself or a care assistant to be able to reach all parts of your body for washing. There is no general agreement about a minimum size of shower area, but a minimum width of 800 mm and length of 1000 mm (31.5–39.4in.) (Kimbell 1999) if you use a drop-down seat, and larger (1000 mm minimum for both width and length,

Harpin 2000) if you use a mobile shower chair have been suggested. It may help you to visualise what space, rails and fitments may be needed if you mime the showering process, especially if you have assistance.

For a person showering seated, a seat height of 480mm, a horizontal rail at 680mm beside the seat and a vertical rail spanning a height of 800–1300mm is recommended (BSI 2001). These should be amended to suit the individual's needs unless the shower is to be used by several people.

A combination of curtains and half-height panel screens is available, usually as a different option supplied with the shower tray, but some screens can be fitted after a shower is installed. The alternative is free-standing screens, which are versatile and easy to move but may be tricky to keep in the place you want them.

Although the process of obtaining these installations can be stressful and lengthy (Picking 2001) they do facilitate independence when used with an appropriate seat or chair (Rhodes 1989; Adams and Grisbrooke 1998).

CUBICLES

An optional small ramp is usually available to enable relatively easy access if you use a mobile shower chair. A cubicle entails less structural work to install, and therefore although the unit may cost more than the materials necessary for other shower installations, the overall cost may be less. There is also less disruption during fitting. The drawback is that cubicles are considered less reliable, but there is currently no published evidence to support or refute this.

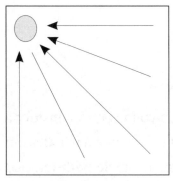

Fan drainage

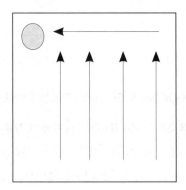

Inclined plane drainage

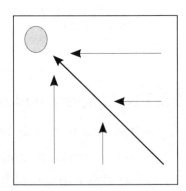

Single valley drainage

Illustration 5.3.3

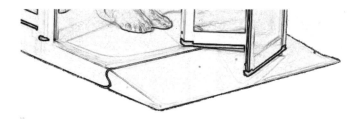

Ramped shower tray

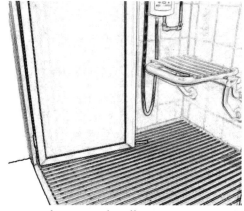

Sunken tray with grille

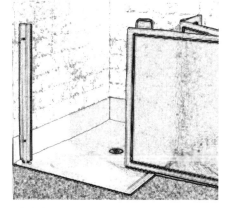

Level-access tray

Illustration 5.3.3 cont'd

If your bathroom cannot be made accessible to you, or you need to retain the bath and the room is not big enough for a shower as well, a cubicle sited in another room is one way of providing a showering facility. In theory the cubicle can be reissued to another person in due course, but in practice this is often not possible.

FINANCIAL HELP

In the UK, some financial help for structural installations such as showers may be available through a grant (the Disabled Facilities Grant) administered by the local authority.

MULTIPLE USERS

For an installation to be suitable for both wheelchair users and those who walk into the shower, an adjustable-height fold-away shower seat and an extended runner (or two shorter ones) for the shower head would be needed. The former is to cater for those who walk in (Pesola 1999), the latter to enable the shower head to be positioned correctly for people seated or standing.

Table 5.3.3 Advantages and disadvantages of level-access and easy-access showers

Feature	Advantages	Disadvantages	★
Ramped tray	Does not have to be let into floor.	Requires effort to get up the ramp. This can be particularly difficult with small castors as there is an initial slight lip.	★
Sunken tray with mat or grille inside so it is level with the floor	Flush, so easy to roll on and off.	Metal grilles can be heavy to lift up for cleaning. Plastic mats are light.	★
Level-access tray	Flush, so easy to roll on and off. No mat or grille to lift when cleaning.		★
Graded floor area	Flush, so easy to roll on and off. A fan gradient or a plane slope to a gully is easier for a mobile chair to negotiate than a single valley.	Fan gradient is technically trickier, and mistakes during installation result in water pooling.	★
Tray set into floor with waterproof flooring over	Technically easier to install than the above; same end result.	Have to select a tray from set range of size and drain position.	★
Panel screens	Contain the water well.	If the shower area is confined, it is easy to bang arms on the panel screens.	★
Curtains	Curtains that extend to the floor of shower tray and have a weighted lower edge should keep inside the lip of the shower tray.	Even with a weighted curtain, more spillage is likely than with panel screens.	★
Siting of shower elsewhere in house	Bath is retained.	Cubicles with ramped access are available for wheelchair users.	★
		Some have seats that slide or swing out to facilitate sideways transfers.	★
Ensuite cubicle	Provides toilet, basin and shower in a small area.	Toilet and shower combined may be culturally unacceptable to some.	★★
Care assistant	Splashing: Half-height panels reduce splashing and still enable assistance to be given from outside the shower area.	Half-height panels impede access by care assistant when washing your lower half.	★

5.3.4 Static and free-standing seats

Seats may either be fixed to the wall or free standing. Free-standing seats without backrests are called stools. Others have backrests, and some are adjustable in height. Separate, wall-fixed backrests are available for use with fixed seats.

When choosing a seat, also ensure there is enough space in the shower area for elbow room, and that a care assistant is able to reach where necessary. Also consider storage of free-standing seats if others in the household will use the shower: these products do not fold (folding shower stools are rare).

THE HEIGHT OF THE SEAT

If you are stepping in, choose a seat height such that your bare feet can rest on the floor, but from which it is easy to get up (using a grab rail if necessary).

If you are transferring sideways, choose the height to match your wheelchair seat (when you are sitting on it). If you want a seat outside the shower area to dry and dress on, fix two seats adjacent to one another, with space for the curtain or panel to pass between them during the shower.

If your needs are likely to change, for instance you can step in now but may have to rely on a wheelchair later, choose an adjustable-height wall-fixed seat so you can have it high at first, but could lower it to level with your wheelchair if you have to use one later. The higher cost of these products would also be justifiable in some other situations, for example for a child.

MULTIPLE USERS

In a residential setting, a level-access shower area with a wall-fixed seat that is adjustable in height and folds away would be appropriate. The seat would then not impede the use of mobile shower chairs (subsection 5.3.5 below) by those residents requiring one.

Table 5.3.4 Advantages and disadvantages of static and free-standing seats

Feature		Advantages	Disadvantages	★
Wall-fixed seat		Can be folded against the wall when not in use, so enabling you to shower standing.	The weight limit for each product must be checked: if you are large or heavy you will need a robust seat, possibly with feet to distribute the load between wall and floor.	★
Static free-standing seat		Can be used for other activities, e.g. at the basin.	Not as stable as wall-fixed; storage space required if others use the shower. Careful selection needed if the tray is plastic (see below under 'Legs/feet').	★
Seat	flat		Can be slippery and less comfortable than other seats.	★
	contoured	More stable to sit on than flat seat (DLF 1998).		★
	padded	More comfortable than flat seat, and conforms slightly to buttocks to give some stability.	May become slippery when wet.	★
	horse-shoe cut out	Easier access around the bottom when washing.	You might catch your legs in the opening if they are prone to spasm (MDA 1994). A new design with smaller split has been described (Nelson *et al.* 2000).	★★ ★★
	plastic seat	Usually has a backrest.	If the holes punched for drainage are of a size that might allow flesh to sink into them, place a towel between seat and buttocks (MDA 1997).	★★
	wooden slats		Less comfortable than other surfaces (MDA 1998a).	★★
Armrests		Give additional security during shower; assist rising to standing.	Should not be used in place of providing trunk support: a more supportive seat is advised (DLF 1998).	★
Legs/feet		Legs joined into a 'U' shape can be used safely on a plastic shower tray. Legs on a drop-down seat reduce the loading on the wall fixing.	Four separate legs may pierce plastic trays in time unless they are broad ended (DLF 1998), hence garden seats are not suitable.	★

Note: Further information from a user evaluation of showers is available (MDA 2002).

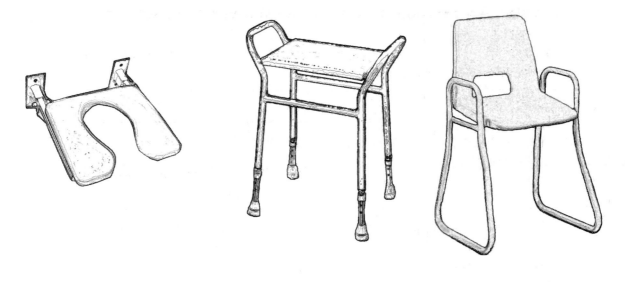

Wall-fixed seat with horseshoe opening

Shower stool

Seat with looped legs for plastic shower tray

Illustration 5.3.4

5.3.5 Mobile shower chairs

This subsection covers a wide range of products: basic shower chairs with castors; chairs with larger wheels for self-propelling; chairs that have multiple functions, such as a sanichair, commode or for bathing; chairs that are more supportive, with features such as reclined backrests, tilt-in-space facility, straps and moulded or mesh support for the body; and cradles. The key difference between shower chairs and products that are not designated for shower use but may look similar is that they are manufactured to withstand rusting and other deterioration due to constant drenching.

Chairs are for the adult market and for children. Supportive seats are mainly for children, although the larger sizes may suit smaller adults, and all cradles are made for adults, but some manufacturers will make to customer requirements. It is therefore necessary to consider products across the child/adult divide to ensure potentially suitable products are not overlooked.

Table 5.3.5 Guidance on mobile shower chair features

Feature	Issues related to yourself (the user)	Care assistant related issues	★
WHEELS			
Four 125 mm diameter castors	Attendant required to propel.	Difficult to negotiate thresholds; harder to push over carpet (DLF1998; Kimbell 1999; MDA 1994).	★★
Two 125mm diameter castors, two larger (314 mm) diameter wheels	Attendant required to propel.	Easier to steer than four small castors (MDA 1999).	★★
Two 125 mm diameter castors, two large (at least 510 mm) diameter wheels	Self propulsion feasible, but products without handrims may feel abrasive to the hands (MDA 1999).	Easy to steer and negotiate small thresholds.	★★
BRAKES			
Foot operated	Some designs can be painful if the ankles are knocked against them. Attendant usually operates the brakes.	Test in usual footwear for ease of applying and releasing (MDA 1994).	★
Two or four brakes?	If you wish to use them they must be on front castors and be tested barefoot for ease of applying and releasing.	Stability better with four brakes, but these take time to apply so care assistants often do not apply all four (MDA 1994).	★★
Central locking		Quick and easy to apply by care assistant. Not yet commercially available (Broadhurst and Grimes 2001).	★
Visual cue for on/off		Able to check instantly, and acts as reminder to apply brakes.	★
Hand operated	Self operated or by attendant.	No need for four brakes.	★
FOOTPLATES			
None	Must be able to keep feet off the floor whilst being pushed.	Chair is more compact, but care must be taken not to injure user's legs and feet.	★

Fixed footplate	Must be within wheelbase if there is any possibility it might be stood on (MDA 1994).	Increases chair's overall length, so manoeuvring will be harder.	**
Flip-up footplate	Not usually adjustable in height.	Cannot be mislaid, but the legs have to be lifted together to swing footplate up if user cannot lift own legs, increasing the manual handling risk.	*
Extra 'arm'	Drop-down footrest to support leg whilst washing foot (Nelson *et al.* 2000).		**
Swing-away detachable footrests	Usually adjustable in height. More liable to break if high pressure applied on them, e.g. extensor spasm (MDA 1999).	Less weight to lift one leg at a time when removing foot from the rest. Risk of mislaying detachable footrests.	**
ARMRESTS	If elbows are sensitive, choose padded armrests. Armrests should be used for safety rather than trunk support (DLF 1998).		*
Fixed	Stable (MDD 1993c).		**
Swing away	Check ease of unclipping.	No risk of mislaying armrests.	
Detachable	Facilitates sideways transfers. Check ease of removing *and* replacing (MDD 1993c). Least stable of armrest types, and durability less than for fixed armrests.	Risk of mislaying detachable armrests.	*
TYPES OF SEAT	See Table 5.3.4 *Advantages and disadvantages of static and free-standing seats.*		
STRAPS	All straps impede washing, so an alternative is to choose a chair that is more supportive (see below).		
Lap strap	Advisable for use whilst the chair is moving.	Loose lap straps are easily mislaid.	*
Harness for body	Good support.	Impedes washing the back.	**

Thigh straps	More comfortable than crotch strap (MDA 1999).		**
Foot straps	Stabilise the feet. A footbox is an alternative.		*
Head pads	Usually adjustable along a Velcro strip.		*
Straps made to customer specification	Several manufacturers are willing to provide straps in differing combinations or to individual specification.		*
ADDITIONAL SUPPORT	If you need additional support, it is expected that you will be hoisted in and out of the shower chair. If independent transfers are feasible it is better to choose an upright (or very slightly reclined) shower chair and use straps (MDA 1999).		**
Reclined backrest	If sitting balance is not very good, a slight recline may mean straps are not needed.	More difficult to lean the person forward to wash his or her back.	*
Tilt-in-space facility	Reclines the body without straightening the hips, so useful if hip extension spasm likely. Several products position you similarly, but do not tilt to an upright position.	Once tilted, the chair's overall length is increased, so more room is required in the shower area.	*
Mesh covering	If mesh not welded, it conforms to your body shape; comfortable and supportive (MDA 1999).	Spray passes through mesh to rinse body; can get 'commode' aperture in some products.	**
Custom-made cradle	Some manufacturers will make cradles to customer specification. Alternatively, consider a trolley or stretcher (subsection 5.3.6 below).		*

Data from MDA 1999 unless otherwise stated.

MULTIPLE FUNCTIONS

Sanichair and/or commode as well as shower

A sanichair that conforms to BS4751 (BSI 1984) will go over a standard British toilet pan. The position of the cistern affects the distance the chair can be pushed back, so push handles that project backwards or a looped push handle may prevent the sanichair from being pushed sufficiently far over the pan (Kimbell 1999; MDA 1994). Straight (vertical) handles would be needed.

If a shower chair also functions as a commode, there will be a detachable rack for a pan. Check the product fits over the toilet once the rack and pan have been removed. This is mentioned in Table 4.1.6 *Guidance on issues related to commode features.*

Sanichairs that provide a high level of postural support are now marketed for all age groups.

Bath and sanichair as well as shower

One product suitable for use in a bath is a cradle that can be attached to a hoist, which also has a mobile base that converts it into a sanichair and shower chair. This is mentioned in slanted box 2 in Figure 5.2.6 *Specialised support in the bath.*

Another is a more standard seat with its own hoist system for lifting the seat into a bath, or on to a mobile base so it can be used as a sanichair or shower chair.

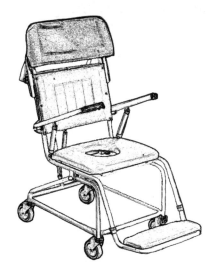 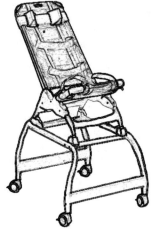 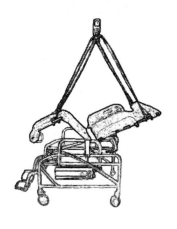

Shower chair with fixed footrest and tilt-in-space facility

Shower chair that can be used in the bath when lifted off the base

Mobile shower/sanichair. The cradle can be detached and hoisted into a bath

Illustration 5.3.6

5.3.6 Shower trolleys and stretchers

You lie recumbent on these devices. The trolleys are mobile bases with or without adjustable-height facility. They are constructed with a polyester cover over a frame and with a drainage collection tray underneath, or a vinyl mattress with low sides resting within metal supports. Currently two products are of more substantial construction. Drainage from the collection tray or mattress is through a single waste opening.

The height of these products should enable a care assistant to wash you without stooping.

The stretchers are wall-fixed, either over a bath (folding upwards) or over a shower area (products will fold up or down but not both). If the stretcher rests on the bath rim, a care assistant will need to kneel when washing you. Some are adjustable in height, and some have drainage collection trays under the polyester cover.

These devices may evoke strong reactions about dignity. Being wheeled along lying down means all feeling of control is relinquished, but from the care assistants' point of view these products minimise manual handling risks and make washing easy.

Drainage is not always considered satisfactory. There may be pooling around the user during the shower, and/or the drainage opening may not cope with the outflow. One user enlarged the holes in the polyester cover of a stretcher (MDA 1999); a trolley can be tilted a little more to encourage drainage although not all products have this facility.

Table 5.3.6 Guidance on shower trolleys and stretchers

Factor		Guideline	★
Yourself (the user)	Support or padding for misshapen spine	Non-bulky cushions (see subsection 5.2.6 above) could be used on the product (MDA 2001). One manufacturer will replace the polyester cover of the stretcher with a mesh material, to accommodate the spine more.	★
	Head support	Most products have optional head or backrests. Alternatively use a moulded head-support cushion (see subsection 5.2.6 above).	★
	Knees should be bent to reduce spasm, or knees cannot straighten out	One manufacturer has a knee rest as an option. Alternatively use a moulded head-support cushion (see subsection 5.2.6 above).	★
	Warmth	The room should be warm. Some surfaces feel warmer than others. If transferring onto the trolley/stretcher when in shower area, warm the surface by running the shower spray over it for a few minutes.	★
	Independent transfers	These products not usually used by those who could transfer independently, unless sharing a residence with people who are more disabled. Choose a product that is adjustable in height.	★
Care assistant	Assisting transfers	Horizontal transfer from bed to trolley can be done with a slide sheet (see Chapter 6). Alternatively, use hoist.	★
	Dual use as drying/dressing area	Choose product that drains well.	★★
	Many care staff	Choose adjustable height product.	★
	Central locking brakes	These ease the process of applying and releasing brakes. Available on some products.	★
	Manoeuvring	All trolleys are awkward to manoeuvre.	★★
Environment	Use of shower area by several users	Fold-away stretcher will enable the area to be used by those with shower chairs too.	★
	Limited space available	Fold-away stretcher allows the shower area to become circulation space when not in use.	★
	Avoiding excessive water spillage	If the stretcher is over a bath, ensure it either has a drainage tray or is narrower than bath to reduce water spillage.	★★

Data from MDA 1999 unless otherwise stated

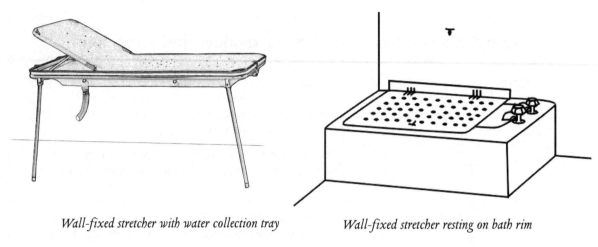

Wall-fixed stretcher with water collection tray *Wall-fixed stretcher resting on bath rim*

Illustration 5.3.6

Key points

This chapter has reviewed evidence concerning assistive devices (ADs) for personal cleanliness.

Although cleanliness may be satisfactorily achieved by strip washing, the option to bath or shower is usually preferred.

- Evidence to guide choice between bath and shower is presented.

- No evidence of formal trials was found on ADs for washing and drying oneself.

Bathing

- Evidence concerning taps and handrails is reviewed.

- Bath boards and seats are frequently used in combination.

- Lifting bath seats enable a user to get nearer the bottom of the bath than standard bath seats.

- Possible products for those who require more support are considered.

- Advantages and disadvantages of special baths are listed.

Showering

- Evidence on showering products is sparse; guidance is mainly drawn from expert opinion.

- There is some evidence to guide the choice of shower chairs.

References

Adams, J. and Grisbrooke, J. (1998) 'The use of level access showers 12 months after installation.' *British Journal of Therapy and Rehabilitation 5*, 10, 504–510.

*Survey: 26 tenants who had a level-access shower fitted in the last 12 months were contacted; 11 agreed to be interviewed. All but 2 were over 60 years old. The benefits they cited were increased safety and reduced pain; easier transfers and less strain for their carers.****

Agree, E. (1999) 'The influence of personal care and assistive devices on the measurement of disability.' *Social Science and Medicine 48*, 4, 427–443.

Survey by interview of 1509 from a larger longitudinal study of people aged 70+ years in Michigan. Statistical tests were applied to model probabilities. No indication of whether interviews were face to face or by telephone. Looked at how effective either personal assistance or assistive devices (ADs) were at removing disability. Examined diagnostic groups rather than types of task, and from the data predicted that ADs alone should be effective in removing disability for 58 per cent of those with arthritis, compared to 29 per cent of those with chronic lung disease. The author also compared those 'less impaired' and those 'severely impaired', and predicted that 76 per cent of the former should experience no residual disability with ADs alone, but this dropped to 52 per cent for those with more impairment. ***

Aitchison, E. (ed) (1999) *Safer handling of people in the community.* Teddington, Middlesex: Backcare.

A consensus of expert opinion, covering the legal framework, handling principles, training and equipment.

Broadhurst, M. and Grimes, R. (Personal communication 2001)

Have designed central locking castors for mobile shower chairs. Regional Medical Physics Department, Newcastle General Hospital, Newcastle-upon-Tyne, NE4 6BE, tel: 0191 273 8811 ext. 22192.

BSI (1984) BS 4751 *Mobile sanitary chairs.* Milton Keynes: British Standards Institution.

BSI (2001) BS9300: 2001 *Design of buildings and their approaches to meet the needs of disabled people – Code of Practice.* Milton Keynes : British Standards Institution.

This standard is for assessing existing buildings and guidance for new buildings for accessibility and usability by disabled people, but is not for buildings exclusively for disabled people. It states that, 'No single layout or design will suit all disabled people.' Its recommendations are therefore useful guidelines from which one builds an individual's requirements.

CAE (Centre for Accessible Environments). Accessed at www.cae.org.uk in November 2001.

Chamberlain, M.A., Thornley, G. and Wright, V. (1978) 'Evaluation of aids and equipment for bath and toilet.' *Rheumatology and Rehabilitation 17*, 187–194.

*The authors surveyed 150 people who had bathing or toileting devices 6–24 months post-discharge from hospital. Sixty-five per cent had arthritis; the remainder had stroke, orthopaedic or neurological conditions; 70 per cent were over 60 years old. They had the following: 115 non-slip bath mats, 85 rails by the bath (but other respondents may have commented on integral bath handles), 72 bath seats, 33 bath boards. Thirty-five per cent had bathroom doors less than 635 mm wide.****

Chronically Sick and Disabled Persons Act 1970 London: HMSO.

Clemson, L. and Martin, R. (1996) 'Usage and effectiveness of rails, bathing and toileting aids.' *Occupational Therapy in Healthcare 10*, 1, 41–59.

*Postal questionnaire sent to 293 former patients who had had rails prescribed. There was a 63 per cent response rate (n=185) of which 144 were analysed. The study findings showed those with lower limb impairments preferred oblique and horizontal rails, and deduced that this may have been because of their need to assist weight bearing.** The numbers were quite low (43 rails by bath with no breakdown of how many were* *oblique/horizontal/vertical) so can only be considered as tentative guidelines. Of the 70 interviewees who had rails by the shower, all but one were satisfied with the height and angle of the rail, but what these were is not described, except that 3 people felt that vertical rails were difficult to reach.*

Cooper, B. A. and Stewart, D. (1997) 'The effect of a transfer device in the homes of elderly women.' *Physical and Occupational Therapy in Geriatrics 15*, 2, 61–77.

A single product trial of a floor-to-ceiling vertical pole in the homes of 30 elderly women for a three-month period. Twenty-one of them chose to have it placed in the bathroom. No negative comments were received about it. ★★

Department of the Environment (1999) Approved document 'Part M: access and facilities for disabled people.' *Building Regulations (Amendment) 1998.* London: The Stationery Office.

Disability North (1998) *Bathing resource pack.* Newcastle upon Tyne: Disability North (in-house publication).

This in-house publication by a Disabled Living Centre represents professional expertise and knowledge. ★

DLF (1998) Disabled Living Foundation factsheets to assist choice of shower equipment accessed via the internet: www.dlf.org.uk/factsheets/ Accessed on 26/01/2001.

Expert opinion. ★

Edwards, N. and Jones, D. (1998) 'Ownership and use of assistive devices among older people in the community.' *Age and Ageing 27*, 463–468.

A random sample of over-65-year-olds from three health authorities in Scotland was surveyed. They found that 50 per cent of the 1405 participants used a non-slip bath mat, 21 per cent used a handrail by the bath, 9 per cent used a bath seat and 8 per cent used a bath board. ★★★

Galer, M. and Feeney, R. (1979) 'Your top ten aids.' *British Journal of Occupational Therapy 42*, 9, 212–213.

A survey showed that non-slip mats, rails, bath boards and seats comprised 98 per cent of bathing equipment issued by the social services departments. ★★ *[Although the source of ADs and range available is more varied now, the percentage of all bathing ADs that these four items represent is probably similar.]*

George, J., Binns, V., Clayden, A. and Mulley, G. (1988) 'Aids and adaptations for the elderly at home: underprovided, underused and undermaintained.' *British Medical Journal 296*, 1365–1366.

Survey in which about 25 per cent of a general practice's patients over 75 years were randomly selected (n=150); 140 agreed to a home interview. Hearing aids, spectacles, walking aids, wheelchairs, toileting, bathing were included in survey. The authors found that 59 per cent had difficulty bathing. ★★ *Only half of those reporting difficulty with bathing were deemed to need assistive devices.*

Gitlin, L. and Corocan, M. (1993) 'Expanding caregiver ability to use environmental solutions for problems of bathing and incontinence in the elderly with dementia.' *Technology and Disability 2*, 1, 12–21.

The authors described interventions with 17 caregiver spouses of people with moderate Alzheimer's disease, who were experiencing problems such as resistance to bathing, unsafe practices and increased agitation. Five visits over a three-month period. All the assistive devices and the majority of the behavioural solutions that the occupational therapist proposed were accepted and incorporated into the daily schedule. ★★★

Gitlin, L., Miller, K., and Boyce, A. (1999) 'Bathroom modifications for frail elderly renters: outcomes of a community-based program.' *Technology and Disability 10*, 141–149.

Longitudinal study in which 34 elderly people were assessed and supplied with bathing devices, and 20 followed up 3 months later. An additional 55 who had previously had bathing devices were surveyed too. Ninety per cent of the first group had difficulty in getting in/out of the bath; provision of the ADs significantly improved this; 85 per cent felt the ADs had made tasks easier, and 63 per cent now required less personal assistance. *** *Cites Hoffman et al. (1996) that 62 per cent of people over 85 years old report difficulty with one or more self-care activity.*

Harpin, P. (2000) *Adaptations manual.* Newcastle upon Tyne: Muscular Dystrophy Group.
Expert opinion derived from her experience with people with muscular dystrophy. *

Hill, G. (1996) 'Bath and shower installations.' *British Journal of Therapy and Rehabilitation 3,* 11, 586–592.
Expert opinion. *

Kelsall, A. and Cochrane, G. (eds) (1996) 7th Edition *Personal care.* Oxford: Disability Information Trust.
Reviewed products but did not formally evaluate them. *

Kimbell, J. (1999) 'When bathing is no longer an option.' *British Journal of Therapy and Rehabilitation 6,* 7, 330–337.
Expert opinion. *

Korpela, R., Seppänen, R-L. and Koivikko, M. (1992) 'Technical aids for daily activities: a regional survey of 204 disabled children.' *Developmental Medicine and Child Neurology 34,* 985–998.
Survey of 752 children with neurological disorders in a region in Finland; 209 used assistive devices (ADs); 49 of these lacked suitable ADs for bathing. Some children's devices could not be used, or were not functioning well, because the child had grown out of them. Eighty-five per cent of the 54 ADs for bathing were in use. *** *The authors comment, 'even though their fitting was not optimal, parents persevered with them longer than with aids for toileting because of the lack of alternatives' (p.995).* **

LBOTM (London Boroughs Occupational Therapy Managers) (2000) *Criteria for the loan of equipment to people with disabilities.* Social Services: Harrow, London.

Mann, W., Hurren, D. and Tomita, M. (1993) 'Comparison of assistive device use and needs of home-based older persons with different impairments.' *American Journal of Occupational Therapy 47,* 11, 980–987.
Survey comprising a single visit to 157 people 60 years and older who used or were waiting for ADs. A questionnaire about ADs was amongst the battery of tests. Those with both cognitive and physical impairments reported dissatisfaction with 33 per cent of their devices. Those with cognitive impairments had fewer devices and used those they had less, compared with the rest of the sample. **

Mann, W., Hurren, D. and Tomita, M. and Charvat, B. (1996) 'Use of assistive devices for bathing by elderly who are not institutionalised.' *The Occupational Therapy Journal of Research 16,* 4, 261–286.
Survey of 319 disabled people from a longitudinal study of elders. They were interviewed about bathing: 294 reported some difficulty bathing; 219 had a bathing device, 177 were satisfied with them. Data on satisfaction were analysed in relation to the users' physical ability and used to develop a model to assist prescription of bathing devices. For those without cognitive impairment, a hierarchy was shown to be statistically significant, in which devices were required as disability increased. The first two items were a non-slip mat then a rail; the other devices were not exactly equivalent to the boards and seats that are commonly used in the UK. The data reliably suggest that with increasing age, the use of a non-slip mat is highly recommended both for safety and to assist users to retain independence. ****

Mann, W. and Tomita, M. (1998) 'Perspectives on assistive devices among elderly persons with disabilities.' *Technology and Disability 9,* 119–148.

Survey by interview of 508 current AD users from a longitudinal study. Some users found difficulty in using washing ADs, so reaching some parts of their body was awkward, and others reported that the devices did not wash effectively. One respondent complained of a bath board taking up too much space. The number of board users was not specified.

A few comments about hoses on taps being unsatisfactory, but it is not clear how many of the 508 AD users had such products. **

MDA (1994) Mobile, *Armchair, folding and bed-attached commodes: a comparative evaluation*, DEA A9. Norwich: Medical Devices Agency, HMSO.

Formal comparative user trial in which 55 people tested up to 6 commodes each. 'Some' of 14 users reported getting a leg trapped in the apertures of horseshoe-shaped seats, especially when in spasm. **

MDA (1997) Safety Notice: *Bath and shower seating equipment: risk of injury*, SN9709. London: Medical Devices Agency.

Reported several instances of men's testicles becoming entrapped in holes in shower seats. Towelling or similar protective material between seat and user's body was recommended.

MDA (1998a) *Bath boards and seats: a comparative evaluation*, EL1. London: Medical Devices Agency.

Formal comparative user trial in which 42 subjects, with a range of disabilities, tested bath boards and seats in pairs, so 10 people tested each pair of products. Ensuring the board does not overhang the bath edge is common sense and a matter of good practice. Weight limits stated by manufacturers are fixed as a result of careful technical testing. Comments that an integral handle on a board may eliminate the need for a wall-fixed rail. A wall-fixed rail could be horizontal or oblique, about 150 mm above the bath rim (opinion not overtly based on the research). * *A mean of 2 out of 10 reported slipping on the surfaces cited. Less than 60 per cent of respondents reported boards with the cited surfaces comfortable (see Table 5.2.3); other surfaces were all reported as comfortable by more than 60 per cent.* *** *Some respondents did not feel the size was correct for those seats deeper than 280 mm, but the majority were satisfied with all depths. Only two (20%) of the testers reported the wooden slats comfortable.* **

MDA (1998b) *Portable bath lifts: a comparative evaluation*, MH1. London: Medical Devices Agency.

Formal comparative user trial in which 12 lifting bath seats were tested by 30 users, mean age 68 years; 67 per cent had rheumatoid arthritis. The products were divided into three groups, and users allocated to one of them to test the two or three products within that group. Each was tested for a week (total of ten users per product). Only one product was padded. It was rated comfortable by 77 per cent, compared with 38–82 per cent for the unpadded seats. **

MDA (1998c) Medical devices and equipment management for hospitals and community-based organisations, DB 9801. London: Medical Devices Agency.

MDA (1999) *Bathing and showering equipment for people with severe disabilities: an evaluation*, EL3. London: Medical Devices Agency.

A number of methods was used to gather information about all bathing and showering products that provided more support than standard seats. Three focus groups were undertaken to explore the experience of disabled people with bathing and showering devices, and review product literature together. Two were with parents of disabled children aged 10–16; one was with 6 disabled children in similar age group.

Current users aged 10–65 years were asked about their products through a postal survey (111 eligible returns), telephone interview (31 of the postal respondents) and personal visit to 12 residential homes. Opinions of staff in a further 13 residential homes were gained by post via a separate questionnaire.

*Two respondents (of 18) had used a towel to protect skin from the mesh; all 4 respondents using a seat with crotch strap complained of their child's discomfort with it.***

*Six of the shower trolley/stretcher users (n=32) commented about poor drainage. Four respondents cited the dual use as drying area an advantage; two found manoeuvring the trolley difficult; one stretcher over the bath extended beyond the bath rim so water spillage occurred.***

MDA (2001) *Bath cushions for people with severe disabilities: an evaluation*, EL6. London: Medical Devices Agency.

Formal comparative user trial in which 56 people tried different combinations of 5 bath cushions, for 1–2 weeks each in their own places of residence.

MDA (2002) *Showers for people with physical impairments: an evaluation.* At www.medical-devices.gov.uk

MDD (1993a) *Tap turners: a comparative evaluation*, DEA A1. Norwich: Medical Devices Directorate, HMSO.

*Formal comparative user trial in which 64 adults (mean age 60 years) tested 2 or 3 of the 11 products under evaluation, i.e. each tap turner was tested by 16 subjects. All had rheumatoid arthritis. Many found the products' appearance unattractive, but the results are not reported fully, so exact proportions cannot be determined.*** *Several products were difficult to attach, in particular the crystal tap turner (all 16 had difficulty) and the Easiturn for cross-head taps (11 of the 16 subjects).****

MDD (1993b) *Lever taps: a comparative evaluation*, DEA A4. Norwich: Medical Devices Directorate, HMSO.

*Formal comparative user trial in which 60 adults (mean age 63 years) tested 3 of the 12 products under evaluation, so each tap had 15 tests. These 12 were a representative sample from the range available on the market at the time. Ninety-seven per cent had rheumatoid arthritis. The shorter (61–71 mm) length lever was preferred to the longer 150 mm length, because although both were easy for most users, the longer ones were considered obtrusive. However, only 2 of the 12 products were 150 mm levers. One product had vertical levers; 14 of 16 testers found them 'awkward' to use.***

MDD (1993c) *Basic commodes: a comparative evaluation*, DEA A5. Norwich: Medical Devices Directorate, HMSO.

*Formal comparative user trial in which 18 commodes were divided into 3 groups; 40 users were allotted to 1 group and tested all 6 commodes in that group. Fifty-six tests of removing and replacing armrests on commodes: 48 per cent found them easy to remove; 36 per cent found them easy to replace.****

Meghani, Z. (1991) 'Study of selfcare and mobility aids and appliances by the elderly.' M.Sc. Gerontology, Kings College, University of London.

*Survey to follow up 29 people, aged 65+ years, who had been issued with 3 or more devices. A home interview was conducted 4–8 months post-discharge. Thirty-six per cent stated they had less instruction than they would have liked.****

Nelson, A., Malassigné, P., Cors, M. *et al.* (2000) 'Promoting safe use of equipment for neurogenic bowel management.' *SCI Nursing 17*, 3, 119–124.

*Developed a sanichair by a series of user-trialled prototypes. Features included deeper footplates with heel cups; 'Footlift' arm to support a leg at seat height during foot washing; sturdy swing-away armrests; larger diameter wheel rims.**

Parker, M. and Thorslund, M. (1991) 'The use of technical aids among community based elderly.' *American Journal of Occupational Therapy 45*, 8, 712–718.

Survey by interview with 57 people aged 75 and over who were selected from a larger study of disabled people because they had ADs or required them. They were interviewed and assessed by an occupational therapist. They

found that 90 per cent had difficulty bathing, but only 4 per cent were unable to wash their face or brush their teeth without assistance.★★★

Parkes, B. (1993) 'What the professionals need to know: to bath or shower.' Surrey: B.Sc. (Hons.) Occupational Therapy.

Survey by interview with 60 residents randomly selected from 126 residents in 2 high-care sheltered housing complexes about bathing and showering, and 33 per cent said they did not shower because they preferred another method, whereas 17 per cent did not bath because of a preference for another method.★★★

Pesola, K. (1999) 'Bathroom – an important detail in designing for older people.' In C. Bühler and H. Knops *Assistive technology on the threshold of the new millennium*, pp.392–396. Amsterdam: IOS Press.

Designed a universal shower room for ambulant or wheelchair users with or without need for personal assistance, and a mock-up was tested by people in a residential home.★★

Pheasant, S. (undated: *c.*1997) 2nd edition *Bodyspace*. London: Taylor & Francis.

Anthropometry, ergonomics and design text book. The 65–80-year anthropometric table is based on the assumption that reduction in stature is similar in the UK to the US, calculated from UK census data. ★★★★

Picking, H. C. (2001) 'Do disabled people believe that they receive appropriate professional support, information and practical help when adapting their homes?' University of Southampton: M.Sc. in Rehabilitation and Research.

Conducted three focus groups with people who had recently had adaptation work done on their home. These included shower provision, and several participants expressed how stressful the process had been.★★

Rhodes, M. (1989) 'A study to examine whether floor drainage showers, installed on the recommendation of the community occupational therapist, satisfy the disabled user.' Univ. of Surrey (Roehampton Institute of Higher Education): B.Sc. Health Studies.

Survey of 25 people who had had a shower installed within the past 12 months by interview. Seventy-two per cent felt that the shower had met their expectations, and independence was achieved by an additional six people following the provision, to forty-four per cent of the sample.★★★

Rogers, N., Ward, J., Brown, R. and Wright, D. (1996) 'Ergonomic data of elderly people and their application in rehabilitation design.' *Disability and Rehabilitation 18*, 10, 487–496.

Short lever taps can be up to three times more effective than crystal-style taps according to ergonomic studies reviewed.★★★

Schemm, R. and Gitlin, L. (1998) 'How occupational therapists teach older patients to use bathing and dressing devices in rehabilitation.' *American Journal of Occupational Therapy 52*, 4, 276–282.

The authors audited the amount of instruction in device use that the OT had given the patient, and the patients' perception of the ADs' usefulness for 86 patients seen by 19 occupational therapists. They concluded that 'More research is needed to determine the long term effectiveness of assistive device training' (p.276) in the hospital setting prior to discharge.★★ *The patients were 55+ years old, and had either a stroke, lower limb amputation or an orthopaedic condition, e.g. a fractured hip.*

Shipman, I. (1986) 'Bath aids – their use by a multi-diagnostic group of patients.' *International Rehabilitation Medicine 8*, 182–184.

Survey by interview with 75 people who had bathing devices (mean age 68 years). Overall 65 per cent were still in use. Joint disease was the only diagnosis that predicted continued use (sample also included fractured leg, stroke and spinal cord injury). Spinal cord injury was found to predict discontinued use but the author noted that the seats did not have backrests and these users may have required back support.★★

Sonn, U., Davegårdh, H., Lindskog, A-C. and Steen, B. (1996) 'The use and effectiveness of assistive devices in an elderly urban population.' *Aging Clinical and Experimental Research 8*, 3, 176–183.

Epidemiological survey to determine assistive device (AD) use amongst all the population over 70 years in a defined urban area. Half of this entire age group (n=140) agreed to participate, and 12 per cent of those 70–79 years were using bathing ADs, compared with 29 per cent of those over 80.*** Those refusing were more likely to be older (85+) or less physically able. This indicates that the results stated may slightly underestimate a general population sample of 70+ year-olds.

Steward, B. (2000) 'Living space: the changing meaning of home.' *British Journal of Occupational Therapy 63*, 3, 105–110.

A review of sociological perspectives on the home.*

Stowe, J., Thornley, G., Chamberlain, M. and Wright, V. (1982) 'Evaluation of aids and equipment for bathing, survey II.' *British Journal of Occupational Therapy 45*, 92–95.

Formal study of 100 people, predominantly aged 60–79 years, who required a bath AD on discharge from hospital. They were randomly allocated to one of two groups. The treatment group were visited ten days after discharge, and appropriate devices demonstrated and loaned until the permanent one was delivered. A further visit was then made to collect the temporary ones and give instruction etc. The follow-up interview for all participants was made at six months post-discharge. The study showed that making the 2 visits post-discharge resulted in 85 per cent of bathing devices being in use 6 months later, in contrast to the control group usage rate of 73 per cent.***

Verbrugge, L., Rennert, C. and Madans, J. (1997) 'The great efficacy of personal and equipment assistance in reducing disability.' *American Journal of Public Health 87*, 3, 384–392.

Survey of 9526 people by telephone interview, 10-15 years after the start of a longitudinal study. They were asked about difficulty with 12 daily living tasks, and the data from those who had much difficulty or were unable to do a task was analysed (n varied between 334 and 1164 depending on the task). Seventy-three per cent reported that they used personal assistance only with upper limb tasks (dressing, opening a jar) compared with equipment only (5% and 8% for the two tasks) or a combination (5% and 10%). Getting in and out of a bath did not show such a marked contrast (35% personal assistance only, 20% equipment only; 16% both). ***

Chapter 6

Assisted Moving and Handling

Introduction

In the course of everyday life, you move around a lot. Even within the home, you need to move between rooms to undertake jobs as different as bathing or preparing food, getting into bed or eating.

Before working through this section, it is important to do the following:

- Consider your (the user's) requirements, and the requirements of the carer and others in the household if applicable (Chapter 1, Stage 1 in Figure 1.3).

- Have in mind the environment(s) in which the assistive device(s) will be used (Stage 2 in Figure 1.3).

This chapter assumes that, in the process of going through the stages described in Chapter 1, section 1.3, decisions and arrangements for any necessary alterations have been made, and the quest for an assistive device (AD) is undertaken in the light of these (Stage 3). If you choose a hoist however, this may entail additional alterations to the home. This chapter guides you through Stage 4 of the process (see Chapter 1, Figure 1.3).

A disability can challenge your ability to move around freely, and the way to solve such problems will depend on how difficult you find any particular task. Each section in this chapter therefore deals with a different level of assistance. But within each section, the key tasks of achieving transfers, climbing stairs, getting onto the toilet, in and out of the bath or shower, and getting in, out of and moving in bed are considered, and presented to help define what features you would want products to possess. The examples give you an idea of how the Figures and Tables are used and may include additional things which could be tested or checked when trying out the two or three potentially suitable products (Stage 5 from the process described in Chapter 1).

Assessment of potential risk to all concerned is necessary for all assistive devices but when you are receiving help to move from one position to another, it is particularly critical. Risk assessment is described briefly in section 6.2. A hoist may be used if you cannot move on your own, but this represents a major shift from you actively initiating a move, to being more passive. The difficulties to which this change may give rise are considered in section 6.3. Finally, cleaning is vital when ADs are used by more than one person, and maintenance is obligatory (HSE 1998) for devices that bear a person's weight. Both these topics are addressed in section 6.5.

This chapter is written with the context of the home in mind rather than an acute hospital, so issues concerning operating theatre or emergency handling are not included. Issues external to the home, such as getting in and out of cars, selecting motor vehicles or scooters, external architectural barriers and boarding ships or aeroplanes are similarly beyond the scope of this book. Mobility problems outside the home are mentioned only briefly.

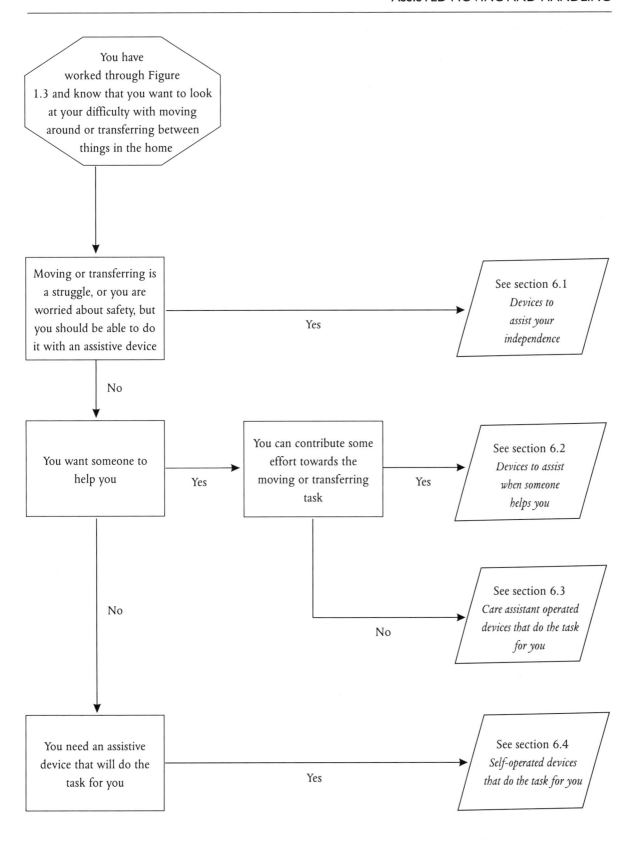

Figure 6 Difficulties with transfers in the home.

6.1 Devices to assist your independence

You have determined that you should be able to do the tasks provided you have the right sort of device to help you. Use Figure 6.1 to decide what sections you need to look at.

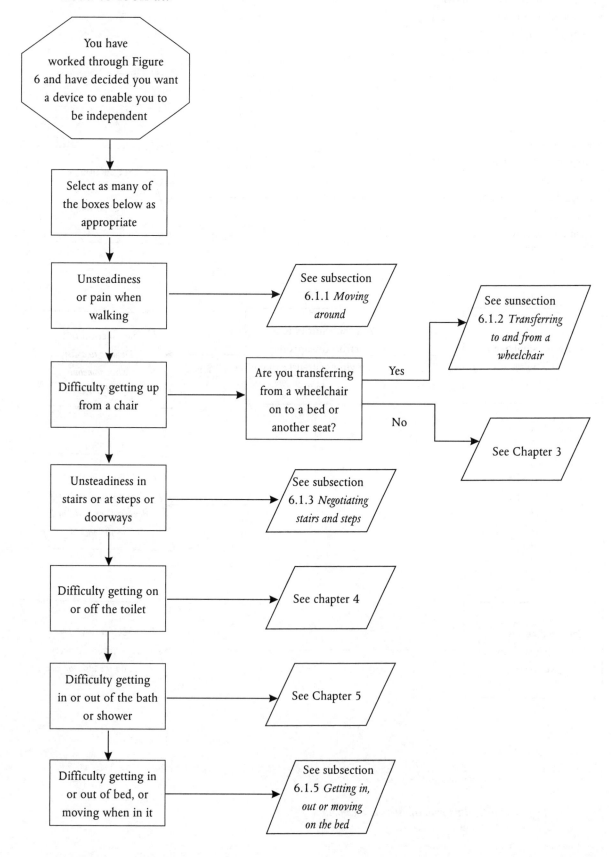

Figure 6.1 Where do difficulties arise?

6.1.1 Moving around

For many people, being unsteady when getting around the house, or a reduction in the length of time one can stand, comes gradually. It is often a fall, increased pain or a near-accident that triggers the search for something to reduce the risk of hurting yourself.

Walking aids are frequently issued by physiotherapists in the community or by hospital staff. Broad guidelines for which type you might find helpful are in Figure 6.1.1, but there will be situations that do not fit into such generalisations.

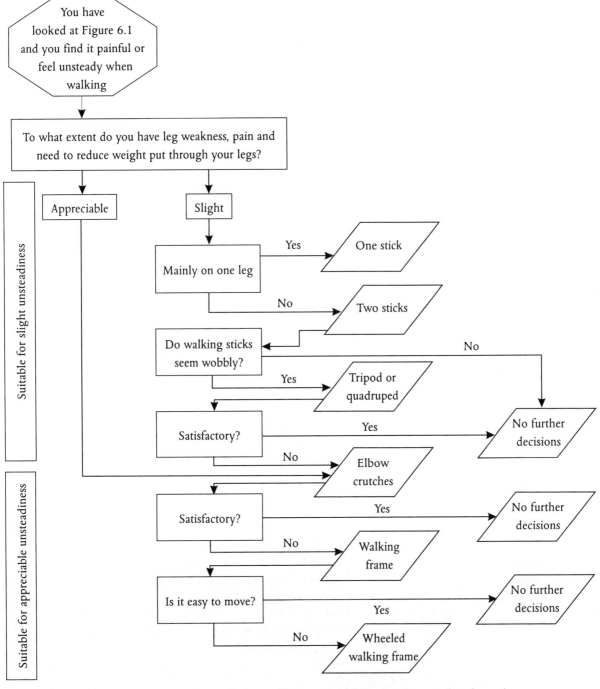

Figure 6.1.1 Choosing walking aids (See Table 6.1.1 for information about product features)

More information about features of different types of walking aids are shown in Table 6.1.1.

Table 6.1.1 Guidance on walking stick, crutch and frame features

Device type	Issue	Guideline	★
All products with feet rather than wheels	Safety	Rubber ferrules must be inspected regularly to ensure they provide good grip. Replace worn ones (Sainsbury and Mulley 1982).	★★★
All	Height correct for you	Metal products are usually adjustable in height, or available in several sizes. Wooden ones have to be cut to size.	★★★
	Handgrips painful or difficult to grasp (Mann and Tomita 1998)	Ergonomically designed handgrips can be obtained for metal products. For those with painful wrists, gutter armrests on crutches or walking frames cradle the forearm.	★
Sticks	Tend to fall to floor – difficult to pick up again	Three possible options: a ferrule with flange so stick can be stood up on its own an attachment to enable the stick to be hung on the edge of a table tripod or quadruped sticks which stand up on their own.	★
Tripod, quadruped stick	Safety	The wider base has to be allowed for when negotiating round furniture.	★
Elbow crutches	Ability to release handgrip temporarily	Cuff should be loose around the forearm, but the gap smaller than the forearm width so the cuff does not slip off when the handgrip is released.	★★
Axillary crutches	Can cause nerve damage if used wrongly	Not usually used except for post-fracture.	★★
Walking frames	Manoeuvrability	Wider base gives more stability but is less manoeuvrable where space is confined.	★★
	Transportability	Folding models are available but this tends to make them less stable as you put weight on them, as their joints give a little.	★★

Wheeled walking frames (continued)	Manoeuvrability	Three-wheelers generally easier to manoeuvre than two- or four-wheelers.	**
	Safety	The locking mechanism to prevent the frame folding must be applied whilst in use and checked regularly (MDA 2001b).	
	Transportability	Most are foldable.	*
	You require rests when walking longer distances	Products with a seat provide facility to rest when no chair readily available.	*
	Use of brakes	You must know how to apply brake lock if the frame has wheels.	*
		Pressure brakes (press down on handles to engage) may not be suitable if you are a slight person, or have painful wrists.	**
		Cable brakes (curl fingers round and squeeze) may be difficult if you have painful arthritic hands.	**
	You need to carry things	A basket or tray enables light objects to be carried. An alternative within the home may be a trolley.	*

Unless otherwise cited, data drawn from Hall, Barton, Clarke *et al.* 1991; Hall and Clarke 1991a, 1991b; MDA 1999b.

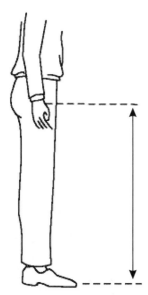

Correct height for walking aids

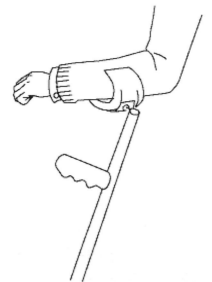

Elbow crutch cuff should hang on arm when handgrip is released

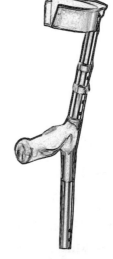

Ergonomic handgrip on elbow crutch

Illustration 6.1.1

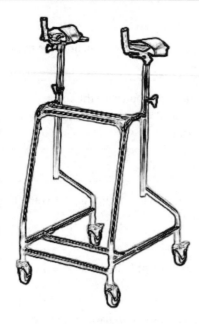

Frame with gutter armrests

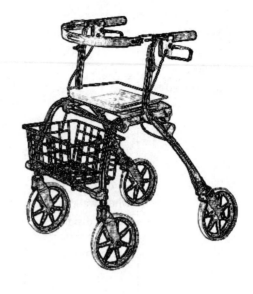

Wheeled frame with seat and basket

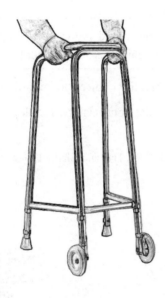

Two-wheeled walking frame

Illustration 6.1.1 cont'd

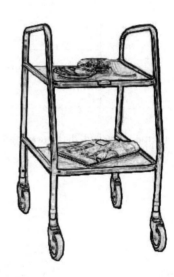

Trolley

With all sticks, crutches or frames, their height is important. The handle should be level with your wrist when you stand with your arm relaxed at your side. It is also important to check that the end of the stick, crutch or frame has a properly fitting rubber tip (ferrule) on it, and that the ferrule has a good tread to prevent the walking aid slipping as you use it.

The design of most of these products has changed little for decades. Recently, there has been a move towards involving designers as well as engineers, and the benefits of this should become evident as new products come onto the market.

This may help people to feel less self-conscious and attract less stigma when they have to use aids (Mann and Tomita 1998).

If you need a wheelchair, it is recommended that you discuss this with your local doctor (GP), an occupational therapist or physiotherapist.

6.1.2 Transferring to and from a wheelchair

If you use a wheelchair, you will need to get from the wheelchair to a chair, bed, or toilet, etc. If standing is difficult, but it is still possible to take weight through your legs, transferring is mainly a matter of technique. The manoeuvre will be made easier if the two seats are roughly the same height, and the height is a suitable one for you (see Chapter 3). When your legs are less reliable, it becomes more critical that the seat heights are identical, and that the big propelling wheels of the wheelchair are of a diameter that do not protrude above the seat level too much.

When little or no weight can be taken through the legs, a transfer board is usually a help. No formal evaluations of these products with independent users have been found, but advantages and disadvantages of different designs of board from a study of their use with assisted transfers are listed in Table 6.2.1a.

6.1.3 Negotiating stairs and steps

Flights of stairs will usually have a banister, but the handrail does not always run the full length of the stairs. Isolated steps within the house normally do not have any rails. If you feel unsteady or nervous negotiating steps, fixing rails by the steps is recommended. For flights of stairs, a rail each side is best.

- Choose a rail that is a comfortable size and shape for your hand.

- A second rail should match the height of the rail already fitted.

- If no rails were previously fitted, ask for a rail roughly at the height of your wrist with your arm relaxed, when standing on the first tread.

- If the stairs fan round a corner, fix a continuous rail round its outer side.

- Avoid gaps in a rail; get the carpenter to join rail sections together.

- If a stair rail does not overcome the problem, a stairlift may be appropriate (see subsection 6.4.2).

Isolated steps within the house can sometimes be removed by raising the floor of the lower room. If this is not possible, one or two vertical grab rails fixed in a position that you can reach going up or down the step should help. A floor-to-ceiling pole also has potential in a variety of situations for pulling or steadying oneself (Cooper and Stewart 1997).

Steps outside the front or back door can usually be altered if rails alone are insufficient for you. Converting the steps to longer (at least 600 mm; 24in.) and shallower steps (see Illustration 6.1.3) enable a person in a wheelchair or with a walking frame to use them. An alternative is a sloped path (ramp) which should have a gradient no steeper than 1 in 12 but preferably be 1 in 20. An outdoor platform lift may be necessary where the site is too steep for a ramp.

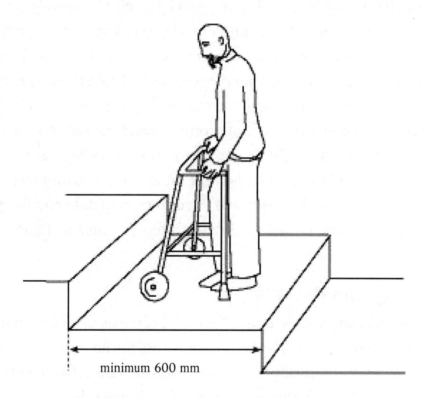

minimum 600 mm

Longer steps provide room for a walking frame and user, or a wheelchair
Illustration 6.1.3

Before embarking on major alterations or installing a stairlift to your property, it is suggested that you consult an occupational therapist who can help you decide what your best option is. In the UK, you can ask the social services department for an assessment of your needs, and advice about eligibility for a grant towards the cost of any work.

6.1.4 Bathing and toileting

Assistive devices to help you with toileting and bathing are described in Chapter 4 and Chapter 5 respectively.

6.1.5 Getting in, out of, or moving on the bed

A duvet tends to be easier to manage than sheets and blankets, because it does not have to be tucked in, and is light. It is therefore easy to fold back to get into bed, and flick over you once you are in.

Table 6.1.5 lists some of the things you may find difficult, with suggestions for how the problems might be solved.

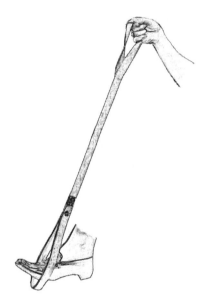

Manual leg lifter with stiffened strap and foot loop

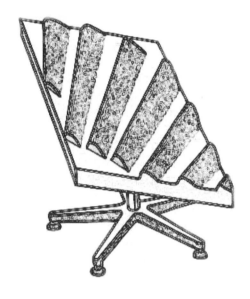

Ribbed slope fixed at an angle to help with getting legs on to bed

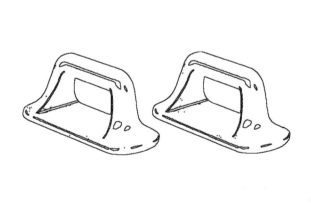

Hand blocks

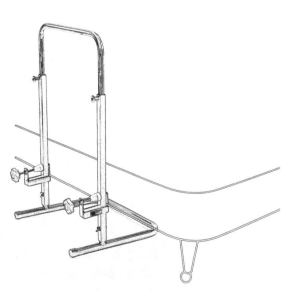

Bed grab handle

Illustration 6.1.5

Table 6.1.5 Guidance on bed mobility

Difficulty	Possible solution	Comments	★
Getting legs into bed	Manual leg lifter	It is easier to get the foot into a stiffened loop, but this is not quite as comfortable as a soft loop (MDA 1999a). If arms are not strong enough, or sitting balance poor, see subsection 6.4.5	★★
	Ribbed slope to 'walk' the legs up (Moy 1987)		★
Shifting hips up the bed	Hand blocks	Should have stable base, and comfortable handgrips (Moy 1987). If arms not strong enough, see subsection 6.3.5.	★★
Lifting hips off the bed	Monkey pole	Useful if a care assistant needs to straighten or change the sheet but not for moving up the bed.	★
Turning over	Smooth sheets and slippery nightwear to minimise friction	Technique: turn head, far hand on chest, far leg bent, and push with that foot as you turn (Aitchison 1999).	★
	Bed grab handle	If not successful, see subsection 6.3.5.	
Sitting up	Rope ladder Bed grab handle	If these are not successful, see subsection 6.4.5.	
Legs off the bed	Not usually a problem. One technique is to turn towards the edge of the bed, bend hips so legs are off the edge, then push up to sitting.	If this is not successful, see subsection 6.3.5.	★
	Manual leg lifter to control speed at which the leg lowers	May help if your leg is painful or a dead weight.	★
Standing up from the edge of the bed	Electrically operated adjustable-height bed	Lower bed when getting in; raise bed when getting out.	★
	Profiling bed (Keogh and Dealey 2001)	See subsection 6.4.5.	★★★
	Bed raising blocks	Eases standing up, but makes getting legs into bed more effort.	★
	Bed grab handle; choose one without gaps large enough for your head to slip through (MDA 2001c).	Or wall-fixed grab rail if bed is positioned appropriately	★

6.2 Devices to assist when someone helps you

Devices such as handling belts, transfer boards and standing aids (products that make it easier for a care assistant to help you as you stand up) can be helpful in many situations, but may not necessarily meet your requirements in particular areas such as the bathroom or toilet. These are therefore considered in separate subsections.

Once you ask someone to assist you, their health and safety must be considered as well as your own. You have to bear in mind that they may view the risks differently from yourself. A discussion together is the best way to avoid misunderstandings that could lead to resentment or missing out an important stage in deciding about how best to undertake the transfer process. When transferring with help, it is vital that you work together with the care assistant as one unit. Agreement must be reached about the method, about what the signal to move is, who gives it, and the destination of the transfer.

RISK ASSESSMENT

Injuries are often sustained when someone moves patients or clients or helps them to move. In the health sector, about half of all reported accidents relate to patient handling (Steed *et al.* 1999). In one survey 27 per cent of nurses stated they had injured themselves during patient handling during their career (Retsas and Pinikahana 2000). In 1987 the prevalence of back injury in the UK was 170 per 1000 nurses (Love 1997). These statistics prompted measures to revamp patient handling policies.

In 1992 regulations were introduced that encompassed all manual handling, including the handling of people (Manual Handling Operations Regulations, HSE 1992). This has obliged employers to avoid requiring their employees to do manual handling tasks where reasonably practicable. If this is not possible:

- a risk assessment must be undertaken

- risks identified must be eliminated or reduced

- training must be provided by the employer for the employees.

A survey conducted soon after 1993 when these regulations came into force showed that very few of the nurses who had suffered injury when undertaking a task had conducted a risk assessment of the task beforehand (Bannister 1996). More recently, systematic risk management has been called 'contentious' (Dale and Woods 2000, p.286), indicating that it is still not global practice, especially in the community.

The incidence of injury amongst informal care assistants, i.e. those who are not paid to look after the person, is also very high, but less well monitored. Two small studies, one with elderly caregivers (Brown and Mulley 1997) and one with parents of disabled children (Nicholson 1999) both reported an injury rate of over three in every four of the respondents.

The Manual Handling Operations Regulations (HSE 1992) do not cover informal care assistants as they are not employees, so grievances would have to be brought under a claim of negligence. To date, courts have been reluctant to find local authorities liable in cases of informal care assistants' back injuries (Mandelstam 2001). Information, risk assessment, training and equipment to manage the safe handling of disabled people should, however, be available via the local social services department, and informal care assistants are advised to ensure they receive these.

WHAT SHOULD BE INCLUDED IN A RISK ASSESSMENT?

The following represents a bare outline of aspects that must be considered. Other publications such as Aitchison (1999) should be referred to for fuller descriptions.

- *Load*: the person's size, ability to co-operate, limitations to movement and likelihood of unpredictable movements (Cook and Nendick 1999).

- *The care assistant*: general fitness and strength, level of training, frequency of manual handling duties (Pearce and Cassar 1999).

- *Task*: can it be avoided? Can it be made easier? How frequent will it be?

- *Environment*: constraints such as confined space, narrow doorways, surfaces at an awkward height; hazards such as steps, loose mats, trailing cables, toddlers or excitable pets.

The outcome of such a risk assessment may be that it would be advisable to choose a device that does the task for you (sections 6.3 and 6.4) rather than you and a care assistant sharing the effort required. This approach may be particularly appropriate for a frail care assistant, frequent transfers, or if your skin is at risk of damage from shearing forces during transfers. The last could result in a pressure sore.

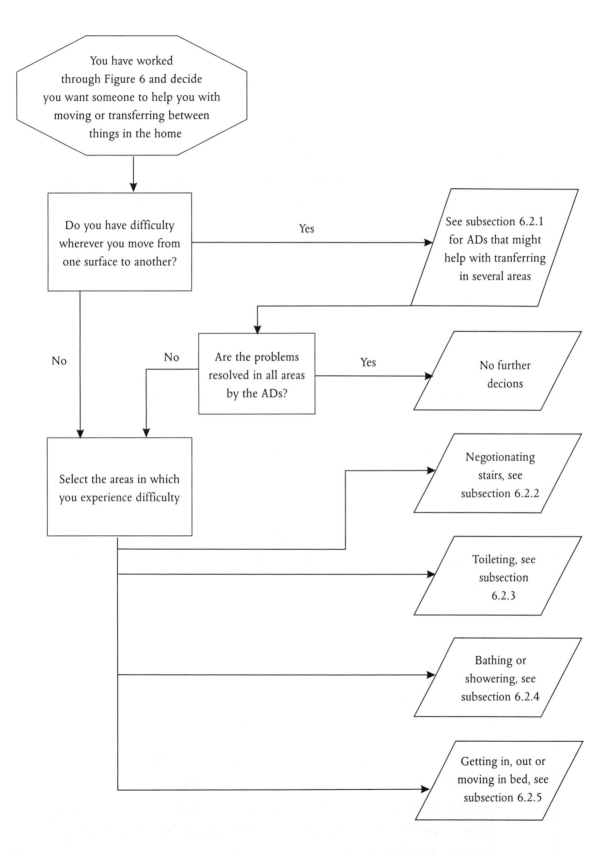

Figure 6.2 Where do you require assistance?

An example

Elaine has rheumatoid arthritis, and now uses a wheelchair indoors that she can just manage to manoeuvre herself, although the narrow bathroom door is always a problem especially as she has to turn to enter it. She has a rail by the toilet and has been transferring without help until a recent bad patch. She now is in a lot of pain and feels unsafe to get on and off the toilet on her own. Her husband Matthew is in full-time employment, so Elaine is alone for several hours every day except for her dog Lucky. Lucky is good company for Elaine, but is quite excitable and very protective of her. Elaine is of medium build and quite tall. She discusses the problem with the home care manager.

- They agree that her care assistant will need to help her on and off the toilet.

- Elaine can still stand up, so the assistance will be mainly steadying and guiding.

- They discuss the bathroom door, and the home care manager offers to ask the occupational therapist to visit and discuss whether the door could be widened and altered to a sliding door.

- The space round the toilet is confined. Elaine sees that she will have to position her chair differently so that the care assistant can get near enough to assist her.

- The home care manager suggests making the toilet seat higher, so that it is easier for Elaine to get up from, and the care assistant will have to stoop less.

- Elaine's care assistant needs to get a firm hold when steadying her. It is agreed that a handling belt will be provided.

- Lucky gets under the home care manager's feet whilst this risk assessment is going on in the bathroom. Although Elaine does not usually close the bathroom door because manoeuvring the wheelchair is such an effort, she sees that the care assistant will have to do so to keep Lucky out.

- Elaine is assigned a new care assistant who has had training in assisting transfers.

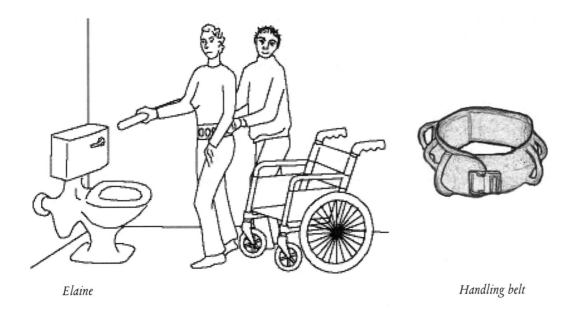

Elaine   *Handling belt*

Illustration 6.2

6.2.1 Transferring

The main assistive devices that can be used by a care assistant to guide and steady you when getting from a wheelchair to another surface are handling belts, transfer boards and standing aids. Handling slings and turntables are used less frequently.

STANDING TRANSFERS

When you can take weight through your legs, transfers from one surface to another can be a process of standing up, turning and sitting down on the new surface. You may need assistance to steady or guide you as you do this, and the assistant will therefore need to feel confident that they can get a firm hold. A handling belt can be used, which usually has handles to give the care assistant a firm grasp, and is put on only for the transfer. Handling slings are less commonly used now, because although they should enable the care assistant to avoid stooping, assistants have reported feeling less in control (MDA 1996b).

If moving your feet is difficult once you are standing, a turntable may prove helpful. You put your feet on it before rising, then the top platform of the turntable rotates on the lower one, so the care assistant can guide your turn without you having to lift your feet. It is best used in conjunction with a belt so the care assistant can get a firm grip.

If you feel you need something to pull on to help you stand up, standing aids are designed for this purpose. They comprise a platform on which the feet are placed, a mast (upright post) and a handle at a height that is easy to grasp. You grasp this to help pull yourself up and steady yourself once standing. Some products are easier to turn once you are standing up on them than others, but no formal evaluation has yet been undertaken. They are often used instead of turntables because of the additional stability they provide for you.

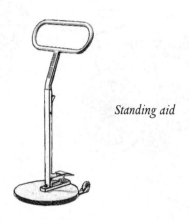

Standing aid

Illustration 6.2.1

LATERAL (SLIDING) TRANSFERS

If little or no weight can be taken through your legs, it may be possible to slide from one surface to another. Transfer boards are used for this, and assistance may be given only to steady you. This is because the twisting movement in the care assistant's spine encouraged by using this device would incur a high risk of injury if any effort were used to move you. The spine is at high risk of damage when exertion is used with such movements (MDA 1996b).

The advantages and disadvantages of transfer board features identified in a study that used them for assisted transfers are presented in Table 6.2.1a.

Table 6.2.1a Advantages and disadvantages of transfer board features

Design feature	Advantages	Disadvantages	★
Long (approx. 700 mm)	More stable	More difficult to position.	**
Wide (more than 250 mm)	More stable	May make positioning more difficult.	**
Curved shape	Can make transfers between two surfaces at an angle to one another easier	More difficult to store as they do not stand upright.	*
With handle loops	Eases carrying	Can catch on brake levers etc. as it is positioned or removed.	*
With integral low friction pad	Eases sliding especially when no clothing between board and skin	Not easy to position correctly under the user.	*

Source: MDA 1996b

A turntable may be used with a transfer board if you are rotating through 90°, for example from wheelchair to bed.

Factors that may guide choice between various types of device are shown in Table 6.2.1b.

6.2.2 Negotiating stairs and steps

Stairs can be daunting when you are not confident that you can manage the whole flight, and sometimes it helps to have a person walk up behind you and down in front of you. It would not be safe for actual physical assistance to be given, as this would put you both at risk of overbalancing, so you may need to look at subsection 6.4.2.

Steadying you at single steps is reasonably safe provided that the assistant is stationary and steady before you negotiate the step, so you can hold a rail fixed to the wall with one hand and the assistant's arm with the other. The alternative is to don a handling belt for the assistant to hold.

Table 6.2.1b Guidance on choosing devices for assisted transfers

Factor	Issue	Product type	Guideline	★
Your muscles are stronger on one side	Asymmetry during the transfer	Turntable	Harder to turn because weight unevenly spread. Position the leg that takes more weight towards the centre.	★★
You have a stoma, or recent abdominal surgery	Discomfort	Handling belt	Not appropriate if it covers the stoma or recent incision site (Cassar and Costar 1998).	★
Your height	Fit	Standing aid	Handle should be at comfortable height to grasp.	★
Your girth	Fit	Handling belt	Should adjust comfortably to your girth.	★
	Comfort and stability	Transfer board	A wider transfer board for a larger person.	★
	Comfort	Handling belt	Padded ones are more comfortable.	★★
Your foot size	Fit	Turntable or standing aid	Diameter should be chosen according to user's foot size so feet just fit inside the edges in usual footwear.	★
Care assistant	Getting a good grip	Handling belt	Handles at back should be horizontal. Padded belts are perceived as giving a more secure grip.	★★

Source: MDA 1996b

6.2.3 Toileting

Similar products to those described in subsection 6.2.1 above will be used for helping you get on and off the toilet, but the factors that make things more complicated are confined space, the need to adjust clothing, and that the assistive device should not get in the way when you adjust your clothing.

Lack of room is known to increase awkward posture or movements in those who assist transfers (McGuire, Moody and Hanson 1996), so extra care in planning the transfer is needed. Needing to adjust clothing also poses an added problem: an assistant should either steady you or adjust your clothing, never try to do both. If you cannot steady yourself using a rail, two assistants may be required, or consider hoisting devices (subsection 6.3.3).

6.2.4 Bathing or showering

Bathing is an activity that poses problems to a large number of people (see Chapter 5, section 5.2). Even using the kind of assistive device described in Chapter 5, you may still need some assistance. The key considerations should be to ensure you will not slip whatever surface you stand or sit on, and that the care assistant minimises stooping and twisted postures.

Subsection 6.3.4 below describes assistive devices that provide mechanical help.

6.2.5 Getting in, out of or moving in bed

Getting in, out of and moving in bed all place different demands on both you and a care assistant.

GETTING IN

If you need help with getting your legs into bed, and a manual leg lifter (see subsection 6.1.5 above) is not successful, often another person is asked to do it. It is worth bearing in mind that your legs themselves are heavy, accounting for 30 per cent of your body weight. The effort involved may be even greater if your legs are stiff. The bending required often makes people lift in a poor position, so increasing the risk of back injury. It may be appropriate to use a powered leg lifter (see subsection 6.4.5), then an assistant using a low friction roller (see subsection 6.3.5) could position you correctly in the bed. Some people find a fabric turntable under their buttocks makes swivelling easier as they get their legs from the side of the bed on to the bed. You would probably need help with removing this.

GETTING OUT

Similar tactics can be used if getting your legs off the bed is difficult. For standing up once you are sitting on the edge, you may need the help of a care assistant using a handling belt, transfer board, turntable or standing aid as described in subsection 6.2.1 above.

MOVING IN BED

The devices described in subsections 6.3.5 and 6.4.5 below are recommended if you cannot sit up, turn or shift yourself up in bed with a bed grab handle or other device mentioned in Table 6.1.5.

6.3 Care assistant operated devices that do the task for you

Introduction

The high incidence of injury amongst those who regularly transfer and lift people, as described in section 6.2 above, has led to much greater use of mechanical devices to relieve the load from care assistants.

Studies have shown that the use of equipment such as handling slings, turntables and handling belts reduced the effort and strain experienced when transferring a person who could not help take any of their weight, but even then the load was still above the recommended level for safe practice (Elford, Straker and Strauss 2000; Ulin *et al.* 1997). This is why such devices should only be used when the person can take a good proportion of their own weight. In contrast, a hoist makes a transfer of a person easy enough that 94–99 per cent of the female population should be able to manage it (Ulin *et al.* 1997). Hoists have been shown significantly to reduce the biomechanical load on care assistants during transfers (Zhuang *et al.* 1999).

Devices that do the lifting for you are collectively called hoists, but the designs now vary considerably according to the transfer undertaken. Further details about the relative merits of the product types can be found in subsection 6.3.1 below.

For some transfers, it may be possible to avoid lifting by sliding instead. Examples include moving in bed, transferring from bed to a trolley, and from one sitting surface to another at the same level. For these, there are devices such as low-friction rollers and sliding sheets, see subsection 6.3.5 below. It is imperative to use such devices when attempting to slide because it reduces the shearing forces on the skin that can cause damage and increase the risk of pressure sores developing. The reduction in friction also lightens the load for the assistant.

If you are unable to assist in your transfer, therefore, a device that avoids or does the lifting for you is the best method. It will not only safeguard the care assistant's health, but also reduce risk of injury to yourself, through mishandling and accidents during manoeuvres.

ATTITUDE TO HOISTS

The process of being picked up may evoke a strong reaction in you, because you do not feel in control, and it may have connotations of being returned to the status of a child. It may also be difficult to acknowledge that the strength you have is not sufficient to lighten the load on your care assistant.

All technology is a means to an end, whether it is using a car to get to a destination more quickly than one could walk, or a telephone to enable conversation with a person who is out of earshot. Assistive devices are no different, except that fewer people need them.

A number of studies has been undertaken to find out more about attitudes to hoists, among both users and care staff. The key findings are set out in Table 6.3 to illustrate possible reasons for negative feelings, and to present factors that could help counterbalance such views.

A five-point plan is quoted as a means of optimising nurses' attitude to handling devices in a hospital setting (Cowell and Shuttleworth 1998, p.129):

- Introduce a planned handling needs assessment for each patient.

- Eliminate all or most ergonomic problems before using new equipment.

- Educate staff thoroughly in equipment use.

- Ensure the equipment is comfortable and well designed.

- Explain to patients the safety rationales for equipment use.

THE ENVIRONMENTAL AND ORGANISATIONAL IMPACT OF HOISTS

Assistive devices have an impact on you, psychologically, environmentally and organisationally. This impact is particularly obvious for hoists. How attitudes and feelings about hoists are intertwined has been touched on in Table 6.3, but the impact on the environment is also important, as hoists are usually quite large. This means that storage space must be found for one, which is commonly in the room where it is used as this is most convenient. Having the device visible all the time is a visual reminder of your disability, which may be unacceptable to you.

The alternative to a mobile hoist is an overhead track. Once fitted this can be much less obtrusive than a mobile hoist, and moving whilst suspended is easier than with a mobile hoist. Installation, however, entails building work, sometimes major, and this is disruptive at the time.

Using a hoist also alters routines. Things usually take slightly longer, but you can be placed more precisely than without a hoist, so should be pulled about less. The introduction of a hoist may also make other activities possible again, such as bathing or using an easy chair. Finally, lightening the physical load on care assistants will often have a positive effect on their own morale and health.

Table 6.3 Factors found to affect attitudes to hoists

Issue	Reasons for negative feelings	Reasons for positive feelings	★
Your (the occupant's) comfort	Product and/or slings do not fit, or do not provide sufficient support. Slings incorrectly positioned around you.	Provision of device and slings that fit the user and provide sufficient support. Operator ensures slings are correctly positioned for every use.	**
Your perception of safety	Operator's confidence is low.	Reduces physical strain on care assistant.	
Your perception of dignity	Significant difference in perceived dignity between hoists, but no indication of factors influencing this (McGuire, Moody and Hanson 1996a).		***
	Some positions may feel undignified		**
Your feelings of control	Lack of involvement in decision concerning the hoist and slings.	Full involvement in consideration of dis/advantages of hoist.	**
Other psychological factors	Frustration with lack of ability, or lack of acceptance of need for hoist (e.g. those whose condition is deteriorating rapidly may be advised to have one, whereas they feel they do not need it).	Feels transfers are easier and enable user to take part in more activities.	**
	Hoist obtrusive, so acts as a constant reminder of disability.		**
Operator's confidence	Lack of training.	Clear handling procedure in care plan (Moody *et al.* 1996).	**
Operator's perception of the occupant's feelings	Considers hoisting undignified.	Considers hoisting is safer and more comfortable for the occupant (McGuire, Moody and Hanson 1996a).	**
Operator's perception of time taken	Perceived lack of time (Duffy, Burke and Dockrell 1999; Green 1996).		**
Environment	Lack of space (Moody *et al.* 1996).		**

Source: Conneely 1998 unless cited otherwise.

Training in the proper use of devices is particularly important when people will be lifted. Those giving instruction should have the requisite knowledge (College of Occupational Therapists 1995), whether the instruction is an informal session within the community or an accredited course.

One of the most frequent reasons given by professional staff for not using a hoist is not feeling confident in its use (McGuire *et al.* 1996b; Retsas and Pinikahana 2000). Training in the use of hoists is often omitted in the community setting (Cowan and Turner-Smith 1999). There are many models of hoist, and each hoist has different slings. It is understandable that a care assistant presented with a hoist and sling with which he or she is unfamiliar feels uncertain, and this anxiety is nearly always transmitted to the user. Your comfort is important, so the correct loops (if the sling has multiple ones) and correct points of attachment must be used. The correct ones, once determined by trial and error, should be marked in some way, and a clear instruction written and drawn in the care plan, so that different care assistants less familiar with the hoist and occupant position the sling and attach it correctly.

6.3.1 Transferring using a hoist

If you cannot assist when transferring from one surface to another, a mechanical hoist will be needed. There are several types of hoist:

- Mobile hoists have two legs fitted with castors on them, attached to a mast. A boom is raised and lowered on the mast, and at the boom's free end is a spreader bar to which the sling is attached. The boom is raised electrically or hydraulically. A person should be transported the minimum distance whilst suspended (DLF 1998).

- Overhead track hoists have similar slings and spreader bars, but the hoist unit is suspended from a ceiling-fixed track. The track can be straight or curved, and junctions are possible. A person can be transported small distances safely on these hoists, because the care assistant can walk beside them to steady and reassure them. A track hoist is easier to move from A to B than a mobile hoist and requires less floor space for its use, but obviously only reaches the area under which the track has been fitted. Alternatively, two tracks each side of the room have a third track across them, which carries the hoist unit so that the whole room is accessible. These are called H or X–Y tracks. Finally, several separate tracks can be installed in different rooms, and the motor (hoisting) unit is attached to any track as desired.

- Standing devices have a foot platform for your feet, and a sling that passes behind your back and attaches to the spreader bar. Once lifted to a standing position, you hold on to the handles on the mast and may be transported small distances. These devices require you to be able to stand with support when used with the sling behind your back, but not necessarily to put any effort into rising. Some products have a divided leg sling option, which would increase versatility. They are mostly considered easy to use (Zhuang *et al.* 2000).

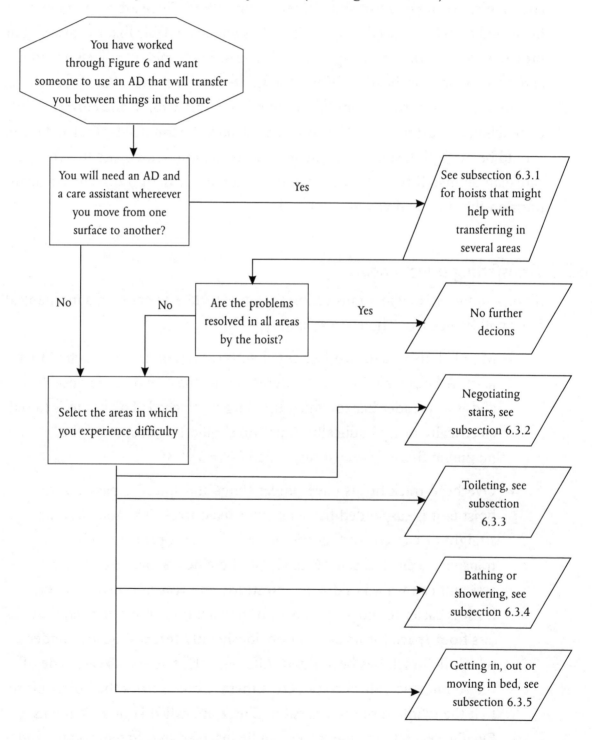

Figure 6.3 Where do you need to be moved?

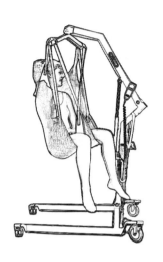

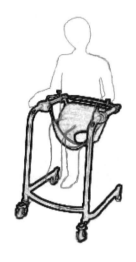

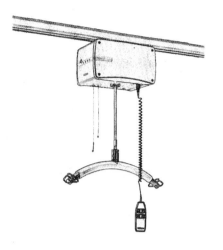

Mobile hoist   *Mobile hoist for seated transfers*   *Overhead track hoist*

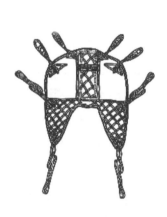

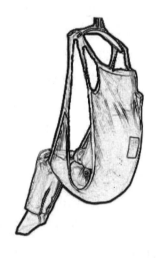

Divided leg sling with head support

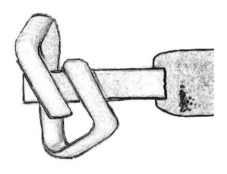

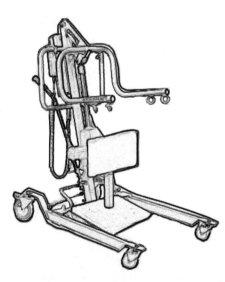

'Tight gap' on sling hook

Standing device

Illustration 6.3.1

There are few products specifically designed for children. Slings of suitable sizes for children are marketed for use with hoists.

Slings are designed by each manufacturer to complement their hoist. The main design is a one-piece sling with two separate leg sections ('divided leg sling') that are passed under the thighs. A one-piece sling like a hammock, which may have a commode aperture, is also available but as it is more difficult to get in place is less used than the divided leg sling. Slings of either design may be made of a netting material for rapid draining for use when hoisting in and out of a bath.

Other slings designed for a specific group of users, for example double amputees, or for a specific purpose such as toileting, are available.

Two-band slings with one band passing behind the back and the other under the thighs used to be marketed, but many users would be at high risk of slipping out between the two bands. This risk increases as the angle between the trunk and thighs gets smaller (Klint Edlund, Harms-Ringdahl and Ekholm 1998), so band slings should not be used. A study that used three sling configurations (one-piece, divided leg and two-band slings) on a number of different spreader bars showed that the spreader bar dimensions affected the occupant's sitting position (Klint Edlund *et al.* 1998). This means that you cannot use slings even of the same general type but made by different manufacturers interchangeably, because you may end up being suspended at an angle that is either uncomfortable, or unsatisfactory for placing you into a good sitting posture in a chair. The other implication is that whilst the manufacturer makes slings to support average people at an acceptable angle, if you are not a standard 'small', 'medium' or large' you will need to find the best sling and loop options by a process of trial and error. The best or 'optimum' configuration should be carefully recorded to ensure it becomes part of your hoisting protocol.

If no available slings meet your needs, some manufacturers will make bespoke (made to order) slings.

Most research studies have been on mobile rather than track hoists, and their findings or recommendations are summarised in Table 6.3.1.

An example

Ian is an engineer, but has had to give up work recently because his motor neurone disease has progressed to the point where he cannot walk, and handling even lightweight things is becoming a problem. He enjoyed the assessment for arm supports and a suitable computer set-up, taking a professional interest in the product design and functioning. His occupational therapist broached the subject of a hoist, to make transferring from powered chair to bed and toilet easier for his wife Jenny. It was too raw a reminder of his increasing weakness, and he shouted her out of the house. The next day he telephoned her, apologised for his reaction, and said that after a long talk with Jenny he now appreciated her needs as well as his own.

The occupational therapist returned with lots of brochures of differing types of hoist. She, Ian and Jenny worked through Ian's current and future possible needs, emphasising what Ian would like to be able to achieve despite increasing paralysis. Once Ian expressed what the most important things were to him, he could begin to see how hoisting could make transfers less of a major anxiety, and that it would reduce the risk of Jenny or care assistants, if they needed them in the future, injuring themselves.

They looked at the types of hoist. Ian thought the overhead hoist looked least obtrusive, but the occupational therapist pointed out that grant assistance for installing these took a very long time, and suggested that she met Ian and Jenny at the local Independent Living Centre (ILC) to try one or two mobile hoists as an interim measure.

After trying the hoists at the ILC that Ian and Jenny felt might be suitable, Jenny asked for one with electrically operated leg-spreader because they had thick carpets and she struggled even on the smooth ILC floor. When the hoist arrived, the occupational therapist came and trained Jenny in its use, and also tried different sling loops on the spreader bar until Ian felt comfortable, and Jenny could lower him into a good position in the powered wheelchair. They marked these loops with tape.

Now they have established their routine, Ian and Jenny feel much better about the hoist, and find they snap at one another less because they are less anxious about the transfers.

Table 6.3.1 Guidance on factors affecting choice of mobile hoist

Factor	Guideline	★
YOURSELF (the occupant)		
Poor head control	Select sling that has head support section.	*
Comfort	The relationship between sling and spreader bar, and the length of the boom need to be checked to ensure your face is not too close to the spreader bar, and that your knees do not bang the mast.	**
	Mesh material has more give, so may be appropriate if comfort is an issue for you.	*
Skin protection	Padded edges to sling, especially under thighs, enhance comfort and reduce risk of skin damage (MDA 1994).	**
Safety	Greater support area increases your feeling of security in a sling (Klint Edlund *et al.* 1998). A more enveloping sling makes adjusting clothing for toileting more difficult, and some manufacturers make a special toileting sling. This should not be used for other transfers unless you are secure in it, and it would be unsuitable if you have poor trunk control (Cassar and Costar 1998).	*** **
	Hoist load capacity must be checked against your weight.	****
	Sling size should be chosen according to your weight and height (Cassar and Costar 1998).	**
Facility to be lifted up from the floor	Some products can only do this if you sit up first; some have sharp edges, knobs or pedals that could catch your legs.	**
OPERATOR		
Overall ease of use	A significant difference between different mobile hoists has been noted, indicating that trial is imperative before a final decision is made (Zhuang *et al.* 2000).	***
Ease of sling attachment	The sling attachment mechanism on the spreader bar should allow ease of getting the sling on and off, without raising the risk of it pulling out inadvertently. More operators found 'tight gap' hooks more difficult to use than other types (see Illustration 6.3.1).	**
Ease of spreading hoist legs	Electrical operation easiest but noisy.	**
	Preference for pedal or hand levers varies (Hignett 1998; MDA 2000).	**
Learnability	Where slings have two or three sized loops, they should be colour-coded for easy identification (McGuire, Moody and Hanson 1996a).	*

Ease of manoeuvring	Larger ones more stable but less manoeuvrable.	**
	Weight of hoist was not found to have a direct relation manoeuvrability.	
	Weight of occupant affects ease of turning more than pushing.	**
Securing the hoist	Kick (push button) brakes preferred, but can be difficult to judge whether on or off.	**
Maintaining a good posture	Handle positions should enable operator to hold them without stooping (Zhuang *et al.* 1999).	**
ENVIRONMENT		
Ease of moving	Larger diameter wheels (min. 75 mm) may cope with carpet better than smaller, but other factors masked the results.	**
	Rubber wheels perform less well on carpet but better on a slope.	**
	Smaller hoists have been considered unstable (MDD 1993; McGuire, Moody and Hanson 1996a).	**
Compatibility with other equipment	Ensure upper limit of hoist's range of lift is high enough to get you on to the bed, and into the bath (if applicable).	**
	Check the legs spread sufficiently wide to fit round the chairs etc. with which the hoist will be used	*

Data drawn from MDA 2000 unless cited otherwise.

6.3.2 Negotiating stairs

If you are not able to operate a lift yourself (see subsection 6.4.2), all models have call and send buttons that a care assistant can operate for you.

6.3.3 Toileting

A hoist would be needed if you require mechanical assistance to transfer to and from the toilet. Special toileting slings for hoists are made that allow freer access to adjust clothing than the standard divided leg slings.

Confined space is usually a complicating factor in the toilet, but the final decision about whether to use a standing device, mobile hoist or track hoist will depend on what device is needed for other transfers during the day. One versatile device in a person's home is usually preferable to several devices each specific to one place or task. In residential accommodation, however, the higher frequency of use in each area such as toilet or bath, and the greater space usually available, makes devices dedicated to one area more cost- and time-effective. One of the reasons frequently given for not using handling devices is that the right equipment was not conveniently to hand (Moody *et al.* 1996), so a full ergonomic assessment of the pattern of handling needs in a residential home would be advisable prior to deciding what devices to purchase.

Hoists often look rather ungainly but improving their appearance is not easy. One attempt at a radically new design (Le Bon and Forrester 1997) was mechanically sound, but proved uncomfortable and undignified for the user, and bulky to store. This exemplifies the importance of including the users at the outset of such a project, and at every stage of development, to ensure that such parameters are built into the specifications for a device (Poulson and Richardson 1998).

Automatic bidet devices to give independence in cleansing after toileting are described in Chapter 4 (subsection 4.1.4).

6.3.4 Bathing or showering

When you need to be raised and lowered into a bath, but can transfer on and off a seat, lifting bath seats should meet your needs (Chapter 5, subsection 5.2.5).

If you need appreciable help with transferring on and off a seat, then a hoist would be recommended. There are several options:

- A mobile hoist can be used with a netting sling that allows water to drain away from it quickly. Sufficient space under the bath is needed to allow the hoist legs to pass under the tub, and the bath panel cut away as appropriate.

- A track hoist system may include accessing the bath.

- A fixed hoist system dedicated to use for the bath, see Chapter 5, subsections 5.2.4 and 5.2.7.

- A spring-assisted lifting platform on which a bath seat is fixed. See Chapter 5, subsection 5.2.6.

- A dedicated hoist system, for example a mobile hoist with a stretcher style chair that is designed to be used in a special bath, see Chapter 5, Table 5.2.7 and Illustration 5.2.7.

- A cradle that can be hoisted in and out of the bath or placed on a mobile base. See Chapter 5, subsection 5.3.5.

There are variations and combinations of products, which provide some flexibility in use, and some advantages and disadvantages of the above options are listed in Table 6.3.4.

Table 6.3.4 Advantages and disadvantages of different options for hoisted bathing

Option	Advantages	Disadvantages
Mobile hoist	Useful for many other transfer tasks.	Requires bath high enough from floor to get hoist legs underneath the tub.
Track hoist	Does not require floor space for manoeuvring. If bedroom wall is adjacent to bathroom a door can be made to allow a direct route.	If bedroom not adjacent, the track has to pass through two doorways (a long, undignified ride when naked, and doorways have to be altered structurally); or a separate track must be installed within the bathroom.
Fixed hoist	No transporting or set-up time required.	You will find the majority of these devices have seats which require you to be able to sit independently. Takes up more space in the bathroom. (See also Chapter 5, subsections 5.2.5 and 5.2.7.)
Spring-assisted lifting platform onto which the cradle is fixed	Mechanical help with lifting you up from the bottom of the bath.	You would still have to be placed in the cradle so it is more appropriate for children (see Chapter 5, subsection 5.2.6).
Stretcher style chair on mobile hoist	Supports you well during transport and the chair lowers directly into the bath. Backrest lowers so *horizontal transfers* are possible.	Can only be used with the manufacturer's special bath, so is more suitable for residential settings. Not suitable for other transfers.
Cradle support within the bath that can be hoisted out	It can be placed on a mobile base to function as a sanichair or shower chair as well, (see Chapter 5, subsection 5.3.5).	You sit quite high in the bath so immersion is limited. The cradle is reclined so takes up more room than an upright chair.

6.3.5 Getting in, out of or moving in bed

IN AND OUT OF BED

If standing aids (subsection 6.2.1 above) are not suitable, a hoist will be needed.

- A standing device (6.3.2 above) may be suitable if you can bear weight through your legs.

- A mobile hoist will require clearance under the bed for its legs.

- A track hoist will mean the bed position cannot be altered. It must pass directly over the position where the hips must be on the bed.

- A special adjustable height chair that can be altered to a flat stretcher configuration (Owen and Fragala 1999; Cowell and Shuttleworth 1998) is an alternative to a hoist for bed to chair transfers. This would require the use of a sliding sheet or low-friction roller (see below) to help you to get from the bed to the chair.

MOVING IN BED

Mechanical assistance with sitting up in bed is described in subsection 6.4.5 below. When others must help you sit up, the use of a profiling bed, sliding sheet or short low-friction rollers is recommended. Profiling beds have been shown to reduce the amount of manual handling required in a hospital setting (Keogh and Dealey 2001).

- Sliding (or glide) sheets are single pieces of slippery material usually with handles. The movement occurs between the bed linen and the sliding sheet.

- Two sliding sheets with the low-friction surfaces together. The movement occurs between the two layers.

- Low-friction rollers are sewn into a tube shape and have the low-friction material on their inner surface. The flattened roller is placed under you, and the movement occurs between the two layers of the roller. One long or two or more short rollers may be used.

- Rigid handling devices have not proved as effective as the above (MDA 1997).

Factors affecting choice of device vary from situation to situation, and guidance concerning these is in Table 6.3.5.

TURNING IN BED

Some top-of-the-range profiling beds are hinged longitudinally so they can turn you from side to side. Some products can be laid under you and operate on a similar principle with the advantage that the existing bed and mattress can be used. A sleeping bag style of product should be selected if there is a risk of rolling too far.

Table 6.3.5 Guidance on choice of care assistant operated device for use in bed

Factor	Product type	Guideline
YOURSELF (the user)		
Weight and size	Low-friction rollers and sliding sheets	Choose a product that fits you. The product should encompass both head and feet if you are recumbent. Too large a product may lead to a less controlled move. If you are light in weight you may feel you slide too easily, and hence feel insecure.
Care of your skin	All	Handles, bulky seams and netting materials should be avoided if you have delicate skin. Heels should be protected from shearing forces as the person is moved.
Comfort	All	If the product is to be next to the skin, choose a material that is not cold or sticky to the touch.
Pain	Low-friction rollers and sliding sheets	If you are post-surgery, with unstable fractures or spinal tumours, you will find it very painful when these devices are positioned. The actual move, however, will be less painful than other methods.
Slipping	One-way glide	Left in situ, helps to prevent slipping when you are sitting up in bed.
CARE ASSISTANT		
Effort in use	Low-friction rollers and sliding sheets	Reduction of effort required to move the person was rated higher for low-friction rollers.
Positioning and removing	Short low-friction rollers	Easiest to position and remove.
Asymmetry of person being moved	Low-friction rollers and sliding sheets	Uneven weight distribution, e.g. following stroke, means one care assistant will have to use more effort than the other, and turning the person may be harder.
Ease of grasping the product firmly	Sliding sheets	Handles not particularly useful, because they are seldom in exactly the right position, but would help care assistants with weaker grip.
Amount of training required	Sliding sheets and slide boards	Require little instruction for use.
	Low-friction rollers	Must be placed so they glide in the right direction and removal of these is greatly eased by use of correct method.
Storage	Padded products	Less easy to carry and store.

Sources: MDA 1997; Pain *et al.* 1999. Evidence **

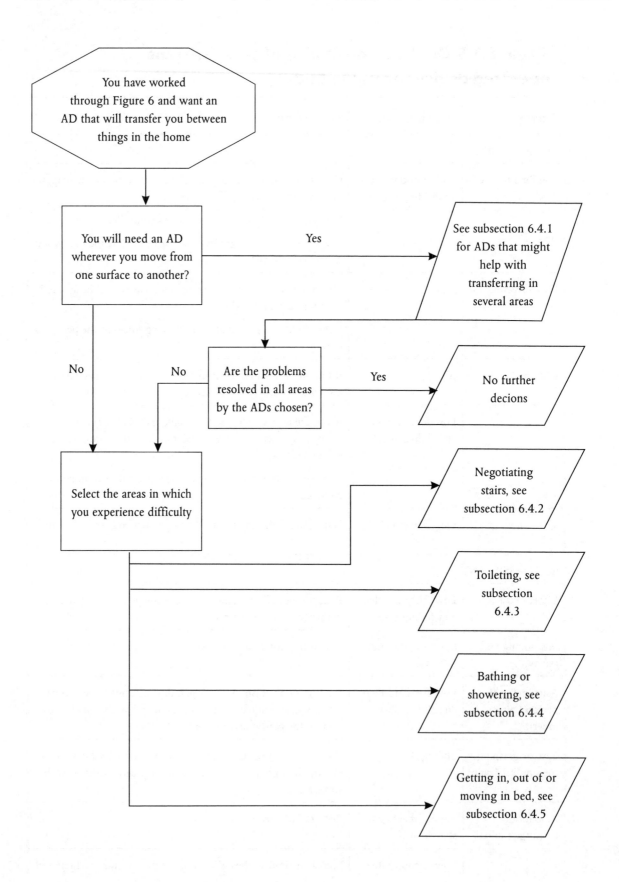

Figure 6.4 What moving or transferring tasks do you want an assistive device to do for you?

More commonly, personal assistance with turning is required, and sliding sheets and long low-friction rollers are the most frequently used devices. Guidance on choice can be found in Table 6.3.5.

Padded rollers are designed to be left in situ under you, so that care assistants do not have to position and remove them at each manoeuvre. Leaving rollers under you is not advisable if you get hot easily, as the quilting acts as an insulator, nor if involuntary movements could cause unwanted shifts in position. If you are on a pressure-distributing mattress, the roller should not be left in situ as the benefits bestowed by the mattress properties will be impaired by the roller.

6.4 Self-operated devices that do the task for you

This section considers the devices that remove the effort in a task, by doing the work for you. In some cases they can be operated by another person, but they are essentially designed for you to operate on your own.

6.4.1 Transferring

If you cannot transfer yourself by using your upper body and arms, it may be possible to use an overhead track hoist independently. However, it is unusual for people to be able to get a sling on and off on their own in such circumstances, so you probably will need some help from another person. See subsection 6.3.1.

6.4.2 Negotiating stairs

If you live in a bungalow you will obviously not need to be able to manage stairs on a day-to-day basis, but most people in the UK live in a house and usually have their bedroom upstairs. Moving the bed downstairs may be feasible if you have toilet and washing facilities downstairs. Another solution is to install a lift.

Lifts can either be fitted on the staircase itself (stairlifts) or move vertically from one floor through to another (vertical lifts). Stairlifts can be straight, curved (to follow turns in the staircase) or have a platform large enough for a wheelchair (platform lift).

The layout of your house and the needs of others in the household also affect the choice of equipment.

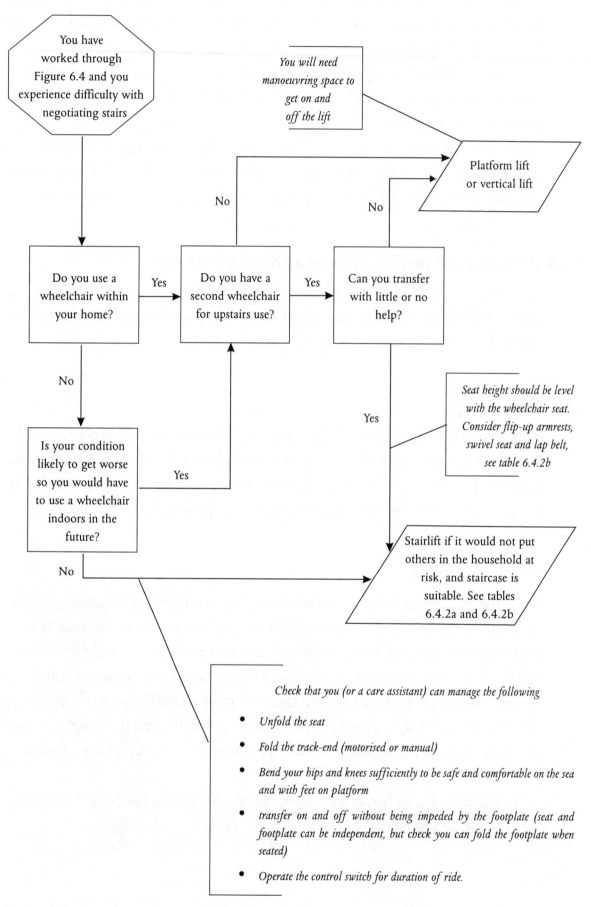

You have worked through Figure 6.4 and you experience difficulty with negotiating stairs

You will need manoeuvring space to get on and off the lift

Platform lift or vertical lift

Do you use a wheelchair within your home?

Yes

Do you have a second wheelchair for upstairs use?

Yes

Can you transfer with little or no help?

No

No

No

Is your condition likely to get worse so you would have to use a wheelchair indoors in the future?

Yes

No

Yes

Seat height should be level with the wheelchair seat. Consider flip-up armrests, swivel seat and lap belt, see table 6.4.2b

Stairlift if it would not put others in the household at risk, and staircase is suitable. See tables 6.4.2a and 6.4.2b

Check that you (or a care assistant) can manage the following

- *Unfold the seat*

- *Fold the track-end (motorised or manual)*

- *Bend your hips and knees sufficiently to be safe and comfortable on the sea and with feet on platform*

- *transfer on and off without being impeded by the footplate (seat and footplate can be independent, but check you can fold the footplate when seated)*

- *Operate the control switch for duration of ride.*

Figure 6.4.2 Choosing a stair or vertical lift

An example

Tina was told she had multiple sclerosis three years ago, and since then has had a really difficult time. Double vision comes and goes. Her legs have been getting progressively worse, so now she has to use a wheelchair around the house. Her four-year-old son Daniel is typically full of energy, which makes Tina feel inadequate as she is always tired. Understandably she is depressed, having despaired of getting the remission that other people keep mentioning. Her occupational therapist has been discussing adaptations to the home to enable Tina to cope on her own for short periods with her son. Today they want to decide how to overcome the stairs, because Tina and her family would rather not have the expense and upheaval of moving house.

- They look at Figure 6.4.2, and as Tina does use a wheelchair indoors and does not have a second one for upstairs use, they see that a platform or vertical lift may be suitable.

- They discuss possible sites for a vertical lift. There is space in Tina and Jason's bedroom if Tina gets the dressing table shifted, but immediately below is a mock fireplace in their through-lounge. No other bedroom is large enough.

- The stairs come straight down into the hall, and at the top there is a half-landing with two steps at a right angle. This means that a platform lift should be feasible provided the stairs are wide enough for Tina to ride facing across the stairs.

- Tina is not very keen on the idea of having a lift in the hall. In Table 6.4.2a she sees that folding platforms are available, and says she would rather take the time to fold the platform away than have it so obvious all the time. The occupational therapist explains the risk should Daniel leave cars or other items in the way of the platform when it lowers, but she is adamant that she would just check, and get Daniel to move them.

- The representatives from a couple of lift firms are asked to visit, so Tina can choose which she prefers. She knows she must choose one with a track that Daniel will not be tempted to drive cars up and down (Table 6.4.2b) so chooses one with a wall-fixed track.

- Jason gets a surveyor to check that the wall will take the weight of the lift. This is confirmed. When an application is made for a Disabled Facilities grant towards part of the cost of the alterations for Tina's needs, the lift will be included.

Table 6.4.2a Advantages and disadvantages of lift designs and features

Lift type	Advantages	Disadvantages	★
Stairlift for standing or perching	Narrower than a standard sitting model	For safety, you must be able to grasp the lift's hand rail firmly. If your ability to stand deteriorates, you will not be able to use it.	★
Stairlift (straight)	Little structural alteration Easy to remove	Blocks part of stair width. Requires sufficient space top and bottom for safe transfer on and off.	★
Stairlift (curved) if staircase has a turn	No structural alterations required to staircase, no need for a folding platform to cover top few steps See Table 6.4.2b.	More expensive than a straight stairlift. May reduce width of staircase too much at corner. See Table 6.4.2b.	★★
Platform stairlift	Can take wheelchair Folding platforms available	Requires plenty of space. Non-folding would have to be sent down when not in use so others can use staircase. If platform is set into floor (to avoid a ramp to get onto it), care must be taken to ensure no items are deposited in the well when lift is up.	★★
Vertical lift	Can take wheelchair	Occupies space in two rooms, one upstairs and one immediately below.	

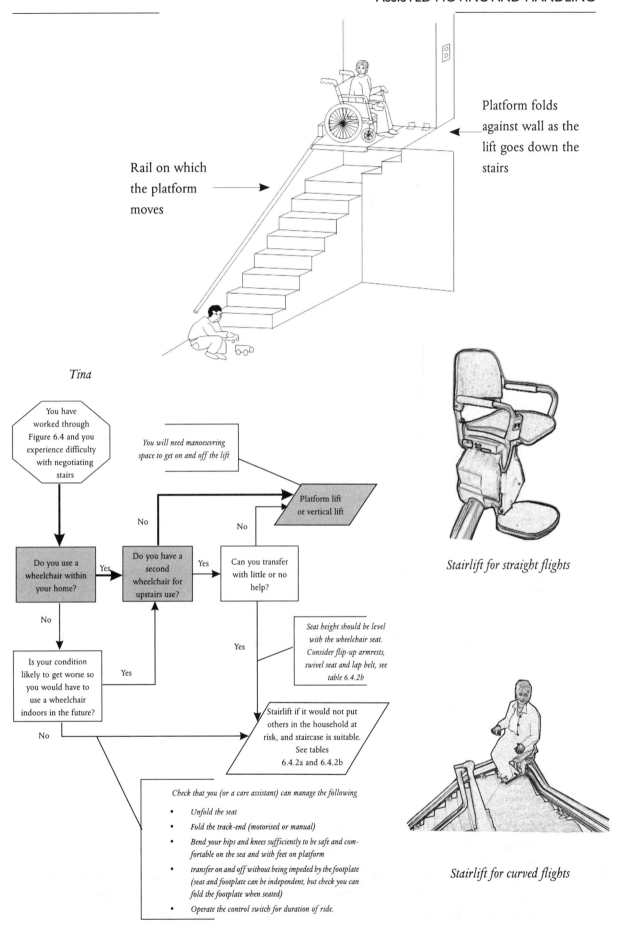

Platform folds
against wall as the
lift goes down the
stairs

Rail on which
the platform
moves

Tina

You have
worked through
Figure 6.4 and you
experience difficulty
with negotiating
stairs

*You will need manoeuvring
space to get on and off the lift*

Platform lift
or vertical lift

No

No

Do you use a
wheelchair within
your home?

Yes

Do you have a
second
wheelchair for
upstairs use?

Yes

Can you transfer
with little or no
help?

No

Stairlift for straight flights

No

Is your condition
likely to get worse so
you would have to
use a wheelchair
indoors in the future?

Yes

Yes

*Seat height should be level
with the wheelchair seat.
Consider flip-up armrests,
swivel seat and lap belt, see
table 6.4.2b*

No

Stairlift if it would not put
others in the household at
risk, and staircase is suitable.
See tables
6.4.2a and 6.4.2b

Check that you (or a care assistant) can manage the following

- *Unfold the seat*
- *Fold the track-end (motorised or manual)*
- *Bend your hips and knees sufficiently to be safe and comfortable on the sea and with feet on platform*
- *transfer on and off without being impeded by the footplate (seat and footplate can be independent, but check you can fold the footplate when seated)*
- *Operate the control switch for duration of ride.*

Stairlift for curved flights

Tina's route through Figure 6.4.2
Illustration 6.4.2

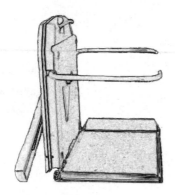

Platform stairlift

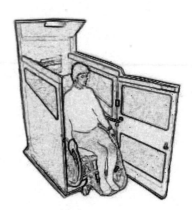

Vertical lift

Illustration 6.4.2 cont'd

Table 6.4.2b Environmental factors affecting choice of lift

Factor	*Issue*	*Guideline*	★
Wall turns away at bottom of staircase	Track has to project into hall: tripping hazard	Hinged track-end; motorised or manual operation available.	★★
Wall turns away at top of staircase	Stair lift stops beside, not over, landing floor	Choose swivel chair and/or flip-up armrests to ease turning prior to getting off: motorised or manual.	★★
Narrow staircase	Stairlift blocks much of stair width	Ensure other householders are able to use stairs safely. Some narrower products available, or choose perch/standing model if appropriate.	★★
Turn in staircase	A step or two at top	An automatic folding platform in conjunction with straight stairlift.	★★
	A step or two at bottom	Remodel staircase at the bottom, then install straight stairlift.	★★
	Two flights or spiral treads at corner	Curved stairlift. A floor-fixed track will take up more space at the corner, so may make use by others unsafe: some products have a wall-fixed track. Some products can be fixed to inner side of curve.	★★
Limited space at top and bottom	Assisted transfers	Ensure sufficient space for care assistants not to compromise their posture.	★
Small children in household	Items left on stair-fixed track	Choose product that has no channels into which items could lodge, for example a wall-fixed track.	★

Source: MDD 1991.

Safety standards for these products are laid down in British and European Standards, and products should be checked for conformance to ISO/DIS 9386-1 and 9386-2 (BSI 1998a). Annual maintenance checks are also required, and a maintenance agreement may sometimes be built into a Disabled Facilities grant or assumed by the social services department.

6.4.3 Toileting

You would probably need someone to help you with transferring on and off the toilet (see 6.3.3 above), but once on, an automatic bidet gives independence with cleaning and drying (see Chapter 4, section 4.1.4).

6.4.4 Bathing or showering

Lifting bath seats, some special baths, and level-access showers (see Chapter 5) can enable you to manage on your own, or with much less help than you would need without these products.

6.4.5 Getting in, out of or moving in bed

There are products that can make things much easier, possibly avoiding the need for someone to help you.

GETTING YOUR LEGS INTO BED

Two types of device are currently available that will address this difficulty, but you may not find they give you complete independence if you have difficulty in shifting your buttocks and legs across the bed.

1. Powered leg lifters are devices that lift the legs from the floor to level with the bed. At the present time, no product also moves the legs from the side of the bed into the centre, so you need to be able to do this, or ask another person to help (using a low-friction roller to reduce the effort required, see subsection 6.3.5 above).

    To use a powered leg lifter, you also need to have fairly good sitting balance, or be well supported at your back. MDA (1999a) has flowcharts to guide you through the decision-making process in more detail.

    If you are a wheelchair user and need the chair close for transferring, choose a leg lifter that is slim when lowered against the bed so the wheelchair can still be positioned close to the bed (MDA 1999a). A narrow profile will also be important when getting onto the bed from a standing position, because your buttocks would otherwise not be far enough onto the bed for safety.

2. Special profiling beds (see Table 6.4.5), in addition to their usual functions, are also designed to convert to a chair shape so that you get in and out of it as you would a chair, rather than having to lift your legs up and on to the bed. They are electrically operated.

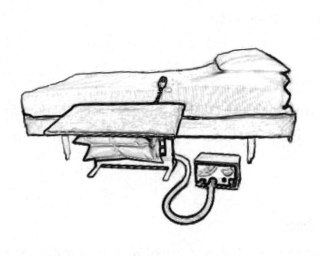

Powered leg lifter

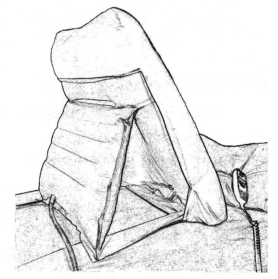

Pillow lift (raised)

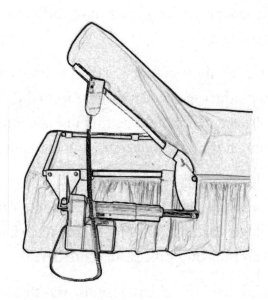

Mattress elevator

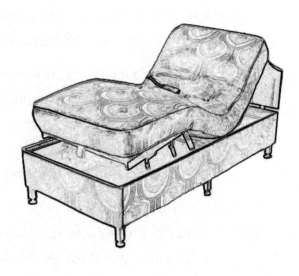

Profiling bed

Illustration 6.4.5

Table 6.4.5 Advantages and disadvantages of mattress elevators, pillow lifts and profiling beds

Product type	Advantages	Disadvantages	★
All	Sit you up and give support in sitting position.		★★★
Mattress elevator	Can be fitted to existing bed.	Not many find it helpful when getting in and out of bed. When elevated, bedside table has to be pulled forward to enable it to be reached.	★★
	A product with a knee break[1] is available, to reduce slipping a little.	You will tend to slip as the elevator rises. If the product does not go completely flat you may tend to slip during the night.	★★
	Less expensive than a profiling bed.	The mattress may be damaged where it bends, over a long period of time.	★
Pillow lift	Easy to fit as it rests on the mattress.	Has to be removed to change sheets.	★★
		Not advisable for those with poor sitting balance. Care must be taken when leaning to one side because of possible instability.	★★
		Slippage as the pillow lift rises was considered greater than with mattress elevators.	★★
Profiling bed	Has knee break to reduce slipping. Some products raise this prior to the section behind back, to reduce slippage further	When elevated, bedside table has to be pulled forward to enable it to be reached, unless a product is chosen whose internal bed frame shifts towards head of bed after elevation.	★
	Can help with getting in and out of bed (Keogh and Dealey 2001).		★★★
	Adjustable-height facility available.		★
	Some products bend to chair position so you can stand up from it as from a chair.		★

Source: MDA 2001a

1. A section rises under knee joint to bend the legs slightly.

SITTING UP IN BED

If you need assistance with sitting up or require support once up, there are three types of device that can be considered. Mattress elevators and pillow lifts are fitted to standard beds; profiling beds are designed so that the mattress base itself moves to a sitting position. The majority of these are electrically operated. It is always important to try products out before choosing which to have, but mattress elevators and pillow lifts should be tested overnight. Whilst the majority of users find these products helpful, a few find them uncomfortable overnight. The products usually cause people to slip down the bed a little, especially if they have a central actuator, and for some this causes a problem (MDA 2001a). Some advantages and disadvantages can be found in Table 6.4.5.

6.5 Cleaning and maintenance

CLEANING

Keeping the products clean is an important part of maintenance, but is especially vital when the devices are used with more than one person. The following guidelines apply in all situations where a product is not exclusively for one person's use (Department of Health 1993; Boden 1999):

- Products that do not come into contact with broken skin or body fluids should be laundered or cleaned when dirty.

- Products that potentially do come into contact with body fluids should be cleaned between users.

- If a user is known to have an infection, disinfection is required.

- Responsibility for ensuring procedures for cleaning are followed should be given to a named person.

In a hospital setting, there was widespread ignorance about how to clean the equipment (Boden 1999). The guidelines above should be customised by each National Health Service Trust (in the UK). These will include procedure, frequency of cleaning, who is responsible for ensuring items are cleaned at the specified times and who should decide when items should be replaced.

Table 6.5 Guidance on cleaning and disinfecting (local cleaning and disinfection policies should be in place and followed)

Factor	Issue	Guideline
Manual cleaning or disinfecting	Prevention of cross-infection	Always wear protective clothing.
Manual cleaning: of washable products	Full immersion	Water cooler than 35C with detergent. Scrub, wipe or spray item. Drain, and rinse in separate clean sink. Dry with absorbent cloth or hot air.
of hard surfaced products	Non-immersion	Use absorbent cloth and water cooler than 35C with detergent. Wipe down thoroughly, using brush if item has crevices. Dry with absorbent cloth or hot air. If alcohol wipe is used to dry the item, this will partially disinfect.
Disinfection	Thermal washing machines	These must rinse at one of the following: 71C for 3 minutes; 80C for 1 minute; 90C for 1 second.
	Chemical washer	
	Ultrasound washer	
	Manual	Immerse the item in the recommended disinfecting solution. Leave for recommended time[1]. Rinse in water of suitable microbiological quality. Dry with clean cloth.

Source: MDA 1996a

1.   Times for HIV or Hepatitus B virus are longer (30 minutes or more, depending on solution used) than for other organisms.

In a residential or hospital setting, hoist slings are frequently at risk of being contaminated with bodily fluid, because a common use is for toileting, so slings should be designated for an individual's sole use (Boden 1999) or disposable ones used. As well as reducing risk of cross-contamination and infection, single-person use would enable hoist slings to be marked with the person's name and the correct loops indicated, making it easier for the succession of staff to be confident in hoisting the patient correctly.

It is also preferable that low-friction rollers or sliding sheets are designated for use by one person only. The advantage of this, as well as reducing risk of cross-infection, is that the product would be stored at the bedside and be readily available, and be the correct size and best match with the person's needs.

Hoist slings and glide sheets should be laundered regularly, even when designated for single-person use. Sufficient numbers of products must be purchased to allow for single-person use and for laundering.

MAINTENANCE

Guidelines to ensure that adequate and regular checks of product safety are conducted should be available in NHS Trusts (UK) and equipment loan stores. There are legal requirements to inspect every six months all devices that lift people, including hoist slings, and that all types of hoist including lifting bath seats should be tested to their maximum load annually (HSE 1998).

Stair and vertical lifts also have to have annual maintenance checks.

Ferrules on walking aids should be inspected regularly and replaced when worn.

Wheeled walking frames should also have regular checks. Castors and, when applicable, brakes and central locking mechanisms, should be secure and functioning satisfactorily (MDA 2001b).

Key points

This chapter has reviewed evidence concerning assistive devices (ADs) for transferring and assisted handling. There is evidence that ADs bestow benefit to those who assist with transfers, but the benefit varies both between product categories and between products within a category.

The ADs have been categorised according to the amount of help you require:

Devices to assist your independence

- Walking aids assist your balance and are an effective way to reduce the weight taken through your legs.

- A number of ADs assist with getting in or moving on the bed.

Devices to assist when someone helps you

- Those helping you to transfer may be at risk of injuring themselves.

- A risk assessment must be done if you have assistance with transfers.

- Use of ADs lightens the load on care assistants but when you (the user) cannot assist, only hoist and sliding devices reduce the strain to below recommended levels.

Devices that do the task for you

- Hoists may be viewed negatively by some, but they are versatile and safe for you (the occupant) and the operator.

- Alternatives to hoists tend to be specific to one transfer type, e.g. bed to chair; in and out of the bath.

- Stairlifts and vertical lifts can solve the problem of negotiating stairs.

- A range of devices is effective in sitting you up in bed and supporting you in that position.

Cleaning and maintenance

- Cleaning procedures in institutional settings must be clear and followed to minimise risk of cross-infection.

- Products that lift people have to be regularly maintained.

References

Aitchison, E. (ed) (1999) *Safer handling of people in the community.* Teddington, Middlesex: Backcare.

> *A consensus of expert opinion, covering the legal framework, handling principles, training and equipment.**

Bannister, C. (1996) 'Learning not to lift.' *Nursing Standard 11, 2, 25–26.*

> *Survey of 1600 registered nurses who had filed a claim for industrial injury: 52 per cent were manual handling incidents; only 13 per cent were whilst using equipment. Risk assessment had been carried out prior to accident in only 20 per cent of cases. ** [These cases probably relate to injuries sustained prior to the Manual Handling Operations Regulations, HSE 1992].*

Boden, M. (1999) 'Contamination in moving and handling equipment.' *Professional Nurse 14*, 7, 484–487.

*Survey with 10 responses from manual handling co-ordinators (62 per cent response rate); ignorance of how to clean and store manual handling equipment was common. Swabs were taken from wards' manual handling equipment (n = 32) and from two wards where equipment was for single-patient use only (n = 8). All of the latter were clear; only 25 per cent of the other wards' swabs were clear.** Author recommends that products are for single-person use, and guidelines for decontamination should be explicit and adhered to.*

British Standards Institution (1998a) ISO/DIS 9386-1 and -2 *Power operated lifting platforms for persons with impaired mobility. Rules for safety, dimensions and functional operations. Part 1: Vertical lifting platforms; Part 2: Powered stairlifts moving in an inclined plane for seated, standing and wheelchair users* (98/706426 DC and 98/706427DC). London: British Standards Institution. Accessed via website www.bsi-global.com

British Standards Institution (1998b) BS EN 10535 *Hoists for the transfer of disabled persons. Requirements and test methods.* London: British Standards Institution. Accessed via website www.bsi-global.com

Brown, A. and Mulley, G. (1997) 'Injuries sustained by caregivers of disabled elderly people.' *Age and Ageing 26*, 21–23.

*Survey by interview of caregivers of people receiving respite care via three consultants (n = 41): 76 per cent reported injuries sustained from manual handling; 46 per cent had received some instruction, mostly during therapy sessions. ** Toileting was frequently considered the most difficult task.*

Cassar, S. and Costar, S. (1998) 'Patient handling aids: prescribing guidelines.' British *Journal of Therapy and Rehabilitation 5*, 3, Suppl. 8–10.

*Expert opinion concerning factors to consider when choosing a product.**

College of Occupational Therapists (1995) *Manual Handling Operations Regulations 1992 and their application within occupational therapy.* London: COT.

Conneely, A. (1998) 'The impact of the Manual Handling Operations Regulations 1992 on the use of hoists in the home: the patient's perspective.' *British Journal of Occupational Therapy 61*, 1, 17–21.

*In-depth interviews with ten hoist users; a second interview was conducted to check findings with users. Acceptance of hoist was promoted by comprehensive assessment, adequate training for carers, involving user and carer in decision-making and consideration of psychological aspects. Important product aspects included comfort, ease of use, compatibility with environment.***

Cook, G. and Nendick, C. (1999) 'Manual handling: what patient factors do nurses assess?' *Journal of Clinical Nursing 8*, 422–430.

*Manual handling risk assessment is multi-faceted, and a flexible approach is probably better than a rigid policy. Postal survey in which 85 of 272 questionnaires distributed to nurses in 7 NHS acute Trusts were completed. They were asked to rate 33 patient-related factors for importance. From these and others that respondents added, a factorial analysis described 5 factors: unpredictable movement, patient's ability to participate, patient's physical and mental condition, limitations to movement, and moving and handling variables. ***

Cooper, B. and Stewart, D. (1997) 'The effect of a transfer device in the homes of elderly women.' *Physical and Occupational Therapy in Geriatrics 15*, 2, 61–77.

*A single product evaluation of a floor-to-ceiling pole which was fitted in 30 women's flats (mean age 77 years). Significant changes in the Canadian Occupational Performance Measure showed the positive impact of having the pole.** All chose to keep the pole. A contrast colour provided a visual reminder of the rail (16 chose to keep the contrast).*

Cowan, D. and Turner-Smith, A. (1999) ' User perspective on the provision of electronic assistive technology: equipped for life?' *British Journal of Occupational Therapy 62*, 1, 2–6.

Postal survey of wheelchair users (predominantly powered) in two health authorities: 135 of 250 were returned. Forty-five per cent had cerebral palsy or multiple sclerosis. Thirty-three per cent were under 25 years old. Fifty-five had hoists; half of these had received training in their use; two rarely used their hoist. Sixty per cent of the whole sample had experienced problems, mainly funding, delay or poor information. **

Cowell, R. and Shuttleworth, A. (1998) 'Equipment for moving and handling patients.' *Professional Nurse 14*, 2, 123–130.

Expert opinion on risk assessment and training and informal appraisal of range of products. *

Dale, C. and Woods, P. (2000) 'A risk assessment and management strategy for community nursing.' *British Journal of Community Nursing 5*, 6, 286–291.

A set of six interrelated components of a risk management strategy proposed: organisational, cultural, clinical, environmental, employee issues and incident reporting. Not exclusively manual handling. *

Department of Health (1993) *Decontamination of equipment prior to inspection, service or repair*, HSG(93)26. London: Department of Health.

DLF (1998) Disabled Living Foundation factsheets to assist choice of shower equipment accessed via the Internet: www.dlf.org.uk/factsheets/ Accessed on 26/01/2001.

Expert opinion. *

Duffy, A., Burke, C. and Dockrell, S. (1999) 'The use of lifting and handling aids by hospital nurses.' *British Journal of Therapy and Rehabilitation.* 6, 1, 20–24.

Eight hospitals (79 wards) were sent questionnaires about use of manual handling devices: 150 of 170 were returned. Hoists were available in 73 per cent of wards. Lack of time was main reason given for not using them (34%). **

Elford, W., Straker, L. and Strauss, G. (2000) 'Patient handling with and without slings: an analysis of the risk of injury to the lumbar spine.' *Applied Ergonomics 31*, 185–200.

Formal trial in which 22 nurses lifted a volunteer from chair to chair with no slings, one sling, two slings. Lumbar motion was monitored and visual analogue scales used for subjective stress on body parts. Overall, use of one or two slings significantly reduced angular displacement *** *so authors conclude their use would reduce risk of back injury. But the nurses were still in high-risk category for injury with regard to spinal flexion.*

Green, C. (1996) 'A study of moving and handling practices on two medical wards.' *British Journal of Nursing 5*, 5, 303–311.

Observational study of ten nurses (five qualified, three unqualified and two students) in two wards. They were observed for a combined total of 30 hours, and interviewed. Concluded that practice still falls short of the guidelines (HSE 1992) and that attitudes unsympathetic to use of mechanical aids are still common. **

Hall, J., Barton, J., Clarke, A. *et al.* (1991) *An evaluation of walking frames* MDD/205/91. London: Medical Devices Directorate.

Formal comparative user trial of 28 walking frames by 86 people, They tested three frames for one week each in their own homes. Wider based frames were more stable but less manoeuvrable. Many folding mechanisms were too difficult for users to manage. **

Hall, J. and Clarke, A. (1991a) *A study to evaluate walking sticks*, MDD/201/91. London: Medical Devices Directorate.

Formal comparative user trial of eight sticks which were divided into two groups. Twenty people tested four or five sticks on a test circuit. Authors recommended training and a short test to determine whether the stick is useful. User must feel it is sturdy enough. Cite one stick relieves approximately 15 per cent of body weight from opposite leg. Two sticks relieve approximately 25 per cent of body weight from either leg (four-point gait), or more from one (three-point gait). See Table 6.1.1.

Hall, J. and Clarke, A. (1991b) *An evaluation of crutches,* MDD/202/91. London: Medical Devices Directorate.

Formal comparative user trial of 6 elbow crutches and 5 axillary crutches. They were tested by 45 users, all except 3 of whom had orthopaedic conditions. They tried all crutches from one group of 3 or 5 products, for 3 days each. See Table 6.1.1

HSE (Health & Safety Executive) (1992) *Manual Handling Operations Regulations* (MHOR). London: HMSO.

HSE (Health & Safety Executive) (1998) *Lifting Operations and Lifting Equipment Regulations* (LOLER). London: HMSO.

Hignett, S. (1998) 'Ergonomic evaluation of electric mobile hoists.' *British Journal of Occupational Therapy 61,* 11, 509–516.

Formal ergonomic evaluation of 12 hoists. They were tested by 16 operators (occupational therapists, nurses) so each hoist tested 8 times on a test circuit. An ergonomist and rehabilitation engineer assessed each hoist for ergonomic, design, manufacture and maintenance issues. ** See Table 6.3.1.

Keogh, A. and Dealey, C. (2001) 'Profiling beds versus standard hospital beds: effects on pressure ulcer incidence outcomes.' *Journal of Wound Care 10,* 2, 15–19.

Formal trial of 2 device configurations with 2 groups of 35 people. One condition was a standard hospital bed with pressure relieving mattress, one was a profiling bed with pressure reducing foam mattress; both were tested for 5–10 days. No pressure sore incidence in either group, but more of those in profiling beds felt it helped them to be independent in and out of bed (P= 0.0001); *** how much the adjustable height and how much the profiling mattress contributed to this is unknown. All the profiling bed group except one were able to change position in bed independently.

Klint Edlund, C., Harms-Ringdahl, K. and Ekholm, J. (1998) 'Properties of person hoist spreader bars and their influence on sitting/lifting position.' *Scandinavian Journal of Rehabilitation Medicine 30,* 151–158.

Formal technical evaluation with 12 healthy volunteers. They were photographed suspended from a jig with each of 7 spreader bars and 3 sling types (21 test configurations per subject, in 2 sessions 6 months apart). They reported an interaction between spreader bar and sling. *** No comfort ratings. The recommendation that trunk-to-thigh angle should be between 60 and 83 * is not supported by data. [A disappointing study except to highlight why slings should not be used indiscriminately on any hoist.]

Le Bon, C. and Forrester, C. (1997) 'An ergonomic evaluation of a patient handling device: the elevate and transfer vehicle.' *Applied Ergonomics 28,* 5/6, 365–374.

A novel design of product for assisting with toilet transfers was evaluated by 11 experts by trial, checklist and discussion. The tests showed that although it was innovative, it was considered low on dignity and comfort for the user.** [The product is not on the UK market.]

Love, C. (1997) 'A Delphi study examining standards for patient handling.' *Nursing Standard 11,* 45, 34–38.

Eleven nurses in an orthopaedic hospital participated in a Delphi survey to agree a hospital policy for patient handling. ** The author notes that different clinical areas would require different policies. Literature review cites prevalence of back injury from Buckle, 1987.

McGuire, T., Moody, J. and Hanson, M. (1996a) 'An evaluation of mechanical aids used within the NHS.' *Nursing Standard 11,* 6, 33–38.

Formal technical evaluation of ten products in a lab setting (seven hoists, one hoist/bathing hoist, one bathing hoist, one standing aid). Unspecified number of nurse pairs, one acting as hoist occupant. Significant difference in effort required to operate electric and hydraulic hoists.*** Smaller hoists were generally less preferred (occupant felt less stable and secure) **.

McGuire, T., Moody, J., Hanson, M. *et al.* (1996b) 'A study into clients' attitudes towards mechanical aids.' *Nursing Standard 11*, 5, 35–38.

Survey and observational study of 20 patients, mean age 85. Number of observation periods were unspecified. Usage of devices was mainly for bathing (n=19), toileting (n=4) or moving from bed to chair (n=5). Seventy per cent of the occupants reported feeling comfortable; only two felt unsafe. Seventy-nine per cent of handling episodes required two nurses to accomplish them. The reason given was that they 'usually' had to lift the patient onto the device! [This would have mainly been the bathing hoist chair.]

Space constraints were observed to have affected operator's posture adversely in 89 per cent of episodes and the spine twisted in 84 per cent (n=16).** McGuire et al. felt that the preconceived ideas that nurses have about patients not accepting mechanical handling devices could be overcome by involving the patient in decisions concerning manual handling needs.

Mandelstam, M. (2001) 'Safe use of disability equipment and manual handling: legal aspects – Part 2, Manual handling.' *British Journal of Occupational Therapy 64*, 2, 73–80.

Mann, W. and Tomita, M. (1998) 'Perspectives on assistive devices among elderly persons with disabilities.' *Technology and Disability 9*, 119–148.

Survey by interview of 508 current AD users from a longitudinal study. At least 8 of 514 walking stick users complained of uncomfortable handgrips, as did some of the 293 walking frame users. Some of the latter had difficulty in transporting their frames. A few comments concerned stigma that the users felt was attached to using walking aids.**

MDA (1994) *Slings to accompany mobile domestic hoists: an evaluation* DEA A10. London: Medical Devices Agency.

Formal comparative user trial of 16 slings for use with 6 mobile domestic hoists by 18 operators and 25 occupants; each sling was tested by 10 pairs. Results for each presented, and guidelines drawn from the results.**

MDA (1996a) *Sterilisation, disinfection and cleaning of medical devices and equipment: guidance on decontamination from the Microbiological Advisory Committee to the Department of Health.* London: Medical Devices Agency.

Provides standards for differing levels of infection risk, and for differing types of surfaces. States that general guidance such as HSG(93)26 (Dept. of Health 1996) 'will need to be interpreted locally' (p.4).

MDA (1996b) *Moving and transferring equipment: a comparative evaluation,* DEA A19. London: Medical Devices Agency.

A biomechanical study was conducted to assess whether any product was associated with harmful movement patterns; none was (***).

Formal comparative user trial of 12 products divided into 4 groups according to design: belts, slings, turntables and transfer boards. All products in 1 group were tested by 12 partnerships of transferrer and user (48 partnerships in total).

MDA (1997) *Handling equipment for moving dependent people in bed: a comparative evaluation,* DEA A23. London: Medical Devices Agency.

Formal comparative user trial of 4 sliding sheets, 8 low friction rollers (4 short and 4 long), 3 other devices were evaluated by a total of 60 lead carers with a varying number of dependent people. Each product was tested by 12–16 lead carers. The handling devices were rated lowest; the low-friction rollers were rated highest.**

MDA (1999a) *Manual and powered leg lifters: an evaluation*, EL4. London: Medical Devices Agency.

*Formal comparative user trial of all leg lifters (4 manual, 5 powered). Thirty-six people tested the products in one category (9–17 trials per product). Manual leg lifters were most useful for those with good general motor function and upper limb strength;** 12 of the 20 who tested powered leg lifters did not find them useful;** this was because it was still difficult or impossible to move the legs across the bed once they were elevated.*

MDA (1999b) *Wheeled walking frames: an evaluation*, MO1. London: Medical Devices Agency.

*Formal comparative user trial using 'lab' and home trials. Circuit trials of 8 wheeled walking frames, with 30 current users each testing 2 frames, then a further 3. One frame was also given some home trials. Two- and four-wheeled frames tend to be more stable than three-wheelers, but less manoeuvrable.** Baskets and seats were considered useful.***

MDA (2000) *Mobile electric hoists: an evaluation*, MH2. London: Medical Devices Agency.

*Ergonomic and technical assessment and formal comparative trial of 12 mobile electric hoists. A panel of experts appraised them, 22 people tested them on a circuit with the same healthy volunteer in the hoist (12 trials per hoist), and technical tests were conducted to determine force required for pushing and turning. Larger wheels and vinyl rather than rubber material usually reduced effort required.** Manoeuvrability variation was not found to have a simple relationship to individual hoist features.*

MDA (2001a) *Mattress elevators and pillow lifts: an evaluation*, EL7. London: Medical Devices Agency. May be accessed via www.medical-devices.gov.uk.

Formal comparative user trial by 56 people who tested up to 4 products from 1 of 3 groups: either mattress elevators, pillow lifts or 2 of each. See Table 6.4.5.

MDA (2001b) *Rollators: risk of collapse and other issues*, SN 2001(16). London: Medical Devices Agency.

Advice concerning regular maintenance of front castor, central locking and cable brakes.

MDA (2001c) *Bed grab handles: risk of head entrapment*, SN 2001(11). London: Medical Devices Agency.

Apertures should not be within a critical range if there is any risk of the user slipping against the bed grab handle.

MDD (1991) *An evaluation of stairlifts for people with disabilities*, MDD/204/91. London: Medical Devices Directorate, Department of Health.

Survey of current users of stairlifts (n=189), interviewed at home. Thirteen straight stairlifts; four curved stairlifts and three platform lifts are reported on, with dis/advantages. See Table 6.4.2a.

MDD (1993) *Mobile domestic hoists: a comparative evaluation*, DEA A3. Norwich: Medical Devices Directorate, HMSO.

*Four electrically operated, five hydraulically operated and three winding gear operated hoists were formally evaluated by technical test, laboratory circuit tests and home trials. Each hoist was tested by ten pairs in lab., nine hoists were trialled by fifteen pairs in the community, testing all hoists in one of three groups of three hoists. Results were presented and guidelines drawn from them.***

Moody, J., McGuire, T., Hanson, M. *et al.* (1996) 'A study into nurses' attitudes towards mechanical aids.' *Nursing Standard 11, 4, 37–42.*

Structured interview with 185 hospital nurses, 25 per cent night staff. Twenty-two per cent had had no training with mechanical aids; 61 per cent informal only. Forty-five per cent felt there was insufficient equipment available. Fifty-nine per cent did not know who was responsible for laundering hoist slings. Forty-nine per cent complained of space constraints when using mechanical aids. Only 67 per cent said they would always adhere to a care plan recommendation to use a mechanical aid.★★

Moy, A. (1987) *Assessment of manual bed aids.* DHSS Disability Equipment Assessment Programme. London: HMSO.

A selection of 13 products was tested by 35 people who tested 1 product each. See Table 6.1.5 for comments about products whose design has not changed.

Nicholson, J. (1999) 'Management strategies for musculoskeletal stress in the parents of children with restricted mobility.' *British Journal of Occupational Therapy 62*, 5, 206–212.

Postal survey to 93 families (146 parents): 118 returned. Sixty-two were carrying 6–10-year-olds much of the time. Back pain complained of by 95. Eleven had hoists; ten felt they eased manual handling load. Sixty-seven per cent found ADs for lifting inconvenient but acknowledged they reduced musculoskeletal problems. Only 38 per cent had received manual handling advice or training in the past 2 years.★★ *Difficulty with stairs was main factor precipitating adaptations to the home.*

Owen, B., and Fragala, G. (1999) 'Reducing perceived physical stress while transferring residents.' *American Association of Occupational Health Nursing Journal 47*, 7, 316–323.

Formal trial of one product but with a comparative group. A 'study' chair that could be straightened out like a stretcher, used with a low friction pad, was tested with 23 residents from one residential home. Staff completed 301 ratings for exertion on shoulders, upper and lower back; 24 reports from residents about safety and comfort. Two other homes that used handling belts or mechanical lifts returned comparable data: 147 ratings from staff, 7 from residents. Study chair showed significantly less exertion for all body parts; ★★★ *it was considered a safe and comfortable means of transfer by residents. [No breakdown of proportion of transfers in comparison homes that were with handling belt, for which one would expect higher exertion ratings, as opposed to mechanical lifts.]*

Pain, H., Jackson, S., McLellan, D.L. *et al.* (1999) 'User evaluation of handling equipment for moving dependent people in bed.' *Technology and Disability 11*, 13–19.

Formal comparative user trial of 15 products selected to represent the products available on the UK market. They were trialled by 60 lead carers who worked either in the community or in a hospital. Each tested all products in one of four groups to which the products had been allotted according to design: sliding sheets, low-friction rollers (one group long, one group short) and miscellaneous. Short low-friction rollers were given highest overall rating. They were considered by 75 per cent to reduce the effort required during handling the patient compared with no equipment.★★ *However, only 47 per cent envisaged frequent use of these products. [MDA 1997 evaluation.]*

Pearce, J. and Cassar, S. (1999) 'Assessing risks.' In E. Aitchison (ed) *Safer handling of people in the community.* Teddington, Middlesex: Backcare.

Poulson, D. and Richardson, S. (1998) 'USERfit – a framework for user-centred design in assistive technology.' *Technology and Disability 9*, 3, 163–171. Full publication: Poulson, D. and Ashby, M. (1996) *USERfit: a practical handbook on user-centre design for assistive technology.* TIDE, European Commission. Brussels-Luxembourg: ECSC-EC-EAEC.

Retsas, A. and Pinikahana, J. (2000) 'Manual handling activities and injuries among nurses: an Australian hospital study.' *Journal of Advanced Nursing 31*, 4, 875–883.

Questionnaires passed to all 523 nurses in one hospital: 269 responded; 108 reported an injury associated with manual handling; 67 per cent of these with direct patient care, and about half of that 67 per cent were connected with lifting patients. Frequency of use of handling devices reported, with reasons for not using them. Not knowing how to use them was cited by 13 per cent.★★ *Authors point out the risks of injury to the patient through poor handling practice.*

Sainsbury, R. and Mulley, G. (1982) 'Walking sticks used by the elderly.' *British Medical Journal* *284*, 1751.

*Survey showed 23 of 62 sticks had worn or loose ferrules.***

Steed, R., Wiltshire, S., Cassar, S. *et al.* (1999) 'Legislation and responsibilities.' In E. Aitchison (ed) *Safer handling of people in the community*. Teddington, Middlesex: Backcare.

Cites prevalence of injury and current UK legal framework concerning manual handling of people.

Ulin, S., Chaffin, D., Patellos, C. *et al.* (1997) 'A biomechanical analysis of methods used for transferring totally dependent patients.' *SCI Nursing 14*, 1, 19–27.

*Formal comparative technical assessment. Two nurses lifted two patients using three manual methods: sling, pivot transfer, sliding board; three mechanical methods: screw, hydraulic and electric hoist. Bed to wheelchair. Video and joint movement analysis; compressive forces at L5/S1 calculated, and subjective ratings of effort taken. All compression forces for manual methods above recommended maximum of 3400N.*** Estimated 94–99 per cent of female population should be able to transfer a person using a hoist. Results did not detect differences between the hoists. Cites literature that describes a relationship between the compressive forces incurred by tasks, and incidence of low back pain.*

Zhuang, Z.,Stobbe, T., Hsiao, H. *et al.* (1999) 'Biomechanical evaluation of assistive devices for transferring residents.' *Applied Ergonomics 30*, 285–294.

*Formal comparative technical trial. Nine nurses transferred two elderly females who were instructed not to assist with the transfer. Twelve conditions: no device, belt, sliding board, standing devices (n = 4), overhead hoist, mobile hoist (n = 4). Force plates and motion analysis used to measure joint movements and calculate compressive forces at L5/S1. Hoists appreciably reduced the strain, but there was a significant difference between their manoeuvrability, mainly the standing devices compared with mobile hoists compared with overhead hoist.*** Authors note that position of the handles when manoeuvring affects force required, and one that places an operator in a poor position may increase risk of musculoskeletal disorders.*

Zhuang, Z., Stobbe, T., Collins, J. *et al.* (2000) 'Psychophysical assessment of assistive devices for transferring patients/residents.' *Applied Ergonomics 31*, 35–44.

Same study as above. Subjective rating for exertion, ease of use by each nurse after each transfer. Devices were ranked by the nurses. Resident rated comfort and security after each transfer. The overhead hoist was not favoured, possibly because it was slow to use and the spreader bar was close to resident's face. Mobile hoists most favoured, significantly more than sliding board, no device, belt and some of the standing devices. But variation within device type was detected, especially the standing devices, the most and least favoured having significantly different (p 0.05) ranking. This is confirmed by significant differences in ease of use and comfort for resident between them. Two of the mobile hoists also varied significantly in ease of use. ***

Part Three

Part Three

Chapter 7

Conclusion

Introduction

Matching equipment to your needs and characteristics as a person with disabilities is sometimes easy but can be intriguingly difficult. It is necessary to understand not only the nature of the task or function you want to perform, but the environment, your preferences, any care assistants who may be involved, and the range of equipment available.

This book has concentrated upon the relatively limited areas in which some systematic research has been done, in order to draw together the lessons that have already been learned and to illustrate the benefits of a systematic approach to decision-making. Good evidence and reliable systems of decision-making are still hard to come by in many areas. This chapter starts by summarising the principles of the process as it might be applied to other areas. It then indicates where and why more research is needed, and ends with a look ahead at what we can expect to be achieved in the future.

7.1 The decision-making process

This book has focused on the provision of information in a format that helps decision-making. All the relevant factors interact, so that each situation poses a unique problem. As more factors enter the equation, so the decision becomes more complex.

Figure 7.1 illustrates the diversity of factors that bring a person to the point of choosing an assistive device (AD), and the components that influence the effectiveness of the choice and the AD's integration into the person's life. Whilst we have addressed part of the process of choosing an AD, it is necessary to see this process in the wider context.

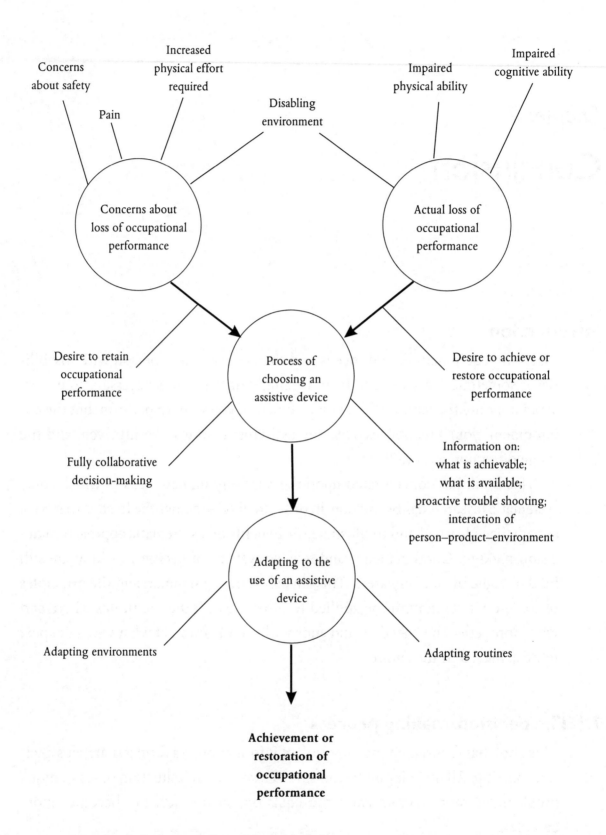

Figure 7.1 Pathway to introduction of an assistive device

Note: Occupational performance refers to the ability to undertake any activity, ranging from daily tasks such as getting out of bed, to hobbies or paid employment.

In Chapter 1, a process for choosing assistive devices was described (see Figure 1.3), but Part 2 addressed only a section of that process, namely selection of a shortlist of products for you to try out (Stages 4 and 5). The following conclusions can be drawn concerning this selection process:

- The safety of yourself (the user) and care assistant is paramount, but care assistants will accept an AD even if it incurs a degree of inconvenience and effort, if they perceive this provides safety for you (MDA 2001a).

- For straightforward problems, elimination of less appropriate products can often be accomplished by a series of fairly clear-cut decisions. For example, Figure 4.1.1 uses pain, paralysis and unsteadiness as the factors in choice of toilet seat and rails. Such guidelines can be used with reasonable confidence provided there is some choice of product within the product type selected. This will allow individual preferences and situations to be catered for.

- Complex problems usually require weighing up the relative advantages and disadvantages of several options. For example, Table 5.2.5 details factors which affect the choice of a bath lifting seat; these may indicate that different products could be suitable, so the decision rests on what is considered higher priority in the given situation.

Trying the product out before making a final decision is essential. Ensuring the AD is safe and easy to use is specifically emphasised by Maczka (1990) and is an essential component in judging the success of an AD when trying it.

7.1.1 Professional advice

In order that complete information is available to inform such a decision, attention given to all the relevant factors has to be well judged and thorough (see Figure 7.1). Those with experience in the field are used to the 'mental juggling' required and are also likely to be familiar with a wider range of products and their features. This is why the help of an experienced practitioner such as an occupational therapist or rehabilitation engineer is advisable (Garner and Campbell 1987). Such professional knowledge complements your knowledge of your goals, preferences and lifestyle requirements (Scherer and Galvin 1994).

7.1.2 Will the best match actually be used?

Using a process such as described in Chapter 1 (see Figure 1.3) will rarely produce a *perfect* match, but the match will usually be sufficiently functional to achieve the purpose for which it was chosen. Even when all elements of the choice of AD have been well matched, the day-to-day outcome thereafter may depend upon how successfully you have been able to adapt to using it in practice. As the old adage has it, 'There's many a slip 'twixt cup and lip!'

Lifestyle and cultural factors have not been addressed in detail in this book. They are topics in their own right, and affect expectations and the motivation for *using* as well as *selecting* ADs. Respectful listening and unpressured discussion are the essence of successful collaboration between you, your family, the practitioner and any care assistants throughout the decision-making process. This is the best way of ensuring that lifestyle and cultural factors will shape the decision that is made. Judge and Parette (1998) remark that it is 'perhaps family and cultural factors that are most susceptible to being overlooked by professionals' (p.200).

Active involvement of yourself as the end user in the process of choosing an AD is known to result in better outcomes than when a decision being presented ready made (Nordenskiöld 1997; Riemer-Reiss 1999). Active involvement can affect the desire to attempt an activity, because it is possible to underestimate the situation, or wrongly assume that no viable solution could be found. The process of working up options can motivate you when seeking a solution; it can enable you to envisage better the purpose of having an AD, and to be realistic about what it can and cannot achieve. All these components will equip everyone concerned (both yourself and your care assistants) when you begin to incorporate the AD into your life (Chen *et al.* 2000). You may need help preparing for possible alterations to the environment and to your routines. The period during which you adjust psychologically to use of the AD and adapt your self-image should be easier if you have been alerted to the need for a learning phase (Hocking 1999; Kronlof and Sonn 1999).

7.2 Product design

Adapting to the use of an AD will of course be easier if the product is well designed. Good design makes products easier to learn how to use, reduces the effort of using them, and minimises stigma that may be attached to their use. The current welcome impetus behind 'Design for All' (INCLUDE(2001); EQUAL; Helen Hamlyn) will benefit many people. Greater ease of use and greater availability of products on the general market will lead to more people incorporating ADs into their lifestyle simply to make life easier or to complete a task more quickly. Inclusive design does not always remove the need for special design for people with disabilities – but it does shift that need further along the spectrum towards more complex and demanding requirements (Küppers 1999).

As impairments increase, small variations in design can have a major influence on whether the product is helpful or not. The increased involvement of consumers in the development of ADs (Poulson and Richardson 1998; Ryan, Rigby and From 1996; Thousand Elders) and more recently computer modelling (EQUAL) are positive moves that should improve products' effectiveness and acceptability.

Improvement in materials and innovations in technology have benefited people with disabilities. Velcro is a celebrated example, but in the past 20 years other materials or designs have been developed that are now used for ADs. Special seating and pressure relief cushions are two examples where innovations have had a particular impact. It is hoped that the move to foster the application of new technologies and materials to 'design for all' products and specialised ADs will yield dividends.

7.3 The impact of the environment

The type of environment will affect the level of disability that impairment brings, and also the need for ADs. Improvements in the design of houses and in the internal access to facilities will help. For example, someone who cannot climb the stairs will not be disabled at home if they live in a bungalow, but would be disabled in a house unless an assistive device such as a stairlift were fitted. As the environment becomes more accommodating, fewer ADs may be needed – or perhaps it will be that a greater range of activities using new generations of assistive devices will become possible.

The requirement to make buildings physically more accessible to disabled people has only recently been extended to private dwellings in the UK (Department of the Environment 1999). The disabling nature of the built environment is slowly reducing. Gone are the days when it was considered reasonable to assume that disabled people would not expect to be able to visit their non-disabled friends, or that working environments would not need to be accessible to disabled people. Increasing awareness of special needs will have an impact on how these regulations are followed. It is not unreasonable to expect that one day no wheelchair user will need a kerb climber because there will be ramped access to all pavements.

7.4 Implications for information providers

Information giving has improved markedly in the past decade, but there is still much more work to be done. For example in a survey by Marks as recently as 1998 (Marks 1998), 13 per cent of respondents did not know where to go for information. In order for an appropriate choice of assistive device (AD) to be made, information about products must be available and easily accessible. Information should include details about the product, how it interfaces with the environment and how it interacts with people who have differing requirements.

7.4.1 Details about the product

Manufacturers usually know their products thoroughly but it is essential for suppliers to have a similar understanding and knowledge. In addition to highlighting their products' key features, they should be able to supply information about measurements, construction, durability and maintenance requirements. In practice, few brochures list all the details that practitioners say they want. Brochures from different companies tend to present information in different ways, almost as if to foil attempts at direct comparison. If an agreed format for presentation of product information could be adopted for each product range, it would greatly facilitate the process of short-listing products for a user to test. Independent AD databases such as ABLEDATA (2001) and DLF-DATA (2001) could adopt a similar format.

7.4.2 How products interface with the environment

Manufacturers supply information about fitting and using their products, and may give some contra-indications for use, but do not provide much additional detail concerning how products interface with the environment. Experienced practitioners hold a wealth of information in their heads, and it is helpful when this is recorded for the benefit of those with less experience.

Some information of this kind can be found in the independent databases referred to above, and within published articles and publications such as the Medical Devices Agency's Disability Equipment Evaluation reports, or shared through training events.

7.4.3 Interactions between the user and the product

In order to choose a product, the pivotal information is how particular features or designs affect the usefulness of that product for an individual. This type of information can gradually be built up by practitioners from their experience, but those with less experience have to glean it from databases such as DLF-DATA factsheets, publications such as those from the Disability Information Trust (Kelsall 2000; Kelsall and Cochrane 1996), the Medical Devices Agency's reports, conference proceedings and published articles. The majority of these will not usually be accessed by users themselves, so practitioners must be able to convey the pertinent details to the user for a given situation to facilitate informed choice (Atkinson *et al.* 1992).

In summary, whilst manufacturers' brochures are freely available to practitioners and end users, they may not contain sufficient information. Actually finding out what products are available will be difficult unless a special database is accessed. Many end users may not yet have the facilities to do this.

Finally, knowledge of how products will fit a person's requirements is gained partly through experience and partly through publications and the other sources of information discussed above. If you are newly disabled you will have little experience on which to draw, and your access to the publications with information about matching person and product may be limited, so the role of the practitioner as an information provider is important. Even though an increasing number of people will undertake their own searches, practitioners will remain key information providers for many users. It is hoped that this book will be used by a practitioner and potential AD user together, so that information can be discussed and a decision reached that fully employs the knowledge of both partners.

7.5 Implications for assistive device providers

7.5.1 Use of guidelines

Providers of assistive devices often produce guidelines that define the eligibility of a client for devices and guide choice according to set criteria (LBOTM 2000). If the guidelines are flexible, they will assist choice whilst allowing individual requirements to be met, but if they are over-prescriptive they will disenfranchise the user. Another potential drawback to over-strict adherence to criteria is that definitions formulated to allocate a person to specific products will be interpreted differently by individual practitioners (Burke 1999), and so may be a source of inequity as well.

7.5.2 Purchasing strategies

Charitable and governmental providers of assistive devices have to balance the needs to supply appropriate devices to their clients, to provide a speedy service and to be cost efficient. Bulk purchase of equipment is attractive as one means of getting value for money. Decisions have to be made concerning what products should be selected for this, and conversely which products can be bought only in small numbers, or even by special order for an individual. There is no such thing as a 'best buy' for *all* the potential users of a service. A range of equipment will inevitably be required in order to meet the differing specific requirements of a range of disabled users living in a range of different environments.

The review of literature conducted for this book supports the current policy of bulk buying a few products that are chosen for their efficiency at meeting the commonest problems, such as walking aids and bath seats. At the other end of the spectrum it will be essential to support special orders for particular individuals in their specific circumstances. Wherever possible, we have highlighted factors that will affect the choice of products to hold in stock, such as the storage space required, ease of cleaning between users, adaptability from one user to the next, multiple functionality or versatility of a product in differing environments.

7.5.3 Information and training

Providers of assistive devices are also information providers, and have a duty to both the users and the practitioners who recommend an AD. Training is frequently cited as an issue in the literature, both for users when they are issued with a product, and for practitioners to enable them to choose products appropriately and inform users accurately. AD providers are in a good position to provide training to practitioners so that they have a broad knowledge of products, their limitations, and for whom the products may be useful. This will equip the practitioners to involve users in the decision-making process, and give adequate instruction in the correct use of the products.

Providers of ADs also have to ensure that each product is delivered with written instructions (MDA 1998), and is properly fitted. Research has shown that a visit to fit and re-demonstrate the use of the product around the time of delivery improves usage (Stowe *et al.* 1982).

Follow-up by letter or visit detects product faults and disuse (e.g. Korpela, Seppänen and Koivikko 1992; Mann and Tomita 1998; Wessels *et al.* 1998) which users may not otherwise report. The reasons for not reporting faults include the users not wanting to be a nuisance, not knowing whom to contact, or being unable to face another 'battle' with the authorities to get what they require. There is a personal cost to the user when the AD is not suitable, which may be out of proportion to its monetary value, so regular follow-up is the ideal. This is already a matter of good practice for more complex or expensive products, and regular follow-up will enhance the recycling of equipment that is now expected (Department of Health 2001).

In summary, the use of guidelines is widespread but they should be applied flexibly and in collaboration with the user. Providers of ADs are well placed to train practitioners in the choice and use of products. Finally, remember that circumstances and individuals change. Regular follow-up of those to whom ADs have been loaned is good practice and is an efficient way to increase the proportion of products that are recycled.

7.6 Implications for research

Much more work needs to be undertaken to describe in more detail how people and assistive devices (ADs) interact. A large proportion of the evidence presented in this book relies upon expert opinion, and for many types of product the voice of the user is still unrecorded. Expert opinion is a valuable source of knowledge but in future it needs to be better supported with systematically gathered evidence. Even for categories such as pressure relief products, within which many studies have been conducted, further work will be required as innovative designs and materials are introduced.

The core factors affecting the relationship between user and product, namely size, safety, ease of use, adjustability, effectiveness, portability, reliability, maintenance arrangements, follow-up, availability and affordability are incorporated in a standardised evaluation measure (Batavia and Hammer 1990; Demers, Weiss-Lambrou and Ska 2000). These are pertinent to most products but not necessarily comprehensive.

The outcomes of AD provision also include reducing the effort required by the user or a care assistant, and preventing an undesired sequel such as a pressure sore or a deformity. It is therefore necessary to have a range of possible measures from which to choose, as each will have its own strengths and weaknesses (Heaton and Bamford 2001), depending upon the questions being addressed.

As well as choosing the appropriate outcome measure, the appropriate method and setting must also be selected. ADs designed to assist a person with fairly straightforward requirements may be studied according to product features, and an examination undertaken of how they affect the user and interact with the environment. The data can often be used to produce recommendations about which features and user requirements combine effectively. Even so, it is advisable for the user to try two or three products to ensure the optimal choice.

The more the AD interacts with the environment, the more important it is to test it within the environment in which it will be used, but even products that do not seem to interact much may benefit from a trial in the appropriate setting. For example, a low-friction roller only interacts with the bedclothes, so could have been functionally tested by users in a 'laboratory' setting. However, ward and nursing home situations provided a more comprehensive and realistic evaluation because the range of staff and users was more diverse than could have been achieved in a 'lab' setting (MDA 1997). Another example is the mattress elevators that proved to have a number of drawbacks for some people and in certain environments (MDA 2001b). These would not have been detected in a 'lab' setting. Environmental information will always be reduced in a 'lab' evaluation, and this has to be carefully considered against the benefits of a more controlled environment.

If the AD requires a long period of time to get used to, or its function reduces the effort required for a task, determining the relative merits of a range of products will require a longer period of testing than is normally possible in a 'lab' setting. If the AD is to prevent deformity or pressure sores, the experimental period has to be sufficiently long to determine how well it achieves this aim against a control group or comparator.

When people have more complex requirements, the possibility of deriving specific recommendations from research studies is lower because the possible combinations of individual requirements are greater. Therefore methodologies such as *case studies* are used, from which one derives guidance rather than specific recommendations regarding choice. However, such guidance is still sparse for most types of AD, so research is much needed despite the challenges of designing a study from which useful information can be drawn.

In summary, more research is needed to explore how people, environments and products interact, particularly for those people who have complex requirements. No single measure will be appropriate for all evaluations, but there is now a number of possible measures to choose from, some of which are standardised. The trial setting and length of trial period also have to be carefully chosen to address the particular product type and research question.

7.7 Implications for education and training

7.7.1 Users

This book has been addressed to users of assistive devices and we hope that the contents of the book give you confidence to find your way through the mass of information needed to make a good choice of AD. Whether you do this with or without a practitioner who has experience in the field will depend on the type of

AD wanted, the source from which you expect to obtain it, and your own experience.

With the increase in private purchases of devices, and the mushrooming of information about products, there will be more demand for impartial advice that is not linked to supply. Some advice centres are already in place, for example the Independent Living Centres (run by the Disabled Living Centres Council, see Chapter 1, subsection 1.4), but people who do not associate their difficulties with being 'disabled' would be unlikely to seek advice through them. A range of information, from leaflets in retail stores to publications such as this one, would go part of the way to bridging the gap in sources of advice and guidance.

Self-help groups will increasingly wish to know more about assistive technology to pass information on to their members. There will also be a need for users to receive training in order to assist one another in choosing appropriate products, and work has been done on training needs and programmes (EUSTAT). We also hope that more people with disabilities will train in the professions involved in assistive technology provision, so that they will bring together the perspectives of adviser and potential user.

7.7.2 Practitioners

Practitioners may fail to listen to clients with sufficient attention because they have already decided on the 'best' solution. ADs promote independence but also symbolise impairment. Some people therefore have a preference to 'manage against the odds' rather than use an AD. Failure to appreciate this can easily result in the over-hasty prescription of an inappropriate AD which is not used, or outright rejection when an AD could have been really helpful.

Professionally trained practitioners assess the multiple factors that impinge on a given situation, and have to consider many possible interventions which may be beneficial, one of which is the provision of ADs. At present, though, there is little published material that plots pathways between the assessment findings and the goal of increased independence through the use of an AD.

Experienced practitioners know many potential pathways towards a successful goal, but this knowledge becomes so second-nature, it is hard to dismantle it into a step-by-step process of logically ordered decisions (see also Appendix I). You may wish to understand the intermediary steps that a practitioner has intuitively taken, and this book has tried to make such steps explicit, using evidence wherever it is available.

Assessment for and provision of many ADs in the UK are now conducted by social services staff who have not had professional training themselves, but who work under a professional's supervision. In-service training and personal development of skills and knowledge in the field of assistive technology are provided for these practitioners, and we hope this book may be of use in this regard, together with other resources designed for the purpose, such as those EUSTAT has developed (EUSTAT).

7.8 Hopes for the future

Now that we are living longer and surviving more serious trauma than in the past, the predictions are that there will be more people who have some degree of disability. The built environment and most products on the general market are designed by the 'average' young adult, traditionally with specifications accordingly, so there are potentially increasing numbers of people who find certain products or services difficult or impossible to use.

The move towards designing for a wider range of abilities is therefore timely and welcome, and is already bearing fruit in many of the products we have seen coming into production recently. People of all abilities enjoy using well-designed products, so some of those initially designed with specific impairments in mind may become part of everyday life. Consider how washing machines have made washing clothes by hand an infrequent chore instead of being a day's task each week!

There is an increasing number of projects that involve collaboration between manufacturers, engineers, users and designers. This joint working at every stage from scoping a project, drawing up specifications, to designing and testing prototypes, is a development that will benefit many people.

The only drawback to this very positive trend is that expert assistance currently available to enable people to acquire these things may become increasingly scarce. More ADs are now available in high street shops or by mail order, but in parallel, statutory and charitable providers are reluctant to include such items in their remit. One way to counteract the disadvantage that this situation imposes on those with disabilities would be to award a grant or vouchers to defray the cost irrespective of the route through which the AD is acquired.

Information for people who have disabilities will continue to multiply, and collation and interpretation of information from many sources will probably become an industry in its own right. This industry will, it is hoped, encompass information to guide choice of ADs as well as medical conditions and treatments. But no matter how ideal information sources become, there will always be the need for someone to be available to advise, who has experience in the field of matching people's requirements and their environments to the product that will best resolve their need. Our hope is that this book will help those with experience in choosing assistive devices to work in partnership with the potential AD user, using the book as a tool to generate ideas and assist the decision-making process.

References

ABLEDATA (2001) www.abledata.com
An American database of assistive devices. Accessed on 25/9/01.

Atkinson, P. *et al.* (1992) *Equipped for independence? Meeting the equipment needs of disabled people.* Department of Health. Heywood: HMSO.
The report includes consideration of information needs, stating that information should be appropriate to facilitate informed choice. Loan services should involve users.

Bain, B. (1998) 'Assistive technology in occupational therapy.' In M. Neistadt and E. Crepeau (eds), 9th edition, *Willard and Spackman's occupational therapy,* pp.498–516. Philadelphia: Lippincott.
Describes a model that places the consumer at the intersection of environment, device and task.

Batavia A. and Hammer, G. (1990) 'Toward the development of consumer-based criteria for the evaluation of assistive devices.' *Journal of Rehabilitation Research and Development 27,* 4, 425–436.
Two focus groups each of six users identified seventeen factors to evaluate concerning ADs.

Burke, C. (1999) 'Summary of reliability study of matrices.' *Technology and Disability 10,* 3, 181–185.
A committee of users and professionals defined criteria to guide choice of seating and wheelchairs. Two therapists used them independently for thirty-five people. Matches were good for wheelchairs (84–100%) but less so for seating devices (64%).

Chen, T-Y., Mann, W., Tomita, M. *et al.* (2000) 'Caregiver involvement in the use of assistive devices by frail older persons.' *The Occupational Therapy Journal of Research 20,* 3, 179–199.
Twenty elders and their caregivers were interviewed. Carers' encouragement affected the user's satisfaction with an AD (p   0.05) and their presence when AD was obtained was associated with their subsequent help as the user became accustomed to using it (p   0.05).

Demers, L., Weiss-Lambrou, R. and Ska, B. (2000) *Quebec User Evaluation of Satisfaction with assistive Technology* (QUEST), version 2.0.
Available from M.Scherer at the Institute for Matching Person and Technology, 486 Lake Road, Webster, NY 14580.

Department of the Environment (1999) Approved document 'Part M: access and facilities for disabled people.' *Building Regulations Amendment 1998.* London: HMSO.

Department of Health (2001) *National Service Framework for older people.* Accessed at www.doh.gov.uk/nsf/olderpeople on 1/10/01.

DLF-DATA (2001) www.dlf.org.uk
A British database of assistive devices available by subscription.

EQUAL – Design for all. Accessed at www.lboro.ac.uk/departments/cd/docs_dandt/research/dfa/data.htm on 11/9/01.

Work is being done to enable new products to be tested in a virtual environment. This will emulate user trials to some extent, and will, it is hoped, lead to products that are effective for people with a wide range of abilities.

EUSTAT (Empowering USers Through Assistive Technology). Accessed at www.siva.it/research/eustat/index.html on 8/12/01.

This European-funded project developed resources for the training of users.

Garner, J. and Campbell, P. (1987) 'Technology for persons with severe disabilities: practical and ethical considerations.' *Journal of Special Education 21*, 3, 122–132.

Literature review and expert opinion. Advocates specialist team to help schools to assess for ADs.

Heaton, J. and Bamford, C. (2001) 'Assessing the outcomes of equipment and adaptations: issues and approaches.' *British Journal of Occupational Therapy 64*, 7, 346–356.

A review of a range of outcome measures.

Helen Hamlyn Research Centre. Accessed at www.rca.ac.uk/schools/research/ hamlyn.html on 10/10/01.

Hocking, C. (1999) 'Function or feelings: factors in abandonment of assistive devices.' *Technology and Disability 11*, 1, 3–11.

A literature review from the psychological perspective.

INCLUDE (2001) www.stakes.fi/include – accessed on 25/9/01.

A project to promote a 'Design for all' approach.

Judge, S. and Parette, H. (1998) 'Family-centred assistive technology decision making.' *Infant-Toddler Intervention: The Transdisciplinary Journal 8*, 2, 185–206.

Literature review and expert opinion.

Kelsall, A. (ed) (2000) 2nd edition *Children with disabilities.* Oxford: Disability Information Trust.

Kelsall, A. and Cochrane, G. (eds) (1996) 7th edition. *Personal care.* Oxford: Disability Information Trust.

Korpela, R., Seppänen, R-L. and Koivikko, M. (1992) 'Technical aids for daily activities: a regional survey of 204 disabled children.' *Developmental Medicine and Child Neurology 34*, 985–998.

Of 752 children with neurological disorders in a region in Finland, 209 used assistive devices (ADs); 80–85 per cent reported a breakdown in use or effectiveness of toileting and bathing devices.

Kronlof, G. and Sonn, U. (1999) 'Elderly women's way of relating to assistive devices.' *Technology and Disability 10*, 3, 161–168.

Eleven women were interviewed. Physical and social factors may force acceptance of an AD if the user does not want to opt out.

Küppers, H-J. (1999) 'A history of AT – critical remarks for the future.' In C. Bühler and H. Knops (eds) *Assistive technology on the threshold of the millennium*, pp.3–6. Amsterdam: IOS Press.

LBOTM (London Boroughs Occupational Therapy Managers) (2000) *Criteria for the loan of equipment to people with disabilities.* Social Services: Harrow, London.

Maczka, K. (1990) *Assessing physically disabled persons at home.* Therapy in Practice Series, No.12. London: Chapman and Hall.

Mann, W., and Lane, J. (1995) 2nd edition *Assistive technology for persons with disabilities.* Bethesda, MD: AOTA.

The assessment process is described as having the person, environment, tasks and devices as components.

Mann, W. and Tomita, M. (1998) 'Perspectives on assistive devices among elderly persons with disabilities.' *Technology and Disability 9*, 119–148.

Five hundred and eight current AD users from a longitudinal study were interviewed. The need for follow-up for review of the person's needs and for maintenance of the devices was highlighted.

Marks, O. (1998) *Equipped for equality.* London: SCOPE.

A postal survey to 4500 people with cerebral palsy had 452 responses. Results included 13 per cent saying they did not know where to go for information, and one recommendation was that a trial period for a device should always be offered.

MDA (1997) *Handling equipment for moving dependent people in bed: a comparative evaluation* DEA A23. London: Medical Devices Agency.

MDA (1998) *Medical devices and equipment management for hospitals and community-based organisations* DB 9801. London: Medical Devices Agency.

MDA (2000) *Equipped to care: the safe use of medical devices in the 21st century.* London: Medical Devices Agency. Accessed at www.medical-devices.gov.uk on 2/1/01.

MDA (2001a) *Bath cushions for people with severe disabilities: an evaluation,* EL6. London: Medical Devices Agency.

MDA (2001b) *Pillow lifts and mattress elevators: an evaluation,* EL7. London: Medical Devices Agency.

Nordenskiöld, U. (1997) 'Daily activities in women with rheumatoid arthritis. Aspects of patient education, assistive devices and methods for disability and impairment assessment.' *Scandinavian Journal of Rehabilitation Medicine 29*, Suppl. 37.

Fifty-three of 73 women with rheumatoid arthritis attended a joint protection course which included use of devices; 663 ADs were issued. Author commented that time for dialogue is needed for people to accept an intervention, and that increased involvement in choice of AD improved satisfaction with it.

Poulson, D. and Richardson, S. (1998) 'USERfit – a framework for user-centred design in assistive technology.' *Technology and Disability 9*, 3, 163–171.

Full publication: Poulson, D. and Ashby, M. (1996) *USERfit: a practical handbook on user-centred design for assistive technology.* ECSC-EC-EAEC. Brussels – Luxembourg: TIDE, European Commission.

Riemer-Reiss, M. (1999) 'Applying Roger's diffusion of innovation theory to assistive technology discontinuance.' *Journal of Applied Rehabilitation Counselling 30*, 4, 16–21.

Telephone interviews with 115 people who had 136 ADs. Method and analysis poorly described. Greater consumer involvement with choice was associated with continued use (p=0.001).

Ryan, S., Rigby, P. and From, W. (1996) 'Understanding the product needs of consumers of assistive devices.' *Canadian Journal of Rehabilitation 9*, 2, 129–135.

Described a process aimed at promoting good design by involving consumers in needs identification, prioritisation, idea generation and design specification.

Scherer, M. and Galvin, J. (1994) 'Matching people with technology.' *Rehabilitation Management 7*, 2, 128–130.

Expert opinion describing a decision-making process: identify goals, gather information, establish criteria for choice. The need for collaboration between consumers and professionals, each acknowledging the other's expertise, is expressed.

Stowe, J., Thornley, G., Chamberlain, M. and Wright, V. (1982) 'Evaluation of aids and equipment for bathing, survey II.' *British Journal of Occupational Therapy 45*, 92–95.

Thousand Elders. Accessed www.bham.ac.uk/gerontology/1000elders.htm on 10/10/01.

Wessels, R., de Witte, L., Weiss-Lambrou, R. *et al.* (1998) 'A Dutch version of QUEST (D-QUEST) applied as a routine follow-up within the service delivery process. 'In I. Placenia Porrero and E. Ballabio (eds) *Improving the quality of life for the European citizen*, pp. 420–424. Amsterdam: IOS Press.

The questionnaire was used in personal interviews with 66 people seven months after issue of a wheelchair, stairlift or shower seat. A further 306 were interviewed who had had their device longer. Commented that this sample had many who suffered less than satisfactory provision, and called for routine follow-up of device users.

Appendix I

Decision-making and Problem-solving

To resolve a difficulty experienced with a task of daily living requires information of many types before possible solutions can considered. Once information has been gathered, the *problem* must be defined, the goal agreed, and then solutions can be generated and evaluated. From the evaluation, the best solution can be selected. This process of problem-solving has been described, with minor variations, by many authors (e.g. Gagné 1977; Hagedorn 1996). Problem-solving could be tackled with very little information, but errors are more likely to ensue because of factors not taken into account. For example, a person experiencing difficulty getting into the bath might decide showering was the only alternative, not realising there were bath boards on the market. Or a bath board might be purchased only to find that the wall was unsuitable to fix a rail, so the board was difficult to use. When the fund of information is fuller, the possibility of innovative and effective solutions is greater (Gagné 1977).

When a difficulty is encountered for which an assistive device might be appropriate the user and practitioner must consider many things during the problem-solving process:

- the user's abilities, preferences, and whether abilities are likely to change with time

- care assistant or family requirements

- the environment

- what approaches to the problem can be taken

- what can realistically be provided

- whether devices are available, or whether alternatives such as custom-made devices are possible.

Once comprehensive information has been gained, the problem defined and the goal agreed, a variety of problem-solving methods may be employed to reach a solution, such as adapting a previously successful strategy (Craik and Tulving 1975), using analogy (Gick and Holyoak 1980) or breaking the problem down into smaller stages and solving each in turn ('difference reduction', see Anderson 1995).

Examples of these are:

- adapting a previous strategy: looking for a similar device but with the feature that was lacking in the previous one

- using analogy: applying a principle that was successful in one situation across to another

- breaking the problem into smaller stages: a complex task will have to be considered component by component.

These strategies will be employed in problem-solving when appropriate, but this book particularly seeks to guide the problem-solving by providing cues and a structure from which to work. Gick and Holyoak (1980, 1985) found that people were more successful at solving a problem if they were given a hint about how to do it, and later work suggested that giving people the explanation about the solution of one problem helped them for analagous ones. Therefore this book provides information that will prompt the problem-solver about things to consider, and worked examples to explain how and why solutions can be achieved.

Being systematic in considering all possible solutions, even those that at first sight seem useless, is a strategy that enhances the likelihood that a decision is optimal rather than 'good enough'. Keeping an open mind and allowing lateral thinking rather than jumping to a solution too soon (premature 'closure', Gagné 1977) are required. This book adopts a structure to encourage consideration of possibilities, using flow charts to guide the order in which things are considered, and tables to set out factors that can be noted or eliminated according to their relevance to the situation in hand.

When problems require simultaneous consideration of many factors, as choosing assistive devices does, the cognitive process has been described under the term 'clinical reasoning'. Clinical reasoning is the process whereby the information gained through assessment of the person's abilities, psychosocial factors, the care assistant's needs, and the environment, is utilised in light of the practitioner's experience and knowledge to 'diagnose' the problems and plan the most appropriate intervention. For simple problems, procedural reasoning will produce a satisfactory solution; these lend themselves to a flow chart with a series of questions to which one answers 'yes' or 'no'. The straightforward nature of these problems means that those without professional qualifications may be able to undertake their analysis (Hagedorn 1996).

But many problems are complex, and require the simultaneous consideration of many factors that impinge. This proactive mental balancing of a raft of factors is termed conditional reasoning (Chopparo and Ranko 1995). This kind of thinking requires a person to have experience as well as knowledge, so that chunks of related information are stored as a single 'schema' (Minsky's frame theory, see Miller 1985). Schemata are then accessed when relevant, and the experienced person brings to the problem-solving process a much richer resource than a novice who would only be able to look at information in a more serial way (Robertson 1996). This book aims to assist the less experienced reader in this process by tabulating a range of factors that need to be addressed, together with possible solutions for each. In essence, it attempts to make experience and research evidence available and usable for those relatively new to the field of choosing assistive technology. Because the suggestions in the book are generalised they may conflict with one another for a given individual, in which case a compromise has to be made. Possible solutions have to be tested out, and if they do not prove satisfactory, the process is revisited to find an alternative to try. This reiteration of part of the process is to be expected with more complex problems, and is described in Chapter 1 (section 1.3).

The decision concerning assistive devices is seldom made by one person in isolation. Often a practitioner assists the user in solving a problem, or the family participates in debating the possibilities and final choice. This complicates the process further, as each person has a different fund of experience and way of thinking. Hewes (1986) felt that tacit group rules determined decisions more than actual discussion; whilst this may be an extreme view, it behoves all partners to value the others' knowledge and skills, so that the decision can truly benefit from the experience of all concerned. It will also help the decision-making partners to follow one another's thinking if they follow the same process; the structure used in this book can facilitate this.

The purpose of this publication is therefore to present information and interpret research evidence about assistive technology in a consistent manner. It can then more easily be used to inform the decision-making process, so enhancing clinical judgements rather than devaluing them.

References

Anderson, J. (1995) 4th edition *Cognitive psychology and its Implications.* New York: Freeman & Co.

Chopparo, C. and Ranko, J. (1995) 'Clinical reasoning in occupational therapy.' In J. Higgs and M. Jones (eds) *Clinical reasoning in the health professionals,* pp.88–102. Oxford: Butterworth-Heinemann.

Craik, F. and Tulving, E. (1975) 'Depth of processing and the retention of words in episodic memory.' *Journal of Experimental Psychology 104,* 268–294.

Gagné, R. (1977) 3rd edition *The conditions of learning.* New York: Holt, Rinehart & Winston.

Gick, M. and Holyoak, K. (1980) 'Analogical problem solving.' *Cognitive Psychology 12,* 1–38.

Gick, M. and Holyoak, K. (1985) 'Analogical problem solving.' In A. Aitkinhead and J. Slack (eds) *Issues in cognitive modelling.* London: Erlbaum Associates.

Hagedorn, R. (1996) 'Clinical decision making in familiar cases: a model of the process and implications for practice.' *British Journal of Occupational Therapy 59,* 5, 217–222.

Hewes, D. (1986) 'A socio-egocentric model of group decision-making.' In R. Hirokawa and M. Poole (eds) *Communication and group decision-making,* pp.265–291. Beverley Hills: Sage Publications.

Miller, G. (1985) 'Trends and debates in cognitive psychology.' In A. Aitkinhead and J. Slack (eds) *Issues in cognitive modelling.* London: Erlbaum Associates.

Robertson, L. (1996) 'Clinical reasoning, Part 2: Novice/expert differences.' *British Journal of Occupational Therapy 59,* 5, 212–216.

Bibliography

Carnevali, D. (1995) 'Self-monitoring of clinical reasoning behaviours: promoting professional growth.' In J. Higgs and M. Jones (eds) *Clinical reasoning in the health professionals,* pp.179–190. Oxford: Butterworth-Heinemann.

Creek, J. (1990) *Occupational therapy and mental health: principles, skills and practice.* Edinburgh: Churchill Livingstone.

Dutton, R. (1995) *Clinical reasoning in physical disabilities.* Baltimore: Williams and Wilkins.

Higgs, J. and Jones, M.(eds) (1995) *Clinical reasoning in the health professionals.* Oxford: Butterworth-Heinemann.

Newell, A. and Simon, H. (1972) *Human problem solving.* Englewood Cliffs: Prentice Hall.

Roberts, A. (1996) 'Approaches to reasoning in occupational therapy: a critical exploration.' *British Journal of Occupational Therapy 59,* 5, 233–236.

Rogers, J. and Holm, M. (1991) 'Occupational therapy diagnostic reasoning: a component of clinical reasoning.' *American Journal of Occupational Therapy 45,* 11, 1045–1053.

Schon, D. (1983) *The reflective practitioner: how professionals think in action.* New York: Basic.

Appendix II

Organisations Involved in Assistive Technology

A number of these organisations is actively involved in research and evaluation. All web addresses were accessed during October–December 2001.

AAATE The Association for the Advancement of Assistive Technology in Europe. www.aaate.org

AARP An American association providing information and resources to people over 50 years. www.aarp.org

CAT Center for assistive technology, University at Buffalo. Research, information and education. www.cat.buffalo.edu

DEACs Disability Equipment Assessment Centres

Three centres funded by the Medical Devices Agency to conduct a rolling programme of evaluations of assistive devices currently on the market.

Access via www.medical-devices.gov.uk or directly at:

Derby: www.ddeac.co.uk

London: www.medphys.ucl.ac.uk/research-groups/incont/incont. htm

Southampton: www.healthehants.org.uk/deac

FAST Foundation for AssiStive Technology, UK. Database of AT publications, research and products. www.fastuk.org

Hjaelpemiddelinstituttet, Denmark. Centre for technical aids for rehabilitation and education. Research, information and education. www.hmi.dk

IRV Centre for rehabilitation and disability. Research, information and education. www.irv.nl

RAATE Recent Advances in Assistive Technology and Engineering. Access via Centre of Rehabilitation Engineering at www.kcl.ac.uk

RADAR Royal Association for Disability and Rehabilitation. An association of and for disabled people, providing advocacy, information and support. www.radar.org.uk

RESNA   Rehabilitation engineering and assistive technology society of North America. Interdisciplinary organisation undertaking research and education in the field of AT. www.resna.org

SIVA Assistive technology research and information, Italy. www.siva.it

Swedish Handicap Institute. Research, information and education. www.hi.se

Appendix III

Glossary

Assessment

> The gathering of information about the person and environment pertinent to the identified problem(s) (see Chapter 1). See also *evaluation*.

Body Mass Index (BMI)

> An index of body proportion calculated by dividing a person's weight (kg) by their height squared (m^2).

Care assistant

> A person who undertakes personal care tasks for people with disabilities, or helps them. The term includes formal care such as in a residential home, paid care staff coming into private homes, and informal helpers such as family members or friends.

Case study

> Detailed report of one (or more) intervention applied in a pre-planned way, using the person's performance prior to intervention as the baseline. Systematic data collection at several points enables change in the person's performance to be studied. Several case studies may be conducted to demonstrate the intervention's effect on people with a range of requirements.

Cross-sectional data

> See *Data*.

Crystal taps

> Large-diameter, spheroid-handled tap fitment with longitudinal ridges to assist grip.

Current user

> A person who is using the assistive device in the course of their daily life at the time.

Custom made

> A product is custom made if it is individually made to specific measurements.

Data

> Pieces of information that are systematically gathered to address a research question. Cross-sectional data is collected at one point in time and provides a 'snapshot'. *Longitudinal data* is gathered at more than one point in time, returning to the same respondents each time, and can therefore show changes. Data may be *qualitative* or *quantitative*, see below.

Evaluation

The gathering of information about the performance and effectiveness of product(s) (see Chapter 2). See also *assessment*.

Evidence

This book classifies evidence as strong (****), some (***), requires care when applying (**), or guidance only (*) (see Chapter 2).

Horizontal transfer

Transfer of person from one surface to another in a lying position.

In-depth interview

An interview with a researcher where a *schedule* (see below) rather than a rigid questionnaire is used, to gain deeper insight into the respondent's experience.

Inter-rater reliability

A measure of the degree to which the test result will be the same when scored by different people on the same subject.

Ischial tuberosities

The bony points on a person's buttocks.

Lateral transfer

A sideways transfer of a person from one surface to another, usually in the seated position.

Longitudinal data

See *Data*.

Non-specialist devices

Products available on the general market. The better their design, the easier disabled people will find them to use.

Orthosis

An appliance worn to support or control joint(s), e.g. a wrist splint protects the wrist during work tasks; a hip abduction orthosis keeps the thighs apart.

Pilot

A formal test of a research protocol to iron out unforeseen problems prior to the main data collection.

Practitioner

A health or social services officer involved in assessing for, and/or advising about suitable assistive devices.

Probability sample

One that is designed to represent certain categories appropriately with regard to their proportion to the overall population, but subjects are randomly selected. Also called a representative sample.

Problem

A difficulty that the user wishes to address.

Protocol

A research 'recipe' constructed for a project.

Qualitative data

Language-based information systematically gathered in a research project. The central purpose of qualitative research is to give insight into processes or attitudes about which little is known. Ideally you need to go to the original publication to find out the characteristics of the subjects and the context in which the data was collected. In practice, you may not be able to do this, so the guideline represents something noteworthy to take into consideration during the selection process.

Quantitative data

Information gathered in a research project using objective ordinal measurements, or information of other types for which there are valid methods for conversion to data that is numerical.

Schedule

A guide for an interviewer containing a list of questions which should be covered and some prompts that may be used if the interviewer wants the respondent to expand on a topic.

Solution

A device or strategy that should solve the identified problem.

System rails

These are formed from a customised selection of rail lengths fixed together with brackets that allow corners in any plane, and right-angled or oblique options.

Test circuit

A defined set of manoeuvres through which products are taken, in order to record performance in a systematic way to allow comparison between products.

Tilt-in-space

A facility on chairs that reclines the occupant whilst keeping the seat-to-backrest angle constant. It means that the hip angle does not change, in contrast to reclining the backrest only, which increases the hip angle.

Tip bars

A projection from the back of a wheelchair to allow a person pushing it to tip it up easily by pressing on the bar with a foot.

User

The person or consumer who has and uses the product in question.

Appendix IV

Literature Search Strategies

The main databases searched online for this book were:

Medline Express	1995-2001
Embase	1994-2001
Cinahl	1982-2001
RCN	1985-2001
BNI	1994-2001
HMIC: DHdata	1986-2001

The terms entered (number of hits) were assistive technology (506), disability equipment (6), seating (326), pressure relief (421), toileting, bathing, showering, patient handling (131), manual handling (303).

In addition, PSYCHinfo was searched for assistive technology, daily living equipment, bathing disabled, toileting disabled, disability equipment, all with no relevant hits; incontinence (706).

Snowballing from article references and from colleagues and a hand search of the *British Journal of Occupational Therapy* 1998-2001 were also undertaken.

Bibliography

Cluzeau, F., Littlejohns, P., Grimshaw, J. *et al.* (1997) *Appraisal instrument for clinical guidelines, Version 1.* London: St George's Hospital Medical School.

Subject Index

abduction orthosis 72, 81
adjustable height ADs
    baths 213, 214
    beds 254
    chairs 65, 101, 107, 276
advice centres 311
air blowers 178
air cushions 92
Amanda, case study 74
anal plugs 159, 160
Andy, case study 83–4
ankle straps 70, 72, 74
appearance, of ADs 22
armrests 59, 87, 226, 229
assessment
    bathing/showering needs 173
    of requirements 20–5, 311–12
    special seating needs 65–6, 67
assisted riser seats
    chairs 57, 60
    toilets 124–5, 126
attitude to ADs 264–6, 295

backrests 62, 68–9, 70, 71, 72, 74,
    75, 76, 79
    bathing/showering 197, 202,
      230
    in leisure seating 64, 87
    toilets 132
Balans chair 61, 62
bath boards 182, 188–92, 193,
    220, 235, 236
bath chairs 205–6, 207–9
bath cradles 205–6, 207–9, 230,
    231
bath cushions 205, 207, 208–9,
    239
bath mats 182, 220
bath plugs 182
bath seats 189, 191, 193–200, 202,
    235, 236
    see also lifting seats
bathing
    aids 182–214
    boards 188–92, 193
    hoists 274–5
    problems 175, 176–7, 236
    seats 182, 189, 191, 193–200,
      202
    special baths 210–14
    specialised support 201–9

transfer to bath 274, 275
bed grab handles 253–4
bed mobility 253–4, 263, 275–6,
    276–9, 294
bed pads 155–6
bidets 136
biofeedback (incontinence) 152,
    159, 163
bladder retraining 152
boards see bath boards; transfer
    boards
'bottom wipers' (toileting) 136
bowel continence 159–60, 160
brakes 147, 229, 249, 290
British Red Cross 13, 16, 26
British Standards
    bathrooms 185
    lifts 285
    sanichairs 231
    shower rooms 214, 221
BRSM seating classification 76
Building Regulations, disabled 16,
    32, 162, 173
buying ADs see purchasing ADs

care assistants 20
    bathing/showering 173, 177,
      182, 209, 224, 232, 233
    health and safety issues 255–6,
      259–63, 284, 291, 292, 297,
      303
    training in use of hoists 267
case studies
    bath boards 190–1
    bath seats 195–6
    bathing 180, 204, 206
    care assistants 258–9
    cerebral palsy, seating 76
    choice of commode 141–3
    flowcharts, toileting 118–19
    getting on and off toilet 122–3
    high muscle tone, seating 70, 73
    hoists 271
    infants, seating 83
    kyphosis, seating 74
    lifting seats, baths 199–200
    low muscle tone, seating 69
    pressure sores 90
    rising from chairs 57–8
    scoliosis, seating 74
    showers 217–18
    stairlift 281–3
    toilet, sitting safely 129–30
castors 55, 85, 290

catheter valves 158–9, 163, 164,
    165
catheters 153, 158
chair raising unit see raising units
chairleg sleeves 57
chest harness, seating 72
children
    bathing 237
    commodes 146
    night-time incontinence 154
    room for growth 54, 237
    seating 54, 80, 82, 83, 107, 108,
      114
    shower seats 227, 239
    toilet aids 129–30, 164, 169,
      314
choice of ADs
    cushions 94
    influencing factors 15, 17, 22,
      301–2
    prioritising features 23–4
    process 20–5, 303
    professional advice 20, 23, 173,
      252, 303
    toilets 127
    see also decision making;
      flowcharts
Chronically Sick and Disabled
    Persons Act 1970 173
cleaning, transfer devices, guidelines
    288–9, 292, 295
clothes, adaptation for toileting
    134–5, 162
comfort, in leisure seating 64
comfort cushions 207
comfort scale 54
commodes 47, 139–47, 165, 166,
    167, 231
confidence levels, in evaluation 36
constipation 160
continence 26, 148–60
Continence Advisory Services (CAS)
    139, 149, 151, 158
contoured seats 79, 104
    toilets 131, 132, 161
conventional seating 67–9, 104
corner seats 83, 84, 108
cradles 274, 275
    see also bath cradles; showers,
      cradles
cross infection, prevention 289
crutches 248, 249
cubicles (showers) 219–20, 222–3,
    224
cushions see pressure relief, cushions

custom moulded supports (toilets) 132
customer support 308
customised seating 76–9

databases, on ADs 306–7, 327
decision making 319
  see also choice of ADs; flowcharts
decubitus ulcers see pressure sores
Delphi technique 38–9
design, of ADs 305
Disability Equipment Register 30
Disabled Living Centres 25
discomfort scale 54
disinfection, of transfer ADs 289
disposable pads 155–6
doorways, regulations 173
drying aids 178–9, 201

easy chairs see leisure seating
effectiveness of ADs 235, 236, 241
Elaine, case study 258–9
electrical stimulation (incontinence) 152
electronic detectors 136, 182
enemas 159, 160
enuresis alarms 154, 166
environment
  assessing requirements 22, 148
  for bathing/showering 177, 233
  effect on disability level 305
  hoists 173, 265
  testing in 309–10
equipment providers 13, 16, 23, 307–8
ergonomic tests 43
evaluation techniques 35–45, 309
exhibitions 26

face-to-face interviews 41–2
female urinals 137–9, 166
ferrules 250, 290
fixed hoists, bathing 274, 275
flaccid muscles *see* low muscle tone
floppy muscles *see* low muscle tone
flowcharts
  assisted moving 245, 246, 247, 268
  bath boards 189
  bath lifting seats 198
  bath seats 194
  bathing 181
  care assistants 257
  choice of children's seating 82
  choice of seating 56

commodes 140, 144
getting on and off toilets 121
incontinence 151
lifts 280
  pressure relief products 98
  showers 216
  toilet seats 128
  toileting needs 117
  transfer devices 268, 278
  walking aids 247
  see also choice of ADs; decision making
fluid intake, continence 148–9
flushing aids 136
foam cushions 92, 102, 110
focus groups 37–8
footrests 87, 228
formal trials 42–5
French knickers 134
funding, of ADs 23, 312

gel cushions 92, 102, 110
getting up, from chairs 55–61
'good fit' in seating 53–4
good posture see posture
grab handles 167, 253–4
guidelines
  cleaning 288–9, 292, 295
  rating system 35–6
  to AD use 307
gussets, in clothing 135

hair washing 180, 215
hand blocks 253, 254
handling belts 259, 262, 263, 298
Harry, case study 118–19
head supports, seating 72
headrests 87
health and safety see care assistants, health and safety
high muscle tone
  bathing/showering 176
  seating 66–7, 70–1, 72
hoists 264–75
Horizontal European Activities in Rehabilitation Technology project (HEART) 14, 32

Ian, case study 271
immobility, consequences 59
incontinence 148–60
  and bathing/showering 176
  treatments 152–3, 163
  types 149–50
indwelling catheters 153, 158

informal evaluations 36–7
information providers 23, 25–7, 306–7, 308, 311
information sources 27–31, 30–1, 311, 312
intermittent catheterisation 86, 153, 158, 169
internet, addresses 30–1, 321–2
internet surveys 40
interviews 40–2
ischial tuberosities 54, 61, 81

Jackie, case study 141–3
James, case study 70, 73, 199–200
jerky movements 73, 75, 176
John, case study 122–3

kitchen tasks, seating 62–3, 105
knee blocks 72, 73

laundering, pads 156
laxatives 159, 160
Lee, case study 90
leg bags 157–8, 163, 165, 166
leg lifters (beds) 253, 254, 285, 296
leisure seating 51, 64–5, 85–7, 106, 109, 112
level access showers 221–4, 235
lifting platforms 206, 274, 275
lifting seats (baths) 197–200, 202
lifts 279–85
liquid pressure relief cushions 92
literature searches 327
location of ADs, and choice 15
low friction rollers 262, 264, 276, 295, 297
  individual use 290
low muscle tone
  bathing/showering 176
  seating 66, 67–9, 71, 72
lumbar support 52, 53, 64, 68, 72, 112

maintenance, of ADs 290
male urinals 137
Manual Handling Operations Regulations 255
Mary, case study 129–30
mattress elevators 46–7, 286, 287, 288
mesh covering, shower chairs 180, 230, 239
mobile hoists 211, 213, 231, 267, 269, 294, 296

choice 43, 272, 274, 275
mobile shower chairs 227–31
mobility around home *see* hoists;
    lifts; transfer devices; walking
    aids
modular products
    seating 76–9
    user trials 44
moist disposable wipes 135–6
monkey pole 254
multiple user ADs 87, 223, 225

National Health Service 16, 23
National Institute for Clinical
    Excellence (NICE) 91–2
night-time incontinence 149, 153
non-slip bath mats 182, 220, 235,
    237

occupational therapists see
    practitioners
office chairs 51, 61–2, 104, 112
one-piece supports (toilets) 132
organisations, for information on
    ADs 25–7, 28, 29–30, 321–2
over-bath showers 220–1
overflow incontinence 150
overhead track hoists 265, 267,
    269, 274, 275, 276

pads (incontinence) 152, 154–7,
    165, 166
pads (seating) 72, 74
pants, adaptations 134–5, 155–6
patient handling 255–79, 292, 294,
    297
patient involvement 304
pelvic floor exercises 152, 164
pelvic straps 68–9, 70, 71, 72, 74,
    81
penile clamps 153
penile sheaths 153, 157, 165, 166
personal hygiene 135–6
Peter, case study 69
pillow lifts 286, 287, 288, 296
pilot studies 38, 172
plugs (bath) 182
poles 162, 236, 254
pommel, seating 72
postal surveys 39–40
posture 52, 61, 66, 68, 91
potty chair 131, 133
power showers 215
practitioners

assessment of needs 20–5,
    311–12
assistance in choice of ADs 20,
    23, 173, 252, 303, 307
evaluation of ADs 37
pressure relief
    cushions 91–6, 98–100, 102,
        105, 108, 110, 111, 207,
        209
    seating 51, 88–100
    strategies 89, 91
pressure sores 88–9, 103, 105, 110,
    111, 256, 264
Primrose, case study 57–8, 190–1,
    195–6
prioritising features needed 23–4
problem solving 317–19
process, for choosing ADs 20–5
product design 304–5
product information 31, 306–7
profiling beds 254, 276, 286, 287,
    288, 294
prone angle seats 79, 81
providers, of ADs 13, 16, 23,
    307–8
pull down rails (toilets) 132
purchasing ADs
    advice 16
    providers strategies 307–8
    trends 312

questionnaires 39, 40

rails
    bathrooms 172, 184–7, 189,
        235, 236, 237
    showers 220, 221, 222
    stairs 251
    toilets 124–5, 126, 132, 136,
        162
raised seats (toilets) 124, 165
raising units 57, 58, 60, 101, 102,
    108, 109, 113, 206, 274, 275
ramped seats 70, 72, 74, 109
ramps 252
recline/tilt 71, 72
recliner chair 57, 60, 86
Red Cross 13, 16, 26, 173
reflex bladder 150
requirements, assessment 20–5,
    311–12
residential care
    and continence problems 148
    rails 185–6
    seating 65, 97, 107

reusable pants 155–6
reviews, use of ADs 17
ribbed slope (beds) 253, 254
riser/recliner chair 57, 60, 108
rising cushion 57, 58
risk assessments
    bathing 174
    patient handling 255–6, 292
    pressure sore scales 89, 99

sacral pad 70, 109
saddle seat 79, 81, 111
safety
    bathing 182, 192, 197, 202–3
    care assistants 177, 182, 209,
        224, 284, 291, 292, 297,
        303
    lifts 282, 284, 285
    mobile hoists 272
    in showers 215, 219, 221
    on toilet 127–33
    of trials 43
    walking aids 248–9
sanichairs 133, 203, 231, 239
seat angle 62, 79, 109, 110, 111
seating
    adaptations 57–8, 105
    assisted riser seats 57, 58, 60,
        101, 102, 108, 109
    BRSM classification 76
    choice flowchart 56
    dimensions 53–4, 110, 113
    kitchen tasks 62–3
    leisure chairs 64–5, 85–7
    modular and customised 76–9
    multiple user chairs 87–8
    non-conventional 80–8
    office tasks 61–2
    posture 52, 61, 68
    pressure relief 88–100, 102, 105
    special needs 65–88, 105–6,
        108, 114
    standard needs 55–65
    see also bath seats; showers, seats;
        toilet seats
second-hand ADs 16, 30, 31
self moulding cushions 207
sexual activity, continence 149
Sharon, case study 204, 206
shower curtains 221
shower trolleys/stretchers 232–4,
    239
showering
    problems 175, 176–7
    safety 215, 219, 221

showers 240
   chairs 217, 227–31
   choice 216
   controls 215, 217
   cradles 227, 230, 231
   cubicles 219–20, 222–3
   financial help 223
   screens 219, 222, 224
   seats 217, 225–7
   trays 219–20, 222–3
side entry baths 211, 212, 213–14
side support, seating 72
single product evaluation 36, 44
skirts, adaptations for toileting 134
sliding sheets 264, 276, 277, 295, 297
   individual use 290
slings 270, 273, 293, 298
   individual use 289–90
slipper bed pans 138
sloped seats 68–9
soap aids 178
social services, as provider 16, 23
solutions 22–3
spa facility (baths) 210
spastic bladder 150
spastic muscles see high muscle tone
special seating needs 65–88, 105–6, 108, 114
sponges 178
spring assisted raising units 57, 58, 60, 101, 108, 109, 113, 206, 274, 275
stairlifts 273, 282–4
stairs 251–2, 261, 279, 297
standard seating 55–65
standing aids 259–60, 262, 263, 268, 269, 275, 294
star rating, AD evaluation 35–6
statistics
   AD evaluation techniques 39–41
   on disability 14, 15, 32, 33, 59, 104
step-in cubicles (showers) 219–20
Stephen, case study 180, 217–18
steps 251–2, 261
stiffening of joints 59, 67
stools, kitchen tasks 62–3, 105
straddle seats 80–1
straps 68–9, 70, 71, 72, 74, 81, 85, 87, 229–30
stress incontinence 149
stretcher chairs (bathing) 211, 213, 274, 275
suppositories 159, 160

surveys 39–41
swivel chair 55
swivel seats (baths) 189, 191, 220

taps 182, 183, 239, 240
technical tests 42–3
telephone surveys 40
tests, AD equipment 42–3, 44, 309–10
thermostatic controls 182, 215, 221
thigh straps, seating 73, 76
tight muscles see high muscle tone
tilt-in-space, seating facility 75, 86, 87, 102, 230
tilting baths 211, 212
Tina, case study 281–3
toe washer 178, 179
toilet frames 124, 126, 162, 167
toilet regime 153
toilet seats 124, 126, 129, 131, 162, 165, 167
toileting 120–47
   help from care assistants 262
toilets
   choice issues 127
   flushing aids 136
   getting on and off 120–7
   hoists for 273–4
   sitting safely 127–33
towelling strap 178, 179
training 240, 267, 309, 311, 315
transfer boards 260–1
transfer devices 260–1, 264–75, 278, 294, 297, 298
   self operated 279–88, 294, 297
trays 76, 80, 85, 86, 87
Trevor, case study 76
trial periods 24, 51, 54, 87, 97, 101, 174, 288, 310
trials 42–5, 44, 309–10
trousers, adaptations 134
turntables 259, 261, 262
   fabric 55, 263

urethral devices 152, 169
urge incontinence 150, 162
urinals 136–9, 166
urine infections 136, 158
user trials 44–5

vacuum moulded cushions 207
vaginal devices 152, 169
vertical lifts 282, 284
video conferencing 41

walking aids 247–51, 290, 295, 298
   height 249, 250
walking frames 248–50, 290, 293–4, 295, 296
washing aids 178–80
wheelchairs 107, 113
   alternative seating 51–2
   transferring from 251
wheels, shower chairs 228
whirlpool facility (baths) 210
wings, in chairs 64
work surfaces 62–3, 71

Yvonne, case study 73–4

Assistive devices are referred to as ADs; organisations and societies are listed collectively under organisations

Author Index

ABLEDATA 306, 313
Abrams, P. 169
Acher, S. 106
Adams, J. 174, 180, 222, 235
Agree, E. 179, 235
Aitchison, E. 197, 235, 254, 256, 291
Åkerlund, J. 163
Akoumianakis, D. 14, 33
Alberg, D. 32
Alexander, N. 64, 101
Ali, M. 32
Alzheimer's Disease Society 161
Anders, K. 152, 161
Anderson, J. 317, 319
Arborelius, V. 113
Arch, M. 125, 167
Armstrong, R. 71, 104
Asbury, N. 115, 149, 150, 161
Atherton, J. 54, 64, 101
Atkinson, P. 307, 313

Bain, B. 18, 32, 313
Ballinger, C. 141, 161
Bamford, C. 309, 314
Bandolier 36, 46
Bannister, C. 255, 291
Bannister, S. 161
Bardsley, G. 132, 161
Barnea, T. 102
Barton, J. 249, 293
Bashford, G. 101, 109
Batavia, A. 313
Bayles, T. 104, 163
Bellin, P. 169
Bentley, A. 159, 160, 163
Bentur, N. 40, 46, 60, 102
Beresford, S. 37, 46, 136, 161
Betz, K. 88, 93, 102
Binns, V. 163, 236
Bishop, S. A. 88, 89, 102
Blake, D. J. 73, 78, 86, 88, 94, 99, 103
Boden, M. 288, 289, 292
Bone, M. 14, 32
Booth, E. 81, 110
Bowes, C. 81, 110
Boyce, A. 236
Brandstater, M. 105
Brienza, D. 102

British Standards Institute 161, 168, 235, 285, 292
Broadhurst, M. 228, 235
Brown, A. 256, 292
Brown, C. 107
Brown, J. 164
Brown, R. 240
Browne, L. 28
Brunswic, M. 62, 102
BSRM 102
Bulla, N. 102
Bundy, A. 110
Burdon, D. 37, 46, 133, 141, 161
Burgh, D. 47
Burgio, K. 152, 162
Burke, C. 266, 293, 307, 313
Burns, S. 88, 93, 102
Butler, P. 114
Butler, R. 168

Campbell, P 303, 314
Carnes, M. 152
Carnevali, D. 320
Carr, J. 88, 111
Cassar, S. 256, 262, 272, 292, 297, 298
Caudrey, D. 75, 111
Centre for Assessible Environments (CAE) 172, 235
Chaffin, D. 298
Chamberlain, M.A. 109, 124, 140, 162, 173, 187, 235, 241
Chan, D. 59, 102, 106
Charvat, B. 32, 237
Chatfield, J. 101
Cheek, L. 114
Chen, T–Y. 304, 313
Chopparo, C. 319
Clark, M 89, 97, 102
Clarke, A. 249, 293, 294
Clarke, A. K. 62, 101, 112
Clarke, S. 110
Clayden, A. 163, 236
Clemson, L. 120, 125, 162, 185, 219, 235
Cluzeau, F. 327
Cochrane, G. 136, 137, 164, 219, 237, 307, 314
College of Occupational Therapists 267, 292
Collins, F. 53, 54, 66, 89, 94, 97, 98, 99, 100, 103, 112
Collins, J. 272, 298
Conine, T. 89, 103
Conneely, A. 266, 292

Cook, G. 256, 292
Cook, T. 91, 112
Cooper, B. 32, 125, 162, 187, 236, 252, 292
Cooper, S. 121, 167
Corocan, M. 174, 236
Cors, M. 239
Costar, S. 262, 272, 292
Cottenden, A. 155, 157, 162
Coury, B. 54, 61, 62, 104
Cowan, D. 267, 293
Cowell, R. 265, 276, 293
Craighead, S. 37, 46, 134, 141, 161
Craik, F. 317, 319
Creek, J. 320
Crepeau, E. 33, 66, 73, 79, 104
Cristarella, M. 80, 103
Cunningham, J. 107
Cusack, C. 164
Cutter, N. 73, 78, 86, 88, 94, 103

Daechsel, D. 103
Dale, C. 255, 293
Dansereau, J. 113
Davegårdh, H. 168, 172, 241
Davey 133, 134, 162
Davila, G. 169
De Witte, L. 316
Dealey, C. 254, 276, 287, 294
Dean, G. 139, 163
Defloor, T. 95, 103
Deitz, J. 66, 73, 79, 104
Delbecq, A. 38, 46
Demers, L. 309, 313
Department of the Environment 16, 32, 162, 173, 236, 305, 313
Department of Health 288, 293, 309, 313
DiLellio, E. 102
Disability North 185, 188, 203, 236
Disabled Living Foundation 94, 104, 215, 226, 228, 236, 267, 293
DLF–DATA 306, 313
Dockrell, S. 266, 293
Drury, C. 54, 61, 62, 104
Duffy, A. 266, 293
Dunlop, D. 59, 104
Dutton, R. 320

Ebe, K. 114
Eckford, S. 169
Edwards, M. 159, 160, 163

Edwards, N. 181, 182, 236
Ekholm, J. 270, 272, 294
Elford, W. 264, 293
Elliott, D. 14, 32
Ellis, M. 64, 104, 109
Elser, D. 152, 163
Empowering Users Through
    Assistive Technology (EUSTAT)
    311, 312, 314
Engberg, S. 148, 149, 153, 163
EQUAL 304, 305, 313

Fader, M 137, 139, 163
Fairgrieve, E. 132, 161
Feeney, R. 121, 167, 182, 236
Fife, S. 65, 67, 71, 104
Finlay, O. 60, 113, 146, 163
Finlayson, M. 40, 46
Finuf, L. 78, 79, 108
Fleckenstein, S. 114
Forrester, C. 274, 294
Forsyth, W. 168
Fragela, G. 276, 297
Frank, G. 24, 32
From, W. 47, 111, 305, 315

Gagné, R. 317, 318, 320
Galer, M. 182, 236
Gallacher, K. 78, 105
Gallo, M. 169
Galvin, J. 303, 315
Garner, J. 303, 314
Garrett, D. 111
Geiger, C. 41, 46, 124, 163
George, J 120, 163, 172, 236
German, K. 159, 163
Geyer, M.J. 102
Gick, M. 317, 318, 320
Gitlin, L. 41, 46, 124, 163, 174,
    236, 240
Glia, A. 159, 163
Goode, P. 162
Goodman, B. 152
Goodman, J. 107
Gore, S. 161
Grandjean, E. 62, 104
Green, C. 266, 293
Green, E. 110, 114
Greenfield, E. 77, 106, 128, 132,
    146, 147, 164
Griffin, M. 114
Griffiths, D. 169
Grimes, R. 228, 235
Grimshaw, J. 327
Grisbrooke, J. 174, 180, 222, 235

Groll, J. 110
Grunawalt, J. 64, 101
Grypdonck, M. 95, 103
Gustafson, D. 38, 46
Gylin, M. 163

Hagedorn, R. 317, 318, 320
Hahn, I. 169
Hall, J. 249, 293, 294
Hammer, G. 309, 313
Hancock, R. 169
Hanson, C. 111
Hanson, M. 262, 266, 272, 273,
    294, 295, 296
Harms-Ringdahl, K. 270, 294
Harpin 175, 214, 219, 221, 237
Harrison, R. 101
Harvey, M–A. 169
Hastings, J. 65, 73, 105
Havixbeck, K. 40, 46
Hawley, M. 42, 46
Health and Safety Executive 244,
    255, 256, 290, 294
Healy, A. 65, 66, 73, 105
Heaton, J. 309, 314
Helander, M 61, 105
Helen Hamlyn Research Centre
    304, 314
Henderson, J. 88, 91, 105
Hershler, C. 103
Hewes, D. 319, 320
Higgs, J. 320
Hignett, S. 43, 46, 272, 294
Hill, G. 177, 237
Hobson, D. 53, 105, 127, 164
Hocking C. 304, 314
Holm, M. 320
Holtendahl, K. 152, 164
Holyoak, R. 317, 318, 320
Hsiaso, H. 298
Hughes, M. 113
Hughes, S. 59, 104
Hulme, J. B. 66, 78, 105, 106
Hurren, D. 32, 174, 237

INCLUDE 304, 314
Incontact 148, 164

Jackson, S. 169, 297
James, L. 114
Jensen, J 41, 46
Jensen, L. 14, 32
Jepson, J. 127, 164
Johnson Taylor, S. 106
Jones, D. 181, 182, 235

Jones, M. 320
Judge, S. 304, 314

Kairsary, A. 164
Karg, P. 102
Kelsall, A. 136, 137, 164, 219,
    237, 307, 314
Keogh, A. 254, 276, 287, 294
Kimbell, J 177, 215, 219, 221,
    228, 231, 237
Kirby, R. 114
Kitzinger, J. 47
Klint Edlund, C. 270, 272, 294
Koester, D. 64, 101
Koivikko, M. 168, 172, 237, 308,
    314
Koo, T. 91, 106
Korpela, R. 168, 172, 174, 237,
    308, 314
Kronlof, G. 304, 314
Küppers, H–J. 305, 314

Lachman, S. 77, 106
Lafayette-Lucey, A. 148, 163
Lane, J. 18, 32, 46, 314
Lange, M. 86, 106
Laporte, D. 59, 102, 106
Law, M. 18, 32
Laycock, J. 152, 164
LBOTM 307, 314
Le Bon, C. 274, 294
le Carpentier, E. 54, 55, 64, 106
LeBlanc, R. 113
Lee, Y. 91, 106
Letts, R. M. 66, 70, 71, 73, 106
Levine, R. 41, 46, 124, 163
Lewington, C. 159, 164
Lewis, P 169
Lindberg, F. 113
Lindskog, A–C. 168, 241
Littlejohns, P. 327
Locher, J. 162
London Boroughs Occupational
    Therapy Managers 173, 237
Lose, G. 169
Love, C. 255, 294

MacLeod, D. 114
Maczka, K. 33, 303, 314
Madans, J. 179, 241
Major, R. 114
Mak, A. 91, 106
Malassigné, P. 239
Mandelstam, M. 27, 28, 33, 256,
    295

Manheim, L. 59, 104
Mann, W. 14, 18, 32, 41, 46, 59, 64, 75, 107, 124, 156, 165, 174, 178, 181, 182, 221, 237, 248, 251, 295, 308, 313, 314, 315
Marks, O. 306, 315
Martin, J. 14, 16, 32, 33
Martin, R. 120, 125, 162, 185, 219, 235
McCafferty, E. 65, 99, 107
McClenaghan, B. 79, 107
McClish, D. 163
McCuaig, M. 24, 32
McDowell, B. 148, 163
McGrath, P. 107
McGuire, T. 262, 266, 267, 272, 294, 295, 296
McIntosh, J. 137, 138, 139, 164
McLellan, D. L. 161, 297
McQuilton, G. 80, 112
Medical Devices Agency 39, 46, 47, 54, 60, 80, 82, 84, 87, 91, 94, 96, 97, 107–8, 140, 141, 154, 155, 156, 157, 175, 177, 188, 192, 197, 202, 203, 207, 213, 226, 228, 231, 232, 238, 239, 249, 254, 259, 260, 272, 285, 288, 290, 295, 296, 303, 308, 310, 315
Medical Devices Directorate 140, 141, 183, 239, 273, 284
Meghani, Z. 120, 166, 174, 239
Megrew, M. 125, 167
Meltzer, H. 14, 32, 33
Miedaner, J. 78, 79, 108
Miller, G. 319, 320
Miller, K. 236
Milling, J. 104, 163
Milne, J. 108, 128, 132, 146, 147, 164
Milson, I. 169
Minkel, J. 77, 89, 108
Mizrahi, I. 102
Molenbroek, J. 53, 105, 127, 164
Moody, J. 262, 266, 272, 274, 294, 295, 296
Moore, C. M. 39, 47
Morgan, M. 164
Moy, A. 254, 297
Mulcahy, C. 67, 70, 71, 73, 109, 110, 128, 130, 166
Mulley, G. 147, 163, 167, 236, 248, 256, 292, 298

Multiple Sclerosis Council 148, 167
Munro, B. 60, 101
Munro, G. 59
Munton, J. 59, 109
Myhr, B. 61, 67, 79, 80, 81, 109, 110
Myhr, U. 114

Naylor, J. 147, 167
Neistadt, M. 33
Nelham, R. 109
Nelson, A. 229, 239
Nendick, C. 256, 292
Nene, A. 114
Newell, A. 3320
NICE 91, 110
Nicholson, J. 297
Nochajski, S. 33
Noone, P. 164
Nordenskiöld, U. 304, 315
Noronha, J. 79, 110
Norrlin, S. 114
Norton, C. 89, 158, 167

O'Mara, N. 75, 111
O'Neill, P. 42, 46
Organist, L. 148, 163
Owen, B. 276, 297

Page, M. 121, 124, 125, 167
Pain, H. 277–8, 297
Parette, H. 304, 314
Parker, M. 173, 239
Parkes, B. 174, 185, 240
Patellos, C. 298
Pearce, J. 256, 297
Pellow, T. 60, 88
Perr, A. 37, 47
Pesola, K. 172, 223, 240
Pettersson, L. 139, 163
Pezzino, J. 105
Pheasant, S. 62, 64, 65, 110, 125, 127, 132, 145, 167, 184, 185, 240
Pickering, R. 161
Picking, H.C. 222, 240
Pinikahana, J. 255, 267, 297
Poll, W. 169
Poor, R. 105
Pope, P. 72, 73, 78, 79, 81, 110
Poulson, D. 274, 297, 305, 315
Pountney, T. 70, 72, 73, 109, 110, 114
Price, S. 105

Promocon 127

Radell, J. 114
Ramsay, C. 65, 105
Ranko, J. 319
RCP 158, 167
Reid, D. 81, 111
Rennant, C. 179, 241
Retsas, A. 255, 267, 297
Reynolds, T. 88, 111
Rhodes, M. 174, 222, 240
RICAbility 150, 160, 167
Richardson, S. 274, 297, 305, 315
Riemer-Reiss 304, 315
Rigby, P. 47, 54, 77, 111, 305, 315
Riley, M. 148, 167
Rithalia, S. 88, 93, 111
Roberts, A. 320
Robertson, L. 319, 320
Roe, B. 158, 167
Rogers, J. 320
Rogers, N. 183, 240
Rosen, C. 104, 163
Rowley, P. 163
Roxborough, L. 104
Russell, L 88, 111
Ryan, S. 47, 111, 305, 315
Ryan-Woolley, B. 154, 167

Sainsbury, R. 248, 298
Sanford, J. 125, 167
Schemm, R. 174, 240
Scherer, M. 303, 315
Schiefloe, A. 164
Schon, D. 320
Schulein, M. 105
Scweitzer, J. 33
Seeger, B. 75, 79, 111
Seppänen, R–L. 168, 172, 237, 308, 314
Sexsmith, E. 65, 105
Shamdasani 47
Shaver, J. 78, 106
Shechtman, O. 96, 111
Shields, R. 91, 112
Shipman, I. 197, 240
Shipperley, T. 53, 89, 98, 103, 112
Shuttleworth, A. 265, 276, 293
Simon, H. 320
Ska, B. 309, 313
Smoth, J. 169
Sonn, U. 14, 33, 120, 168, 172, 241, 304, 314
SPOD 168
Steed, R. 255, 298

Steele, J. 59, 60, 101, 109

Steen, B. 168, 241

Stephanidis, C. 14, 33

Steward, B. 173, 241

Stewart, D. 47, 125, 162, 187, 236, 252, 292

Stewart, P. 80, 112

Stobbe, T. 298

Stockton, L. 112

Stone, D. 163

Stone, V. 46

Stowe, J. 174, 241, 316

Straker, L. 264, 293

Strauss, G. 264, 293

Strong, S. 32

Sumison T. 47

Sveistrup, H. 59, 102, 106

Swedberg, L. 73, 112

Sweeney, G. 62, 64, 112

Taylor, S. 65, 66, 72, 73, 77–8, 86, 113

ten Haar, B. 52, 60, 65, 68, 70, 71, 73, 75, 112

Thornley, G. 162, 173, 187, 235, 241, 316

Thorslund, M. 173, 239

Thyssen, H. 169

Tobin, G. 148, 167

Tomita, M. 32, 41, 46, 64, 75, 107, 124, 156, 165, 174, 178, 221, 237, 248, 251, 295, 308, 313, 315

Trefler, E. 65, 66, 72, 73, 77–8, 86, 113

Tremblay, C. 113

Tulving, E. 317, 319

Turner, C. 68, 113

Turner-Smith. A. 267, 293

Ulin, S. 298

Usiak, D. 46

Van der Veen, A. 38, 46

Vebrugge, L. 179, 241

Verelst, M. 152, 164

Vernardakis, N. 14, 33

Versi, E. 169

Vickerman, J. 139, 168

von Wendt, L. 61, 67, 79, 80, 81, 110, 114

Wall, J. 89, 113

Walsh, J. 105

Ward, J. 240

Warren, J. 157, 158, 168

Waterlow, J. 89, 99, 113

Watret, L. 107

Webb, L. 42, 46

Weidenhielm, L. 113

Weinberger, M. 152, 168

Weiner, D. 113

Weiss-Lambrou, R. 75, 113, 309, 313, 316

Wessels, R. 308, 316

White, A. 14, 33

White, H. 115, 149, 150, 161

Whitehead, J. 168

Wiltshire, S. 298

Woods, P. 255, 293

Wrench, A. 77, 106

Wretenberg, O. 113

Wright, D. 240

Wright, V. 109, 162, 173, 235, 241, 316

Wyman, J. 163

Zhang, L. 61, 105

Zhuang, Z. 264, 268, 273, 298

Zollars, J. 73, 114